Hidden Histories of the Dead

In this discipline-redefining book, Elizabeth T. Hurren maps the post-mortem journeys of bodies, body parts, organs and brains, inside the secretive culture of modern British medical research after WWII as the bodies of the deceased were harvested as bio-commons. Often the human stories behind these bodies were dissected, discarded or destroyed in death. *Hidden Histories of the Dead* recovers human faces and supply-lines in the archives that medical science neglected to acknowledge. It investigates the medical ethics of organ donation, the legal ambiguities of a lack of fully informed consent and the shifting boundaries of life and re-defining of medical death in a biotechnological era. Hurren reveals the implicit, explicit and missed body disputes that took second place to the economics of the national and international commodification of human material in global medical sciences of the Genome era. This title is also available as open access.

ELIZABETH T. HURREN is Professor of History at the University of Leicester.

Hidden Histories of the Dead

Disputed Bodies in Modern British Medical Research

Elizabeth T. Hurren

University of Leicester

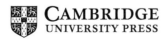

CAMBRIDGE
UNIVERSITY PRESS

CAMBRIDGE
UNIVERSITY PRESS

University Printing House, Cambridge CB2 8BS, United Kingdom

One Liberty Plaza, 20th Floor, New York, NY 10006, USA

477 Williamstown Road, Port Melbourne, VIC 3207, Australia

314–321, 3rd Floor, Plot 3, Splendor Forum, Jasola District Centre,
New Delhi – 110025, India

79 Anson Road, #06–04/06, Singapore 079906

Cambridge University Press is part of the University of Cambridge.

It furthers the University's mission by disseminating knowledge in the pursuit of
education, learning, and research at the highest international levels of excellence.

www.cambridge.org
Information on this title: www.cambridge.org/9781108484091
DOI: 10.1017/9781108633154

First published 2021

A catalogue record for this publication is available from the British Library.

ISBN 978-1-108-48409-1 Hardback

Dedicated with love
To my uncle and godparent
John Joseph Patterson Esq
(1945–2019)
and
To my hairdresser
Sharron Elizabeth Tomlin
(1973–2019)
and
In memory of a shared friendship for history
Lin Ross of Nevill Holt Hall

Contents

Illustrations

Figures

Tables

Acknowledgements

This book has been written with the generous support of the Wellcome Trust in London, to whom I am very grateful for the financial funding they awarded to me in the past five years. I hope that the new research it contains is a fitting tribute to the extraordinary legacy and personal vision of Sir Henry Wellcome. He sought during his lifetime to engage the curiosity of the public with the fascinating hidden histories of the body in the twentieth century, and beyond. It thus contains wide-ranging new research material assembled as part of a major transdisciplinary, large Programme Grant: WT RA15G2019 on which I have been a Joint Principal Investigator, exploring 'Disputed Bodies in Modern Medical Research'. In so many respects, what has been accumulated represents the culmination of over two decades' archival research. This has meant that in two previous books, I have been able to explore the 1750 to 1830 as well as 1830 to 1930 phases of body supply in human anatomy. Now these are extended in this third monograph by exploring the neglected period of 1930 to 2000. This sort of historical perspective over the *longue durée* has never before been feasible in a history of the body in Britain. I am therefore very appreciative of all the kind assistance given to me by the dedicated staff working in county records offices, university libraries and national medical institutions, across the UK. Although they are too numerous to list here, I did want to pay a short tribute to their collective expertise. It remains remarkably open to enquiry, for it is admirable how they continue to maintain the highest professional standards against the backdrop of exceptional budget cutbacks in local government services and the heritage sectors. It therefore affords me enormous pleasure to be able to place this book once again on open access thanks to a Wellcome Trust publishing subvention. In so doing, I hope its contents will promote around the world the remarkable archival collections that are available to academics in Britain.

This book has also been written against the backdrop of far-reaching changes happening in the academic sector, many of which are undermining the foundation of scholarship. It has been thought-provoking to complete a trilogy of books and to contemplate that beyond REF2020 many fewer historians will have the same opportunities to publish high-quality outputs in the near future. I am therefore appreciative of those colleagues who have retained a commitment to collegiality in the face of the commercialisation of education, its mushrooming bureaucracies and a fees culture that encourages instrumentality amongst the student body. Having had a former career in finance for ten years and left it to embrace life-enhancing educational values, it is unsettling to find oneself back in such a profit-driven environment awash with management-speak of questionable value. Thankfully, academics continue to care and speak out about these worrying cultural trends. That they do so attests to one of the most engaging aspects of being a historian – the recognition that history is not just in our keeping, but in our making too. If this book, and those like it, can make a contribution to a larger conversation about the importance of high-quality research to shape our medical world for the next generation, then it will have succeeded in its central purpose.

At the same time, I continue to be inspired by the kindness of strangers. The hospitality that has been shared as I journeyed around Britain doing public engagement for this book has been a wonderful experience. I would in particular like to pay a short tribute to those hospices that opened their doors to my research enquiries. Inside I encountered patients, friends and families who spoke so movingly about end-of-life experiences. I unquestionably came away a different person from what I learned from those contemplating death. Hospices not only do remarkable work but have an ethos that is so life-enhancing. On a daily basis they defy clichés about them being either sad or scary places – they are the opposite. In their architecture, staffing and general facilities, I discovered light-filled places where people were making the most of life however limited their prognosis. It has been a privilege to be part of such a constructive, holistic and welcoming community. I discovered consensual medical ethics, practical support and dignified choices. Along the way, I also learnt afresh the central importance of regenerating the legacy of love. Thank you therefore to all those who peopled this book, many of whom are not named to protect patient confidentiality. I hope that in some small way that what is written reflects an extraordinary energy of purpose that was shaped by all those patients who spoke to me.

It is a fact of life that no academic book makes it out of the study without the loving support of friends and family. This book (like the others that precede it) reflects the delicious cooking and generosity of spirit of Professor Steven King. His commitment to the female principle is one, amongst a number, of his special character traits. For this book is ultimately about something he exudes – compassion. It is dedicated therefore to three special people who died in 2019 just as the revisions for this book were being finished. My uncle and godparent John Patterson spoke movingly to me, as did my hairdresser Sharron Tomlin and friend Lin Ross. They shared what compassion meant to them after their respective cancer diagnosis and painful treatments, and the pivotal role that it plays in all our lives wherever we experience medicine and the body in a global community. Thanks to them, *Nunc scio quid sit amor* – Virgil *Eclogues, VIII.*

PROFESSOR ELIZABETH T. HURREN

Lammas, Rutland.

Abbreviations

AA1832	Anatomy Act (2 & 3 Will. 4 c. 75: 1832)
AA1984	Anatomy Act (Eliz. 2 c. 14: 1984); see also HTA1984
ACPO	Association of Chief Police Officers, UK
AHCBD	Ad-Hoc Committee on Brain Death, convened at Harvard University, 1968
ALCOR	Alcor Life Extension Foundation
AMI	Acute Myocardial Infection
ARA1988	Anatomy Act Regulation Act (Eliz. 2 c. 44: 1988)
BD&RA1953	Births, Deaths, and Registrations Act (1 & 2 Eliz. 2 c. 20: 1953)
BLAA1880	Burial Laws Amendment Act (43 & 44 Vict. c. 42: 1880)
BMA	British Medical Association
BMJ	British Medical Journal
CA1952	Cremations Act (15 & 16 Geo. 6 & 1 Eliz. 2 c. 31: 1952)
CAA1926	Coroners Amendment Act (16 & 17 Geo. 5 c. 59: 1926)
CAA1956	Clean Air Act (4 & 5 Eliz. 2 c. 52: 1956)
CCA1888	Council Councils Act (51 & 52 Vict. ch. 41: 1888)
CCF	Congestive Cardiac Failure
C&FCASS	Children and Family Court Advisory Service, UK
CJA2009	Coroners and Justice Act (Eliz. 2 c. 25: 2009)
CMO	Chief Medical Office, UK
COAD	Chronic Obstructive Pulmonary Disease
CPA1974	Control of Pollution Act (Eliz. 2 c. 40: 1974)
CPR	Cardiopulmonary Resuscitation
CR1984	Coroners Rules (SI 1984 No. 552)
CSE&W	Coroners Society for England and Wales
CUH	Croydon University Hospital
DofH,UK	Department of Health, UK
DofH	Declaration of Helsinki
DofLS	Deprivation of Liberty Safeguard
DHSS	Department of Health and Social Security
DofG1948	Declaration of Geneva, 1948
DS0	Distinguished Service Order

EC1979	Medical Research Council Ethics Code, 1979
EPA1990	Environment Protection Act (Eliz. 2 c. 43: 1990)
FAA	Federation of Associations of Anatomists
fMRI	Functional Magnetic Resonance Imaging
GHD	Growth Hormone Deficiency
GMP	Greater Manchester Police Force
HF&EA1990	Human Fertilisation and Embryology Act (Eliz 2 c. 37: 1990)
HOTA1989	Human Organ Transplant Act (Eliz. 2 c. 31: 1989)
HTA	Human Tissue Authority
HTA1961	Human Tissue Act (9 & 10 Eliz. 2 c. 54: 1961)
HTA1984	Human Tissue Act (Eliz. 2 c. 14: 1984); also called AA1984
HTA2004	Human Tissue Act (Eliz. 2 c. 30: 2004)
IHD	Ischemic Heart Disease
LGA1894	Local Government Act (56 & 57 Vict. c. 73: 1894)
LVF	Left Ventricular Failure in the Heart
MA1752	Murder Act (25 Geo. 2 c. 37: 1752)
MA1858	Medical Act (21 & 22 Vict. c. 90: 1858)
MDA1913	Mental Deficiency Act (3 & 4 Geo. 5 c. 28: 1913)
MDDS	Mitochondrial DNA Depletion Syndrome
MID	Mentioned in Despatches
MRC	Medical Research Council
NC1947	Nuremberg Code, 1947
NCEPOD	National Confidential Enquiry into Patient Outcome and Death, 2006
NET	National Ethics Trust
NHS	National Health Service, UK
NGNI	Next Generation Neural Interfaces, Imperial College London
NPL1834	New Poor Law Amendment Act (4 & 5 Will. 4. c. 76: 1834)
NPSA	National Patient Safety Agency
ODR2020	Organ Donation Register, NHS strategy 2020
PGP	Pituitary Gland Programme
P&CEA1996	Police and Criminal Evidence Act (Eliz. 2 c. 25: 1996)
RCP	Royal College of Pathologists
RSM	Royal Society of Medicine
SA1961	Suicide Act (9 & 10 Eliz. 2 c. 60: 1961)
TEPARC	Trans-European Pedagogic Anatomical Research Group
TRA1884	Third Reform Act (48 & 49 Vict. c. 3: 1884)
UCHL	University College Hospital, London
UDDA1981	Uniform Determination of Death Act, USA, 1981
UMDS	United Medical and Dental Schools of Guy's and St. Thomas' hospitals
WMA	World Medical Association

Ethical Note

This book complies with the Data Protection Act (1988) and recent GDPR (2018) in the UK. Anonymous names feature throughout the chapters. Each dissection case was given a unique identifier, known only to the author for ethical reasons. The new data is based on anatomical case material collected in the archives from 1945 to 2000. It is therefore beyond the one-hundred-year rule that historians often work with. All named cases have a unique set of letters. Each alphabetical description does not relate to the original names in the case files. This is to ensure that should there be any living relatives of the dead, their family name is not revealed. Sometimes, aspects of people's personal backgrounds are additionally disguised to ensure privacy is not breached. Those names that are cited in full, as per the original files, have come from primary research material already in the public domain. These are often newspaper reports and media interviews where relatives chose to speak openly. They are set out in the footnotes. At all times, the author has sought to maintain confidentiality. Over a three-year period of research, extensive record linkage work checked each case file's circumstances carefully. Anatomy records have therefore only been summarised and general statistics produced. If a representative case is cited, it has always been de-identified in such a way that it would be difficult to re-identify it. The author has tried to ensure that there are not any discrepancies or errors. If any have inadvertently arisen, then do please contact them on – eh140@le.ac.uk

Part I

Relocating the Dead-End

Our Dead Are Never Dead To Us,

Until We Have Forgotten Them

[*Adam Bede*, George Eliot, 1819–1880]

Introduction: A Consignment for the Cul-de-Sac of History?

At the heart of modern conceptions of biomedicine sits a core narrative of 'progress', one in which profound scientific breakthroughs from the nineteenth century onwards have cumulatively and fundamentally transformed the individual life course for many patients in the global community. Whilst there remain healthcare inequalities around the world, science has endeavoured to make medical breakthroughs for everybody. Thus for many commentators it has been vital to focus on the ends – the preservation or extension of life and the reduction of human suffering emerging out of new therapeutic regimes – and to accept that the accumulation of past practice cannot be judged against the yardstick of the most modern ethical values. Indeed, scientists, doctors and others in the medical field have consistently tried hard to follow ethical practices even when the law was loose or unfocussed and public opinion was supportive of an ends rather than means approach. Unsystematic instances of poor practice in research and clinical engagement thus had (and have) less contemporary meaning than larger systemic questions of social and political inequalities for the living, related abuses of power by states and corporate entities in the global economy, and the suffering wrought by cancer, degenerative conditions and antibiotic resistant diseases. Perhaps unsurprisingly given how many patients were healed, there has been a tendency in recent laboratory studies of the history of forensic science, pathology and transplant surgery, to clean up, smooth over and thus harmonise the medical past.[1] Yet, these processes of 'progress' have also often been punctuated by scandals (historical and current) about medical experimentation, failed drug therapies, rogue doctors and scientists and misuse of human research material.[2] In this broad context, while the living do have a place in the story of 'progress', it is the bodies of the dead which have had and always have a central role. They are a key component of medical training and anatomical teaching, provide the majority of resources for organ transplantation and (through the retention and analysis of organs and tissue) constitute one of the basic building blocks of modern medical research. For many in the medical sciences field, the dead could and should become bio-commons given the powerful impact of modern degenerative and other diseases, accelerating problems linked to lifestyle, and the threats of current and future pandemics. Yet, equally inside the medical research community there remain many neglected hidden histories of the dead that are less understood than they should be in global medicine, and for this reason they are central to this new book.

Such perspectives are important. On the one hand, they key into a wider sense that practice in medical science should not be subject to retrospective ethical reconstruction. On the other hand, it is possible to trace a range of modern challenges to the theme of 'progress', the ethics of medical research and practice, as well as the scope and limits of professional authority. This might include resistance to vaccination, scepticism about the precision of precision medicine, an increasing willingness to challenge medical decisions and mistakes in the legal system, accelerating public support for assisted dying, and a widening intolerance of the risks associated with new and established drugs. Nowhere is this challenge more acute than in what historians broadly define as 'body ethics'. By way of recent example, notwithstanding the provisions of the Human Tissue Act (Eliz. 2 c. 30: 2004) (hereafter HTA2004), the BBC reported in 2018 that the NHS had a huge backlog of 'clinical waste' because its sub-contracted disposal systems had failed.[3] Material labelled 'anatomical waste' and kept in secure refrigerated units contained organs awaiting incineration at home or abroad. By July 2019, the *Daily Telegraph* revealed how such human waste, including body parts and amputations from operative surgeries, was found in 100 shipping containers sent from Britain to Sri Lanka for clinical waste disposal.[4] More widely, the global trade in organs for transplantation has come into increasingly sharp relief, while the supply of cadavers, tissue and organs for medical research remains contentious. Some pathologists and scientists, for instance, are convinced that HTA2004 stymied creative research opportunities.[5] They point out that serendipity is necessary for major medical breakthroughs. Legislating against kismet may, they argue, have been counterproductive. Ethical questions around whose body is it anyway thus continue to attract a lot of media publicity and often involve the meaning of the dead for all our medical futures.

Lately these ethical issues have also been the focus of high-profile discussion in the global medical community, especially amongst those countries participating at the International Federation of Associations of Anatomists (hereafter FAA). It convened in Beijing, China, in 2014, where a new proposal promised 'to create an international network on body donation' with the explicit aim of providing practical 'assistance to those countries with difficulties setting up donation programmes'.[6] The initiative was developed by the Trans-European Pedagogic Anatomical Research Group (TEPARC), following HTA2004 in Britain that had increased global attention on best practice in body donation. Under the TEPARC reporting umbrella, Beat Riederer remarked in 2015: 'From an ethical point of view, countries that depend upon unclaimed bodies of dubious provenance are [now] encouraged to use these reports and adopt strategies for developing successful donation programmes.'[7] Britain can with some justification claim to be a global leader in moving away from a reliance on 'unclaimed' corpses for anatomical teaching and research to embracing a system of body bequests based on informed consent. Similar ethical frameworks have begun to gain a foothold in Europe and East Asia, and are starting to have more purchase on the African[8] and North and South American subcontinents too.[9] Nonetheless, there is a long way to travel. As Gareth Jones explains, although 'their use is far less in North America' it is undeniable that 'unclaimed corpses continue to constitute … around 20 per cent of medical schools' anatomical programmes' in the USA and Canada.[10] Thus, the *New York Times* reported in 2016 that a new City of New York state law aimed to stop the use of 'unclaimed' corpses for dissection.[11] The report came about because of a public exposé that the newspaper ran about the burial of a million bodies on Hart Island in an area of mass graves called Potter's Field. Since 1980, the Hart Island Research project has found 65,801 'unclaimed' bodies, dissected and buried anonymously.[12] In a new digital hidden history project called the 'Passing Cloud Museum', their stories are being collected for posterity.[13] And with some contemporary relevance, for during the Covid-19 pandemic the Hart Island pauper graveyard was re-opened by the New York public health authorities. Today, it once more contains contaminated bodies with untold stories to be told about the part people played in medical 'progress'. For the current reality is that 'in some states of the US, unclaimed bodies are passed to state anatomy boards'. Jones thus points out that:

When the scalpel descends on these corpses, no-one has given informed consent for them to be cut up. … Human bodies are more than mere scientific material. They are integral to our humanity, and the manner in which this material is obtained and used reflects our lives together as human beings. The scientific exploration of human bodies is of immense importance, but it must only be carried out in ways that will enhance anatomy's standing in the human community.[14]

In a global medical marketplace, then, the legal ownership of human material and the ethical conduct of the healthcare and medical sciences can twist and turn. But with the increasing reach of medical research and intervention, questions of trust, communication, authority, ownership and professional boundaries become powerfully insistent. As the ethicist Heather Douglas reminds us: 'The question is what we should expect of scientists *qua* in their behaviour, in their decisions as scientists, engaged in their professional life. As the importance of science in our society has grown over the past half-century, so has the urgency of this question.' She helpfully elaborates:

The standard answer to this question, arising from the *Freedom of Science* movement in the early 1940s, has been that scientists are not burdened with the same moral responsibilities as the rest of us, that is, that scientists enjoy 'a morally unencumbered freedom from permanent pressure to moral self-reflection'. . . . Because of the awesome power of science, to change both, our world, our lives, and our conception of ourselves, the actual implementation of scientists' general responsibilities will fall heavily on them. With full awareness of science's efficacy and power, scientists must think carefully about the possible impacts and potential implications of their work. . . . The ability to do harm (and good) is much greater for a scientist, and the terrain almost always unfamiliar. The level of reflection such responsibility requires may slow down science, but such is the price we all pay for responsible behavior.[15]

Whether increasing public scepticism of experts and medical science will require a deeper and longer process of reflection and regulation is an important and interesting question. There is also, however, a deep need for historical explorations of these broad questions, and particularly historical perspectives on the ownership and use of, authority over and ethical framing of the dead body. As George Santanyana reminds us, we must guard against either neglecting a hidden scientific past or embellishing it since each generic storyline is unlikely to provide a reliable future guide –

Progress, far from consisting in change, depends on retentiveness. When change is absolute there remains no being to improve and no direction is set for possible improvement: and when experience is not retained . . . infancy is perpetual. Those who cannot remember the past are condemned to repeat it.[16]

Against this backdrop, in his totemic book *The Work of the Dead,* Thomas Laqueur reminds us how: 'the dead body still matters – for individuals, for communities, for nations'.[17] This is because there has been 'an indelible relationship between the dead body and the civilisation of the living'.[18] Cultural historians thus criticise those in medico-scientific circles who are often trained to ignore or moderate the 'work of the dead for the living' in their working lives. Few appreciate the extent to which power relations, political and cultural imperatives and bureaucratic procedures have shaped, controlled and regulated the taking of dead bodies and body parts for medical research, transplantation and teaching over the *longue durée.* Yet our complex historical relationships with the dead (whether in culture, legislation, memory, medicine or science) has significant consequences for the understanding of current ethical dilemmas. Again, as George Santayana observed: 'Our dignity is not in what we do, but in what we understand' about our recent past and its imperfect historical record.[19] It is to this issue that we now turn.

History and Practice

To offer a critique of the means and not the ends of medical research, practice and teaching through the lens of bodies and body parts is potentially contentious. Critics of the record of medical science are often labelled as neo-liberals, interpreting past decisions from the standpoint of the more complete information afforded by hindsight and judging people and processes according to yardsticks which were not in force or enforced at the time. Historical mistakes, practical and ethical, are regrettable but they are also explicable in this view. Such views underplay, however, two factors that are important for this book. First, there exists substantial archival evidence of the scale of questionable practice in medical teaching, research and body ethics in the past, but it has often been overlooked or ignored. Second, there has been an increasing realisation that the general public and other stakeholders in the past were aware of and contested control, ownership and use of bodies and body parts. While much weight has been given to the impact of very recent medical scandals on public trust, looking further back suggests that ordinary people had a clear sense that they were either marginalised in, or had been misinformed about, the major part their bodies played in medical 'progress'. In see-saw debates about what medicine did right and what it did wrong, intensive historical research continues to be an important counterweight to the success story of biomedicine.

Evidence to substantiate this view is employed in subsequent chapters, but an initial insight is important for framing purposes. Thus, in terms of ownership and control of the dead body, it is now well established that much anatomy teaching and anatomical or biomedical research in the Victorian and Edwardian periods was dependent upon medical schools and researchers obtaining the 'unclaimed bodies' of the very poor.[20] This past is a distant country, but under the NHS (and notwithstanding that some body-stock was generated through donation schemes promoted from the 1950s) the majority of cadavers were still delivered to medical schools from the poorest and most vulnerable sectors of British society until the 1990s. The extraordinary gift that we all owe in modern society to these friendless and nameless people has until recently been one of the biggest untold stories in medical science. More than this, however, the process of obtaining bodies and then using them for research and teaching purposes raised and raises important questions of power, control and ethics. Organ retention scandals, notably at Liverpool Children's Hospital at Alder Hey, highlighted the fact that bodies and body parts had been seen as a research resource on a considerable scale. Human material had been taken and kept over many decades, largely without the consent or knowledge of patients and relatives, and the scandals highlighted deep-seated public beliefs in the need to protect the integrity of the body at death. As Laqueur argues: 'The work of the dead – dead bodies – is possible only because they remain so deeply and complexly present' in our collective actions and sense of public trust at a time of globalisation in healthcare.[21] It is essentially for this reason that a new system of informed consent, with an opt-in clause, in which body donation has to be a positive choice written down by the bereaved and/or witnessed by a person making a living will, was enshrined into HTA2004. Even under the terms of that act, however, it is unclear whether those donating bodies or allowing use of tissue and other samples understand all the ways in which that material might be recycled over time or converted into body 'data'. Questions of ownership, control and power in modern medicine must thus be understood across a much longer continuum than is currently the case.

The same observation might be made of related issues of public trust and the nature of communication. There is little doubt that public trust was fundamentally shaken by the NHS organ retention scandals of the early twenty-first century, but one of the contributions of this book is to trace a much longer history of flashpoints between a broadly conceived 'public' and different segments of the medical profession. Thus, when a *Daily Mail* editorial asked in 1968 – 'THE CHOICE: Do we save the living ... or do we protect the dead?' – it was crystallising the question of how far society should prioritise and trust the motives of doctors and others involved in medical research and practice.[22] There was (as we will see in subsequent chapters) good reason not to, something rooted in a very long history of fractured and incomprehensible communication between practitioners or researchers and their patients and donors. Thus, a largely unspoken aspect of anatomical teaching and research is that some bodies, organs and tissue samples – identified by age, class, disability, ethnicity, gender, sexuality and epidemiology – have always been more valuable than others.[23] Equally, when human harvesting saves lives, questions of the quality of life afterwards are often downplayed. The refinement of organ transplantation has saved many lives, and yet there is little public commentary on the impact of rejection drugs and the link between those drugs and a range of other life-reducing conditions. It was informative, therefore, in the summer of 2016 that the BBC reported on how although many patients are living longer after a cancer diagnosis, the standard treatments they undergo have (and always have had) significant long-term side effects even in remission.[24] These are physical – a runny nose, loss of bowel control, and hearing loss – as well as mental. Low self-esteem is common for many cancer sufferers. A 2016 study by Macmillan Cancer Support, and highlighted in the same BBC report, found that of the '625,000 patients in remission', the majority 'are suffering with depression after cancer treatment'. We often think that security issues are about protecting personal banking on the Internet, preventing terrorism incidents and stopping human trafficking, but there are also ongoing biosecurity issues in the medical sciences concerning (once more) whose body and mind is it anyway?[25]

Other communication issues are easily identifiable. How many people, for instance, really understand that coroners, medical researchers and pathologists have relied on the dead body to demarcate their professional standing and still do?[26] In the past, to raise the status of the Coronial office (by way of example) there was a concerted campaign to get those coroners that were by tradition legally qualified to become medically qualified. But to achieve that professional outcome, they needed better access and authority over the dead. And how many people – both those giving consent for use of bodies and body parts and those with a vaguer past and present understanding of the processes of research and cause of death evaluation – truly comprehend the journey on which such human material might embark? In the Victorian and Edwardian periods, people might be dissected to their extremities, with organs, bodies and samples retained or circulated for use and re-use. Alder Hey reminded the public that this was also the normative journey in the twentieth century too. Even today, Coronial Inquests create material that is passed on, and time limits on the retention of research material slip and are meant to slip, as we shall see in Part II. The declaration of death by a hospital doctor was (and is) often not the dead-end. As the poet Bill Coyle recently wrote:

> The dead, we say, are departed. They
> pass on, they pass away, they leave behind
> family, friends, the whole of humankind –
> They have gone on before. Or so we say.[27]

But, he asks, 'could it be the opposite is true?' To be alive is to experience a future tense 'through space and time'. To be dead is all about the deceased becoming fixed in time – 'while you stay where you are', as the poet reminds us. Yet, this temporal dichotomy – the living in perpetual motion, the dead stock-still – has been and remains deceptive. Medical science and training rely, has always relied, on the constant movement of bodies, body parts and tissue samples. Tracing the history of this movement is a key part in addressing current ethical questions about where the limits of that process of movement should stand, and thus is central to the novel contribution being made in this book.

A final sense of the importance of historical perspective in understanding current questions about body ethics can be gained by asking the question: When is a body dead? One of the difficulties in arriving at a concise definition of a person's dead-end is that the concept of death itself has been a very fluid one in European society.[28] In early modern times, when the heart stopped the person was declared dead. By the late-Georgian era, the heart and lungs had to cease functioning together before the person became officially deceased. Then by the early nineteenth century, surgeons started to appreciate that brain death was a scientific mystery and that the brain was capable of surviving deep physical trauma. The notion of coma, hypothermia, oxygen starvation, resuscitation and its neurology entered the medical canon. Across the British Empire, meantime, cultures of death and their medical basis in countries like India and on the African subcontinent remained closely associated with indigenous spiritual concepts of the worship of a deity.[29] Thus, the global challenge of 'calling the time of death' started to be the subject of lively debates from the 1960s as intersecting mechanisms – growing world population levels, the huge costs of state-subsidised healthcare, the rise of do not resuscitate protocols in emergency medicine, and a biotechnological revolution that made it feasible to recycle human material in ways unimaginable fifty years before – gave rise to questions such as when to prolong a whole life and when to accept that the parts of a person are more valuable to others. These now had more focus and meaning. Simultaneously, however, the reach of medical technology in the twentieth century has complicated the answers to such questions. As the ability to monitor even the faintest traces of human life – chemically in cells – biologically in the organs – and neurologically in the brain – became more feasible in emergency rooms and Intensive Care Units, hospital staff began to witness the wonders of the human body within. It turned out to have survival mechanisms seldom seen or understood.

In the USA, Professor Sam Parnia's recent work has highlighted how calling death at twenty minutes in emergency room medicine has tended to be done for customary reasons rather than sound medical ones.[30] He points out, 'My basic message is this: The death we commonly perceive today . . . is a death that can be reversed' and resuscitation figures tell their own story: 'The average resuscitation rate for cardiac arrest patients is 18 per cent in US hospitals and 16 per cent in Britain. But at this hospital [in New York] it is 33 per cent – and the rate peaked at 38 per cent earlier this year.'[31] Today more doctors now recognise that there is a fine line between *peri-mortem* – at or near the point of death – and *post-mortem* – being in death. And, it would be a brave medic indeed who claimed that they always know the definitive difference because it really depends on how much the patient's blood can be oxygenated to protect the brain from anoxic insults in trauma. Ironically, however, the success story of medical technology has started to reintroduce medical dilemmas with strong historical roots. An eighteenth-century surgeon with limited medical equipment in his doctor's bag knew that declaring the precise time of death was always a game of medical chance. Their counterpart, the twenty-first-century hospital consultant, is now equipped with an array of technology, but calling time still remains a calculated risk. Centuries apart, the historical irony is that in this grey zone, 'the past may be dead', but sometimes 'it is very difficult to make it lie down'.[32]

In so many ways, then, history matters in a book about disputed bodies and body disputes. Commenting in the press on controversial NHS organ donation scandals in 1999, Lord Winston, a leading pioneer of infertility and IVF treatments, said:

The headlines may shock everyone, but believe me, the research is crucial. . . . Organs and parts of organs are removed and subjected to various tests – They are weighed and measured, pieces removed and placed under the microscope and biochemically tested. While attempts can be made to restore the external appearance of the body at the conclusion of a post-mortem, it is inevitable some parts may be occasionally missing.[33]

Winston admitted that someone of Jewish descent (as he was) would be upset to learn that a loved one's body was harvested for medical research without consent and that what was taken might not be returned. As a scientist, he urged people to continue to be generous in the face of a public scandal. He was, like many leading figures in the medical profession, essentially asking the public to act in a more enlightened manner than the profession had itself done for centuries. The sanctions embodied in HTA2004 – the Human Tissue Authority public informa-tion website explains for instance that: 'It is unlawful to have human tissue with the intention of its DNA being analyzed, without the consent of the person from whom the tissue came' – are a measure of the threat to public trust that Winston was prefiguring.[34] But this was not a new threat. As one leading educationalist pointed out in a feature article for the BBC *Listener* magazine in March 1961: 'Besides, there are very few cultural or historical situations that are inert' – the priority, he pointed out, should be dismembering medicine's body of ethics – comparable, he thought, to 'corpses patiently awaiting dissection'.[35] By the early twenty-first century it was evident that medical ethics had come to a crucial crossroads and the choice was clear-cut. Medicine had to choose, either 'propri-etorial' or 'custodial' property rights over the dead body, and to concede that the former had been its default position for too long.[36] Phrases like 'public trust' could no longer simply be about paying lip service to public sensibilities, and there had been some recognition that the medical sciences needed to make a cultural transition in the public imagination from an ethics of conviction to an ethics of responsibility.[37] Yet this transition is by no means complete. New legislation crossed a legal threshold on informed consent, but changing ingrained opinions takes a lot longer. And wider questions for both the public and scientists remain: Is the body ever a 'dead-end' in modern medical research? At what end-of-life stage should no more use be made of human material in a clinical or laboratory setting? Have the dead the moral right to limit future medical break-throughs for the living in a Genome era? Would you want your body material to live on after you are dead? And if you did, would you expect that contribution to be cited in a transcript at an award ceremony for a Nobel Prize for science? Are you happy for that *gift* to be anonymous, for medical law to describe your dead body as *abandoned* to posterity? Or perhaps you agree with the former Archbishop of Canterbury, Dr. Rowan Williams, Master of Magdalen College Cambridge, who believes that 'the dead must be named' or else we lose our sense of shared humanity in the present?[38]

In this journey from proprietorial to custodial rights, from the ethics of conviction to an ethics of responsibility, and to provide a framework for answering the rhetorical questions posed above, history is important. And central to that history are the individual and collective lives of the real people whose usually hidden stories lie behind medical progress and medical scandal. They are an intrinsic aspect of a medical mosaic, too often massaged or airbrushed in a history of the body, because it seemed harder to make sense of the sheer scale of the numbers involved and their human complexities. Engaging the public today involves co-creating a more complete historical picture.

Book Themes

Against this backdrop, the primary purpose of this book is to ask what have often been uncomfortable questions about the human material harvested for research and teaching in the past. It has often been assumed (incorrectly) that the journey of such material could not be traced in the historical archives because once dead bodies and their parts had entered a modern medical research culture, their 'human stories' disappeared in the name of scientific 'progress'. In fact, the chapters that follow are underpinned by a selection of representative case-studies focussing on Britain in the period 1945 to 2000. Through them, we can reconstruct, trace and analyse the multi-layered material pathways, networks and thresholds the dead passed through as their bodies were broken up in a complex and often secretive chain of supply. The overall aim is therefore to recover a more personalised history of the body at the end of life by blending the historical and ethical to touch on a number of themes that thread their way throughout Parts I and II. We will encounter, inter alia, notions of trust and expertise; the problem of piecemeal legislation; the ambiguities of consent and the 'extra time' of the dead that was created; the growth of the Information State and its data revolution; the ever-changing role of memory in culture; the shifting boundaries of life and death (both clinically and philosophically); the differential power relations inside the medical profession; and the nature and use of history itself in narratives of medical 'progress'. In the process, the book moves from the local to the national and, in later chapters, to the international, highlighting the very deep roots of concerns over the use of the dead which we casually associate with the late twentieth century.

  Part II presents the bulk of the new research material, raising fundamental historical questions about: the working practices of the medical sciences; the actors, disputes and concealments involved; the issues surrounding organ donation; how a range of professionals inside dissection rooms, Coronial courts, pathology premises and hospital facilities often approached their work-flows in an ahistorical way; the temporal agendas set by holding on to research material as long as possible; the extent to which post-war medical research demanded a greater breaking up of the body compared to the past; and the ways that the medical profession engaged in acts of spin-doctoring at difficult moments in its contemporary history. Along the way, elements of actor network theory are utilised (an approach discussed in Chapter 1). This is because the dead passed through the hands and knowledge of a range of actors, including hospital porters, undertakers, ambulance drivers, coroners, local government officials registering death certificates, as well as those cremating clinical waste, not all of whom are currently understood as agents of biomedicine. The chapters also invite readers of this book to make unanticipated connections from core questions of body ethics to, for instance: smog, air pollution, networks between institutions and the deceased and the cultural importance of female bodies to dissection. These perspectives are balanced by taking into account that medical scientists are complex actors in their own right too, shaped by social, cultural, political, economic and administrative circumstances, that are sometimes in their control, and sometimes not. In other words, this book is all about the messy business of human research material and the messy inside stories of its conduct in the modern era.

In this context, three research objectives frame Chapters 4 to 6. The first is to investigate how the dead passed along a complex chain of material supply in twentieth-century medicine and what happened at each research stage, high-lighting why those post-mortem journeys still matter for the living, because they fundamentally eroded trust in medicine in a way that continues to shape public debates. We thus begin in Chapter 4 with a refined case-study analysis of the human material that was acquired or donated to the dissection room of St Bartholomew's Hospital in London from the 1930s to the 1970s. Since Victorian times, it has been the fourth largest teaching facility in Britain. Never-before-seen data on dissections and their human stories reconnect us to hidden histories of the dead generated on the premises of this iconic place to train in medicine, and wider historical lessons in an era when biomedicine moved centre-stage in the global community.

Second, we then take a renewed look at broken-up bodies and the muddled bureaucracy that processed them. This human material was normally either dis-patched using a bequest form from the mid-1950, or, more usually, acquired from a care home or hospice because the person died without close relatives in the modern era and was not always subject to the same rigorous audit procedures. What tended to happen to these body stories is that they arrived in a dissection room or research facility with a patient case note and then clinical mentalities took over. In the course of which, little consideration was given to the fact that processes of informed consent (by hospitals, coroners, pathologists and transplant teams) were not as transparent as they should have been; some parts of the body had been donated explicitly (on kidney donor cards) and others not (such as the heart). Effectively, the 'gift' became piecemeal, even before the organ transplantation, dissection or further research study got under way. Frequently, bureaucracy de-identified and therefore abridged the 'gift exchange'. Human connections were thus consigned to the cul-de-sac of history. This is a physical place (real, rather than imagined) inside medical research processes where the human subjects of medical 'progress' often got parked out of sight of the general public. The majority were labelled as retentions and refrigerated for a much longer period of time than the general public generally realised, sometimes up to twenty-five years. This is not to argue that these retentions were necessarily an inconvenient truth, a professional embarrassment or part of a conspiracy theory with Big Pharma. Rather, retentions reflected the fact that the promise of 'progress' and a consequent augmentation of medico-legal professional status and authority proved very difficult to deliver unless it involved little public consultation in an era of democracy. Thus Chapter 5 analyses questions of the 'extra time' for the retention of bodies and body parts created inside the working practices of coroners and which are only drawn out through detailed consideration of organ donation controversies. A lack of visibility of these body parts was often the human price of a narrative of 'progress' and that invisibility tended to disguise the end of the process of use, and larger ethical questions of dignity in death. Likewise, a publicity-shy research climate created many missed research opportunities; frequently, coroners' autopsies got delayed, imprecise paperwork was commonplace at post-mortems and few thought the bureaucratic system was working efficiently. As we will see in Chapter 5, frustrated families complained about poor communication levels between the police, coroners and grieving relatives, factors that would later influence the political reach of HTA2004. Paradoxically, the medical sciences, by not putting their ethics in order sooner, propped up a supply system of the dead that was not working for everyone involved on the inside, and thus recent legislation, instead of mitigating against the mistakes of this recent past, regulated much more extensively. In so doing, serendipity – the opportunity costs of potential future medical breakthroughs – took second place to the need for an overhaul of informed consent. Hidden histories of the dead therefore proved to be tactical and not strategic in the modern era for the medical research community.

Finally, the book culminates by examining the complex ways that bodies could be disputed, and how the body itself was in dispute with, the best intentions of new medical research after 1945. It focusses specifically on the work of pathologists in the modern era and their extensive powers of retention and further research. Unquestionably, many patients have benefitted from brain banking and the expansion of the science of neurology, a central thematic focus of Chapter 6. Yet, this innovative work was often conducted behind the closed doors of research facilities that did not see the need for better public engagement, until recently. As we shall see, that proved to be a costly error too, both for levels of professional trust in pathologists and better public understanding of what patients could expect of medicine in painful end-of-life situations. For many patients, meanwhile, the side-effects of drug development for brain conditions have sometimes been downplayed with detrimental outcomes for their sense of well-being. Quality-of-life 'gains' did contrast with the claims of 'progress' that underpinned a furtive research climate, and this resulted in a public stand-off once NHS scandals about brain retention started to emerge in 1999. On the one hand, in an ageing population research into degenerative diseases had and has a powerful role to play in global medicine. On the other hand, medicine still needs to learn much more about the complex and interconnected relationship between brain, emotion and memory formation as lived experiences. Few in the medical professions appreciated that missed body disputes – misinformation by doctors about lengthy retentions of human material – could create a countermovement that disputed medicine's best intentions. Disputes about the body can go both ways – forwards and backwards – grateful and resentful – accepting and questioning – and it is this Janus-like approach that the book in part recounts.

To enter into this closed world of medico-legal actors and their support staff without setting their working-lives in context would be to misunderstand this fascinating and fast-moving modern medical research culture from 1945 in Britain. In Part I, therefore, Chapter 1 outlines the key historical debates there have been about this complex medical community of competing interest groups and their focus on the need to obtain more human research material. It concentrates on the main gaps in our historical knowledge about their working-lives. To fully appreciate that backdrop, Chapter 2 reviews the broad ethical and legal frameworks that regulated the use of the dead for research purposes locally, nationally and internationally. In this way, Chapter 3 illustrates, with a selection of representative human stories, the main cultural trends and threads of the central argument of the book that will be developed in Part II. We end this Introduction, therefore, with a thought-provoking encounter on the BBC imagined for us by Christopher Hitchens – talented journalist, public intellectual and writer, science champion, prominent atheist and cancer sufferer. He reminded his worldwide audience in *Mortality* (2012) why hidden histories of the dead matter to us all in a global community. His body had disputed chemotherapy's 'kill or cure venom' that made him 'a passive patient in a fight he did not pick' with cancer. He disputed the 'battle' he was expected to wage when the disease was battling him, and praised the promise of precision medicine to retrieve out of the cul-de-sac of history, lost or neglected parts of this dreaded human experience, to be fused with new knowledge and creative-thinking.[39] He hoped that superstitions surrounding cancer (what he called 'its maladies of the mind and body') would eventually 'yield to reason and science' not just in the laboratory but by co-creating with patients, both the living and the dead. For Hitchens died on 15 December 2011. The final deadline that he met was to sequence his genome. It remains deposited for posterity at the

American National Institutes of Health. He pushed past the dead-end one last time, into scientific eternity – *Eram quod eros quod sum – I am what you are; you will be what I am.*[40]

Notes

1. See, by way of example, Duncan Wilson, *Tissue Culture in Science and Society: The Public Life of Biological Technique in Twentieth Century Britain* (Basingstoke: Palgrave Macmillan, 2011); and Wilson, *The Making of British Bioethics* (Manchester: Manchester University Press, 2014); Michael Brown, 'Book review section', *History*, 98 (2013), 330: 302–304.
2. See notably, Peter Gøtzsche, *Deadly Medicines and Organised Crime: How Big Pharma Has Corrupted Healthcare* (London & New York: Radcliffe Publishing, 2014).
3. See, 'NHS waste backlog: what are the rules on disposal?', BBC News, 24 July 2019, accessed 24/7/2019 at: www.bbc.co.uk/news/health-45760576
4. James Rothwell, Qadijah Irshad and Bill Gardner, 'Human remains found in 100 containers of exported recycling sent from UK to Sri Lanka', *Daily Telegraph*, News, 23 July 2019, p. 1.
5. Evidence about this concern, by Sir Mark Wolpert and others, was submitted on behalf of the Royal College of Surgeons and Wellcome Trust to the House of Commons reading on the most recent Human Tissue Bill (15 January 2004). The particular issues were then highlighted in *Hansard*, vols. 40115–16, col. 995, speech at 2.31 p.m., 15 January 2004, Mr Andrew Landsley's evidence, Conservative MP for South Cambridgeshire, at the reading of the clauses in the Human Tissue Bill (15 January 2004), of the new relating to scientists being subject to criminal charges for breach of the HTA guidelines, accessed 17/01/17 at: www.publications.parliament.uk/pa/cm200304/cmhansrd/vo040115/debt ext/40115-16.htm
6. Beat M. Riederer and José L. Bueno-López, 'Anatomy, respect for the body and body donation – a good practice guide', *European Journal of Anatomy*, 18 (December 2014), 4: 361–368, quote at p. 361.
7. Beat M. Riederer, 'Body donations today and tomorrow: what is best practice and why?' *Clinical Anatomy*, 29 (October 2015), 1: 11–18.
8. The African continent underwent a survey in 2010 and the majority of donations in South Africa and Zimbabwe came from the white community, whereas in Libya (a Muslim country) 'unclaimed' bodies are imported from India. Refer, Hope Gangata, Patheka Ntaba, Princess Akol and Graham Louw, 'The reliance of unclaimed cadavers for anatomical teaching by medical schools in Africa', *American Sciences Education, Journal of the American Association of Anatomists*, 3 (July–August 2010), 4: 174–183; Emeka G. Anyanwu, Emmanuel N. Obikili and Augustine U. Agu, 'The dissection room experience: a factor in the choice of organ and whole body donation – a Nigerian survey', *Anatomical Sciences Education*, 7 (2014), 1: 56; Erick J. Mazyala, Makaranga Revocatus, Mange Manyama, et al., 'Human bodies bequest program: a wake-up call to Tanzanian medical schools', *Advances in Anatomy* (2014), 1: 1; Beverley Kramer and Erin F. Hutchinson, 'Transformation of a cadaver population: analysis of a South African cadaver program, 1921–2013', *Anatomical Sciences Education*, 8 (2015), 5: 445.

9. See, for example, Peter A. Khan, Thomas H. Champney and Sabine Hildebrant, 'The incompatibility of the use of unclaimed bodies with ethical anatomical education in the United States: letters to the editor', *Journal of Anatomical Sciences Education* (December 2016), Letter, p. 1.

10. Gareth Jones, 'Unclaimed bodies are anatomy's shameful inheritance', *Scientist*, 2965 (15 April 2014), Comment section, p. 1.

11. Nina Bernstein, 'Unearthing the secrets of New York's mass graves', *New York Times*, 15 May 2016. See also follow-up articles in the *New York Times*: 'Bill would require relatives' consent for schools to use cadavers', 26 June 2016; 'New York's city medical schools will stop using unclaimed bodies', 10 August 2016; 'New York State bans use of unclaimed dead as cadavers without consent', 19 August 2016.

12. See, The Hart Island Project, accessed 9/2/2017 at: www.hartisland.net/

13. Refer also, E. Halperin, 'The poor, the black, and the marginalized as the source of cadavers in United States anatomical education', *Clinical Anatomy*, 20 (2007): 489–495.

14. Ibid., 1.

15. Heather E. Douglas, 'The moral responsibilities of scientists: tensions between autonomy and responsibility', *The American Philosophical Quarterly* (5 December 2012), accessed 13/10/2016 at: www.academia.edu/987446/The_moral_responsibilities_of_scientists_tensions_between_autonomy_and_responsibility

16. George Santayana, *The Life of Reason and Common Sense; The Phases of Human Progress (1905–6): The Age of Reason*, volume 1 (New York & London: Scribner's & Constable, 1905), p. 82.

17. Thomas Laqueur, *The Work of the Dead: A Cultural History of Mortal Remains* (Princeton: Princeton University Press, 2018 edition), p. 1.

18. Ibid., p. 84.

19. George Santayana, *Winds of Doctrine: Studies in Contemporary Opinion* (New York & London: Scribner's & Dent, 1913), p. 199.

20. On the historic scale of harvesting the bodies of the poor for medical teaching and research see Elizabeth T. Hurren, *Dying for Victorian Medicine: English Anatomy and Its Trade in the Dead Poor, c. 1834–1929* (Basingstoke: Palgrave Macmillan, 2012).

21. Laqueur, *The Work of the Dead*, p. 79.

22. *Daily Mail*, Health section, 4 May 1968, issue 22396, p. 8.

23. See, Elizabeth T. Hurren, '"Abnormalities and deformities": the dissection and interment of the insane poor, 1832–1929', *Journal of the History of Psychiatry*, 23 (2012), 89: 65–77.

24. 'Cancer: thousands surviving in the UK decades after diagnosis', BBC News, 1 August 2016, accessed 2/8/2016 at: www.bbc.co.uk/news/health-36925974

25. See, for instance, Hannah Landecker, 'Between beneficence and chattel: the human biological in law and science', *Science in Context*, 12 (1999): 203–225; Veena Das, 'The practice of organ transplants: networks, documents, translations', in Margaret Lock, Allan Young and Alberto Cambrosio (eds.), *Living and Working with the New Medical Technologies: Intersections of Inquiry* (Cambridge: Cambridge University Press, 2000), pp. 263–287; Nancy Scheper-Hughes, 'The ends of the body – commodity fetishism and the global traffic in organs', *SAIS*

Review, 22 (2002): 61–80; Catherine Waldby and Robert Mitchell, *Tissue Economies: Blood, Organs, and Cell Lines in Late Capitalism* (Durham, NC: Duke University Press, 2006); Susan Lederer, *Flesh and Blood: Organ Transplantation and Blood Transfusion in Twentieth Century America* (Oxford: Oxford University Press, 2008), notably chapter 'Banking on the body', pp. 68–106; Farhat Moazam, Riffat Moazam Zaman and Aamir M. Jafarey, 'Conversations with kidney vendors in Pakistan: an ethnographic study', *Hastings Centre Report*, 39 (May–June 2009), 3: 29–44; Michele Goodwin (ed.), *The Global Body Market: Altruism's Limits* (Cambridge: Cambridge University Press, 2013).

26. Refer, Hurren, *Dying for Victorian Medicine.*

27. A poem titled 'Leave Taking' in Bill Coyle, *The God of This World to His Prophet* (Chicago: Ivan R. Dee Publishers, 2006), p.7.

28. Medical experiences detailed in Elizabeth T. Hurren, *Dissecting the Criminal Corpse: Staging Post-Execution Punishment in Early Modern England* (Basingstoke: Palgrave Macmillan, 2016).

29. See, notably, William Dalrymple, *Nine Lives: In Search of the Sacred in Modern India* (London: Bloomsbury, 2009).

30. See https://medicine.stonybrookmedicine.edu/medicine/sleep/resuscitation – Professor Sam Parnia's clinical and research areas are in cardiac arrest resuscitation, brain resuscitation and the cognitive sequelae of surviving cardiac arrest including near death experiences. He is Director of Resuscitation Research at the State University of New York at Stony Brook, USA and an honorary fellow at Southampton University Hospital, UK. Refer, Sam Parnia, *What Happens When We Die?* (Carlsbad, Calif. & London: Hay House, 2005); Sam Parnia with Josh Young, *Erasing Death: The Science That Is Rewriting the Boundaries Between Life and Death* (London & New York: HarperOne Books, 2013); Sam Parnia, *The Lazarus Effect: The Science That Is Rewriting the Boundaries between Life and Death* (London & New York: Rider Books, 2014).

31. 'We'll soon be able to bring the dead back to life – Dr Sam Parnia', *Daily Mail*, 30 July 2013, accessed 3/8/2016 at: www.dailymail.co.uk/health/article-2381442/Dr-Sam-Parnia-claims-corpses-soon-revived-24-hours-death.html

32. John Hale, 'Forcing the young into the past', *BBC Listener*, 1667 (Thursday, 9 March 1961), pp. 1–2, quote at p. 2.

33. Lord Winston interview, Good Health opinion section, response to 'The organ snatchers in the NHS', *Daily Mail*, 5 December 2000, p. 50.

34. Refer, HTA website, accessed 2/11/2016 at: www.hta.gov.uk/policies/human-tissue-act-2004. It explains that there is separate Scottish legislation, the Human Tissue (Scotland) Act 2006. For Wales, see the Human Transplantation (Wales) Act 2003 that amended HTA2004 'to allow for consent to deceased organ donation to be deemed in certain circumstances when a person both lived and died in Wales'. Otherwise, HTA2004 covers England, Wales and Northern Ireland. We return to this context in Chapters 1 and 2.

35. Hale, 'Forcing the young into the past', p. 1.

36. See, notably, Prue Vines, 'The sacred and the profane: the role of property concepts in disputes about post-mortem examination', *Sydney Law Review*, 29 (2007): 235–261. We will later be looking in closer detail at this 'ethical turn' in modern medical research.

37. I am very grateful to Professor Thomas Sokoll for this conceptual framework in Thomas Sokoll, 'The moral foundation of modern capitalism: towards an historical reconsideration of Max Weber's "Protestant Ethic"', in Stefan Berger and Alexandra Przyrembel (eds.), *Moralizing Capitalism, Agents, Discourses and Practices of Capitalism and Anti-Capitalism in the Modern Age* (Basingstoke: Palgrave Macmillan, 2019), pp. 79–108.

38. Dr. Rowan Williams, 'Thinking Anglicans: Easter sermon', Canterbury Cathedral, 11 April 2004, accessed 17/01/2017 at: www.thinkinganglicans.org.uk/archives/0 00556.html

39. Christopher Hitchens, 15 October 2015, interviewed for *BBC Newsnight* by Jeremy Paxman, accessed 22/2/2020 at: www.youtube.com/watch?v=LIVEsa2g4ag

40. Christopher Hitchens, *Mortality* (London & New York: Atlantic Books, 2012), p. 1 & pp. 40–41. Hitchens admired ancient Greece for its secular values and love of beauty in nature, learning and architecture. This inscription was often written in Latin on the gravestones of its fallen heroes who lived and died for humanity.

1   Disputed Bodies and Their Hidden Histories

Introduction

In January 2001, the famous English sportsman Randolph Adolphus Turpin was elected into America's International Boxing Hall of Fame. The celebration marked fifty years since he had defeated Sugar Ray Robinson to win the world middle-weight boxing title in 1951.[1] Older fans of boxing appreciated that Turpin would not be present at the US inauguration. He had committed suicide aged just 38, in 1966. Few, however, knew that the fatal decision to end his life had caused considerable controversy in British medical circles. His boxer's brain became the subject of professional debates and medical research disputes between a coroner, pathologist, senior neurologists and heart specialists, as well as his family and the popular press. In 1966, the tragic events were opened up to public enquiry and exposed medico-legal tensions about who owned a body and its parts in death. In neglected archives, forgotten medical stories like that of Turpin reveal narratives of the dead that often question the global picture of a medico-scientific consensus which argued that the accumulation, deidentification and retention of human material was necessary for 'progress'. We rediscover, instead, faces, people, families and communities whose loved ones became the unacknowledged bedrock of modern British medical research. These missing persons relocated in the historical record exemplify that medical breakthroughs could have been part of an important and ongoing public engagement campaign in a biomedical age.

On Friday 22 July 1966, the lead sports writer of the *Daily Mail* featured the sad death of Turpin. The ex-boxer 'shot himself with a .22 pistol in an attic bedroom over his wife's Leamington Spa café on May 17'.[2] The case looked like a straightforward suicide, but was to prove to be more complicated and controversial. Turpin died 'after wounding his daughter, Carmen, aged two' (although critically injured, she survived the violent attack by her father). At the Inquest, medical evidence established how: 'Turpin fired at himself twice. The first bullet lodged against his skull but was not fatal. The second passed through his heart.' The coroner, however, came in for considerable criticism in the press about his conclusions. It was noted that 'Dr. H. Stephens Tibbits did not call for the brain tests that could have decided if brain damage caused by Turpin's 24 years of boxing (including his amateur days) might have contributed to his state of mind on the day he died'. The pathologist who conducted the post-mortem on behalf of the Coronial hearing expressed the prevailing medical view that: 'An examination by a neuropathologist using a fine microscope could have disclosed any tell-tale symptoms of brain damage such as a boxer might suffer.' In particular, more medical research would have pinpointed 'traces of haemorrhage in the tiny blood vessels of his brain'. But Dr Barrowcliff (pathologist) was not permitted to proceed because Dr Tibbits (coroner) would not authorise him to do so. The pathologist regretted that: 'There was a certain amount of urgency involved here' because of the fame of the suicide victim 'to which academic interest took second place'. The press thus noted: that 'the opportunity had been missed to carry out this study was received with dismay from a physician concerned with the Royal College of Physicians Committee on Boxing'. Its 'eight leading specialists on the brain, heart and eyes' were very disappointed that the pursuit of medical research that was in the public interest had been overridden by a coroner's exclusive powers over the dead. The family meanwhile were relieved to have been consulted at all, since it was not a legal requirement at the time. They were anxious that the Coronial hearing should take into account Turpin's suicide note. His last words, in fact, revealed disagreement between medical personnel, the family and suicide victim about the cause of death and therefore the potential of his brain for further research. To engage with this sort of hidden history of the dead and its body parts dispute, which is normally neglected in the literature, we need to trace this human story in greater archival depth.

Thus, Turpin left a handwritten note which stated that the Inland Revenue were chasing him for a large unpaid tax bill. He claimed this was levied on money he had not actually earned, and this was the chief cause of his death – 'Naturally they will say the balance of my mind was disturbed but it is not', he wrote; 'I have had to carry the can.'[3] Money troubles since his retirement from boxing in 1958 certainly seemed to have mounted. Four years previously the *Daily Mail* had reported on a bankruptcy hearing which established that 'Turpin who earned £150,000 from his boxing career, now tussles for £25 a bout as a wrestler'.[4] At a tax hearing at Warwick it was reported that: 'His main creditor is the Inland Revenue. It claims £17,126 tax for boxing earnings between 1949 and 1958.' He still owed '£15, 225' and could only offer to pay back the tax bill 'at £2 per week' – a repayment schedule which would take '153 years'. Turpin had earned about £750 in 1961–2, but paid back a loan to a friend of £450 and £300 to his wife in cash, rather than the taxman. He was essentially broke and a broken man. The press, however, did not let the matter of his perilous financial situation or mental health condition rest. And because they did not, we can retrace the human circumstances of a controversial Coronial case concerning his valuable brain material: an approach this book will be following in subsequent chapters. For the aim is to uncover the sorts of human faces that were subsumed inside modern British medical research cultures.

In a hard-hitting editorial, the *Daily Mail* insisted that: 'two questions must be answered about Randolph Turpin's wretched life whilst boxing – Was he the lingering victim of punch drunkenness? What happened to the £585,439 paid to see his four title fights?' Here was a 'back-street kid who was a wealthy champion at 23, bankrupt at 34, and demented and dead at 38'.[5] His 'first marriage broke up, there were stories of assaults all pointing to a diminishing sense of social responsibility. A second marriage was to bring him happiness but his career... never recovered'. The newspaper asked why his family GP was not called as a medical witness at the Inquest. When interviewed by the press, the family doctor said that although 'I do not like using the phrase, I would say that Turpin was punch drunk. He was not the sort of man to worry about financial matters or about people who had let him down. In my opinion boxing was responsible for his death.' It was revealed that Turpin was 'part deaf from a childhood swimming accident' and he became 'increasingly deaf through the years'. The GP, however, believed his hearing impairment had not impacted on either his physical balance or the balance of his mind. His elder brother and a family friend, nevertheless, contradicted that statement, telling the press that Turpin had 'eye trouble' and 'double vision' from his boxing days. He often felt dizzy and disorientated. The difficulty was that only Turpin's 4-year-old daughter, Charmaine, and his youngest child, Carmen, aged 17 months (she sustained 'bullet wounds in her head and chest'[6]) really knew what happened at the suicidal shooting. They were too young and traumatised to give evidence in the coroner's court.[7] In the opinion of Chief Detective-Inspector Frederick Bunting, head of Warwickshire CID, it was simply a family tragedy.[8] Turpin had risen from childhood poverty and fought against racial discrimination (his father was from British Guyana and died after being gassed in WWI; his mother, almost blind, brought up five children on an army pension of just 27s per week, living in a single room).[9] Sadly, 'the money came too quickly' and his 'personality did not match his ring skill', according to Bunting. Even so, by the close of the case what was noteworthy from a medico-legal perspective were the overarching powers of the coroner once the corpse came into his official purview. That evidence hinted at a hinterland of medical science research that seldom came into public view.

It seems clear that the pathologist commissioned to do Turpin's post-mortem was prepared to apply pressure to obtain more human material for research purposes. Here was a fit young male body from an ethnicity background that could provide valuable anatomical teaching and research material. This perspective about the utility of the body and its parts was shared by the Royal College of Physicians, who wanted to better understand the impact of boxing on the brain. This public interest line of argument was also highlighted in the medical press, notably the *Lancet*. The family, meanwhile, were understandably concerned with questions of dignity in death. Their priority was to keep Turpin's body intact as much as possible. Yet, what material journeys really happened *in death* were never recounted in the Coronial court. For, once the Inquest verdict of 'death by suicide' was reached, there was no need for any further public accountability. The pathologist in court did confirm that he examined the brain; he said he wanted to do further research, but tellingly he stated that he did not proceed 'at that point'. Crucially, however, he did not elaborate on what would happen beyond 'that point' to the retained brain once the coroner's case was completed in court.

As all good historians know, what is not said, is often as significant as what is. Today historians know to double-check on stories of safe storage by tracing what really happened to valuable human material once the public work of a coroner or pathologist was complete. The material reality was that Turpin's brain was refrigerated, and it could technically be retained for many years. Whilst it was not subdivided in the immediate weeks and months after death, the fact of its retention meant that in subsequent years it could still enter a research culture as a brain slice once the publicity had died down. As we shall see, particularly in Chapter 6, this was a common occurrence from the 1960s onwards. At the time, it was normal for family and friends to trust a medico-legal system that could be misleading about the extra time of the dead it created with human research material. This neglected perspective therefore requires framing in the historiography dealing with bodies, body donations and the harvesting of human material for medical research purposes, and it is this task that informs the rest of the chapter.

The Long View

Historical studies of the dead, anatomisation and the use of bodies for research processes have become increasingly numerous since the early 2000s.[10] Adopting theories and methodological approaches drawn from cultural studies,[11] ethnography,[12] social history, sociology, anthropology and intellectual history, writers have given us an increasingly rich understanding of cultures of death, the engagement of the medical professions with the dead body and the wider culture of body ethics. It is unfeasible (and not desirable) here to give a rendering of the breadth of this field given its locus at the intersection of so many disciplines. To do so would over-burden the reader with a cumbersome and time-consuming literature review. Imagine entering an academic library and realising that the set reading for this topic covered three floors of books, articles and associated reading material. It could make even the most enthusiastic student of the dead feel defeated. Two features of that literature, however, are important for the framing of this book.

First, we have become increasingly aware that medical 'advances' were intricately tied up with the power of the state and medicine over the bodies of the poor, the marginal and so-called 'ordinary' people. This partly involved the strategic alignment of medicine with the expansion of asylums, mental hospitals, prisons and workhouses.[13] But it also went much further. Renewed interest in 'irregular' practitioners and their practices in Europe and its colonies highlighted how medical power and professionalisation were inexorably and explicitly linked to the extension of authority over the sick, dying and dead bodies of 'ordinary' people.[14] More than this, the development of subaltern studies on the one hand and a 'history from below' movement on the other hand has increasingly suggested the vital importance for anatomists, medical researchers and other professionals involved in the process of death, of gaining and retaining control of the bodies of the very poorest and least powerful segments of national populations.[15] A second feature of the literature has been a challenge to the sense and ethics of medical 'progress', notably by historians of the body who have been diligent in searching out the complex and fractured stories of the 'ordinary' people whose lives and deaths stand behind 'great men' and 'great advances'. In this endeavour they have, inch by inch, begun to reconstruct a medico-scientific mindset that had been a mixture of caring and careless, clinical and inexact, dignified and disingenuous, elitist and evasive. In this space, ethical dilemmas and mistakes about medicine's cultural impact, such as those highlighted in the Turpin case with which this chapter opened, were multiple. Exploring these mistakes and dilemmas – to some extent explicable but nonetheless fundamental for our understanding of questions of power, authority and professionalisation – is, historians have increasingly seen, much more important than modern 'presentist' views of medicine would have us believe.[16]

These are some of the imperatives for the rest of Parts I and II of this book. The remainder of this first chapter develops some of these historiographical perspectives. It does so by focussing on how trends in the literature interacted with social policy issues in the modern world. What is presented is not therefore a traditional historiographical dissection of the minutiae of academic debates of interest to a select few, but one that concentrates on the contemporary impact of archival work by historians as a collective. For that is where the main and important gap exists in the historical literature – we in general know some aspects of this medical past – but we need to know much more about its human interactions. Before that, however, we must engage with the question of definitions. Thus, around 1970 a number of articles appeared in the medical press about 'spare-part surgery' (today called organ transplantation). 'Live donors' and 'donated' cadavers sourced across the NHS in England will be our focus in this book too. To avoid confusion, we will be referring to this supply system as a combination of 'body donations' (willingly done) and 'mechanisms of body supply' (often involuntary). The former were bequested before death by altruistic individuals; the latter were usually acquired without consent. They entered research cultures that divided up the whole body for teaching, transplant and associated medical research purposes. This material process reflected the point at which the disassembling of identity took place (anatomical, Coronial, neurological and in pathology) into pathways and procedures, which we will be reconstructing. In other words, 'pioneer operations' in transplantation surgery soon 'caught unawares the medical, legal, ethical and social issues' which seemed to the media to urgently require public consultation in Britain.[17] As one contemporary leading legal expert explained:

This is a new area of medical endeavour; its consequences are still so speculative that nobody can claim an Olympian detachment from them. Those who work outside the field do not yet know enough about it to form rational and objective conclusions. Paradoxically, those who work in the thick of it ... know too much and are too committed to their own projects to offer impartial counsel to the public, who are the ultimate judges of the value of spare-part surgery.[18]

Other legal correspondents pointed out that since time was of the essence when someone died, temporal issues were bound to cause a great deal of practical problems:

For a few minutes after death cellular metabolism continues throughout the majority of the body cell mass. Certain tissues are suitable for removal only during this brief interval, although improvements in storage and preservation may permit a short delay in actual implantation in the recipient. Cadaver tissues are divided into two groups according to the speed with which they must be salvaged. First, there are 'critical' tissues, such as the kidney and liver, which must be removed from the deceased within a matter of thirty to forty-five minutes after death. On the other hand, certain 'non-critical' tissues may be removed more at leisure. Skin may be removed within twelve hours from time of death. The cornea may be taken at any time within six hours. The fact is, however, that in all cases action must be taken promptly to make use in a living recipient of the parts of a non-living donor, and this gives rise to legal problems. There is but little time to negotiate with surviving relatives, and waiting for the probate of the will is out of the question.[19]

Transplant surgeons today and anatomists over the past fifty years shared an ethical dilemma – how to get hold of human research material fast before it decayed too much for re-use. It was this common medico-legal scenario that scholars were about to rediscover in the historical record of the hidden histories of the body just as the transplantation era opened.

Ruth Richardson's distinguished book, *Death, Dissection and the Destitute*, was first published in 1987. It pioneered hidden histories of disputed bodies.[20] In it, she identified the significance of the Anatomy Act of 1832 (hereafter

AA1832) in Britain, noting that the poorest by virtue of pauperism had become the staple of the Victorian dissection table. As Richardson pointed out, that human contribution to the history of medical science had been vital but hidden from public view. Those in economic destitution, needing welfare, owed a healthcare debt to society in death according to the New Poor Law (1834). Having identified this class injustice, more substantive detailed archive work was required to appreciate its cultural dimensions, but it would take another twenty-five years for the next generation of researchers to trace what exactly happened to those dying below the critical threshold of relative to absolute poverty.[21] The author of this new book that you are currently reading for the first time (and three previous ones) has been at the vanguard of aligning such historical research with contemporary social policy issues in the medical humanities.

Once that research was under way, it anticipated several high-profile human material scandals in the NHS. These included the retention and storage of children's organs at Alder Hey Children's Hospital, the clinical audit of the practice of Dr Harold Shipman, and the response to the inquiry into the children's heart surgery service at Bristol Royal Infirmary. Such scandals brought to the public's attention a lack of informed consent, lax procedures in death certification, inadequate post-mortems and substandard human tissue retention paperwork, almost all of which depended upon bureaucracy developed from Victorian times. Eventually, these controversies would culminate in public pressure for the passing of HTA2004 to ensure that a proper system of informed consent repealed the various Anatomy Acts of the nineteenth and twentieth centuries, as we will go on to see in Chapter 2. Recent legislation likewise provided for the setting up of a Human Tissue Authority in 2005 to license medical research and its teaching practices in human anatomy, and more broadly regulate the ethical boundaries of biomedicine. As the Introduction suggested, it seemed that finally the secrets of the past were now being placed on open access in the public domain. Or were they?

Today, studies of the cultural history of anatomy and the business of acquiring the dead for research purposes – and it has always been a commercial transaction of some description with remarkable historical longevity – have been the focus of renewed scholarly endeavours that are now pan-European and postcolonial, and encompass neglected areas of the global South.[22] In part, what prompted this genre of global studies was an increasing focus on today's illegal trade in organs and body parts that proliferates in the poorest parts of the world. The most recent literatures on this subject highlight remarkable echoes with the increasingly rich historical record. Scott Carney, for instance, has investigated how the social inequalities of the transplantation era in a global marketplace are prolific because of e-medical tourism. In *The Red Market* (the term for the sale of blood products, bone, skulls and organs), Carney explains that on the Internet in 2011 his body was, and is, worth $200,000 to body-brokers that operate behind an antivirus firewall to protect them against international law.[23] He could also sell what these e-traders term 'black gold' – waste products like human hair or teeth – less dangerous to his well-being to extract for sale but still intrinsic to his sense of identity and mental health. Carney calculates that the commodification of human hair is a $900 billion worldwide business. The sacred (hair bought at Hindu temples and shrines) has become the profane (wigs, hair extensions and so on) whether it involves 'black gold' or 'Red Market' commodities, in which Carney's original phrasing (quoted in a *New York Times* book review) describes:

an impoverished Indian refugee camp for survivors of the 2004 tsunami that was known as Kidneyvakkam, or Kidneyville, because so many people there had sold their kidneys to organ brokers in efforts to raise desperately needed funds. 'Brokers,' he writes, 'routinely quote a high payout – as much as $3,000 for the operation – but usually only dole out a fraction of the offered price once the person has gone through it. Everyone here knows that it is a scam. Still the women reason that a rip-off is better than nothing at all.' For these people, he adds, selling organs 'sometimes feels like their only option in hard times'; poor people around the world, in his words, 'often view their organs as a critical social safety net'.[24]

Having observed this body-part brokering often during his investigative journalism on location across the developing world, Carney raises a pivotal ethical question. Surely, he asks, in the medical record-keeping the term 'organ donor' in such circumstances is simply a good cover story for criminal activity? When the poorest are exploited for their body parts, eyes, hair and human tissues – dead or alive – the brokers that do this turn the gift of goodwill implied in the phrase 'organ donor' into something far more sinister, the 'organ vendor'. This perspective, as Carney himself acknowledges, is deeply rooted in medical history.

In the past, the removal of an organ or body part from a dissected body involved the immediate loss of a personal history. Harvesting was generally hurried and the paperwork done quickly. A tick box exercise was the usual method within hours of death. Recycling human identity involved medical bureaucracy and confidential paperwork. This mode of discourse mattered. Clinical mentalities soon took over and this lesson from the past has considerable resonance in the present. Thus, by the time that the transplant surgeon talks to the potential recipient of a body donation 'gift', involving a solid organ like the heart, the human transaction can become (and often became) a euphemism. Importantly, that language shift, explains Carney, has created a linguistic register for unscrupulous body traders too. Thus, when a transplant surgeon typically says to a patient today '*you* need a kidney' – what they should be saying is 'you need *someone else's* kidney'. Even though each body part has a personal profile, the language of 'donation' generally discards it in the desire to anonymise the 'gift'. Yet, Carney argues, just because a person is de-identified does not mean that their organ has to lose its hidden history too. It can be summarised: male, 24, car crash victim, carried a donor card, liked sports – female, 35, washerwoman, Bangladeshi, 3 children, healthy, endemic poverty. It might be upsetting on a post-mortem passport to know about the human details, disturbing the organ recipient's mental position after transplant surgery, but modern medical ethics needs to be balanced by declaring the 'gift' from the dead to the living too. Instead, medical science has tended to have a fixed mentality about the superior contribution of bio-commons to its research endeavours.

Historians of the body that have worked on the stories of the poorest in the past to learn their historical lessons for the future, argue that it would be a more honest transaction to know their human details, either post-mortem or post-operative. Speaking about the importance of the 'gift relationship' without including its human face amounts to false history, according to Carney and others. In this, he reflects a growing body of literature on medical tourism, which challenges the prevailing view that medical science's neglected hidden histories do not matter compared to larger systemic questions of social, medical and life-course inequalities for the living. Instead, for Carney and his fellow scholars, the hidden histories of 'body donations' were a dangerous road to travel without public accountability in the material journeys of human beings in Britain after WWII. They created a furtive research climate that others could then exploit. Effectively, unintended consequences have meant that body-brokers do buy abroad, do import those organs and do pass them off as 'body donations' to patients often so desperate for a transplant that medical ignorance is the by-product of this 'spare-part' trade. Just then as the dead on a class basis in the past lost their human faces, today the vulnerable are exploited:

Eventually, *Red Markets* have the nasty social side effect of moving flesh upward – never downward – through social classes. Even without a criminal element, unrestricted free markets act like vampires, sapping the health and strength from ghettos of poor donors and funneling their parts to the wealthy.[25]

Thus, we are in a modern sense outsourcing human misery in medicine to the poorest communities in India, Africa and China, in exactly the same way that medical science once outsourced its body supply needs in the past to places of high social deprivation across Britain, America and Australia, as well as European cities like Brussels and Vienna.[26] The dead (in the past), the living-dead (in the recent past) and those living (today) are part of a chain of commodification over many centuries. In other words, what medical science is reluctant to acknowledge and which historians have been highlighting for thirty years is that a wide variety of hidden histories of the body have been shaped by the 'tyranny of the gift', as much as altruism, and continue to be so.[27]

Unsurprisingly, then, the complexities surrounding this 'gift relationship' are an important frame for this book.[28] Margaret Lock, for instance, has explored *Twice Dead: Transplants and the Reinvention of Death* (2002) and 'the Christian tradition of charity [which] has facilitated a willingness to donate organs to strangers' via a medical profession which ironically generally takes a secular view of the 'donated body'.[29] One reason she notes that public confidence broke down in the donation process was that medical science did not review 'ontologies of death' and their meaning in popular culture. Instead, the emphasis was placed on giving without a balancing mechanism in medical ethics that 'invites an examination of the ways in which contemporary society produces and sustains a discourse and practices that permit us to be thinkers at the end-of-life' and, for the purpose of this book, what we do with the dead-end of life too.[30] Lock helpfully elaborates:

Even when the technologies and scientific knowledge that enable these innovations [like transplant surgery] are virtually the same, they produce different effects in different settings. Clearly, death is not a self-evident phenomenon. The margins between life and death are socially and culturally constructed, mobile, multiple, and open to dispute and reformulation. ... We may joke about being brain-dead but many of us do not have much idea of what is implicated in the clinical situation. ... We are scrutinising extraordinary activities: death-defying technologies, in which the creation of meaning out of destruction produces new forms of human affiliation. These are profoundly emotional matters. ... Competing discourse and rhetoric on the public domain in turn influences the way in which brain death is debated, institutionalised, managed and modified in clinical settings.[31]

Thus, for a generation that donated their bodies after WWII questions of reciprocity were often raised in the press but seldom resolved inside the medical profession by co-creating in medical ethics with the general public. There remained more continuity than discontinuity in the history of body supply, whether for dissection supply or transplant surgery, as we shall see in Part II. The reach of this research culture hence remains overlooked in ways that this book maps for the first time. Meanwhile, along this historical road, as Donna Dickenson highlights, often 'the language of the gift relationship was used to camouflage ... exploitation'. This is the common situation today when a patient consents to their human tissue donation, but it is recycled for commercial gain into data-generation. For the donor is seldom part of that medical choice nor shares directly in the knowledge or profits generated.[32] In other words: 'Researchers, biotechnology companies and funding bodies certainly don't think the gift relationship is irrelevant: they do their very best to promote donors' belief in it, although it is a one-way gift-relationship.'[33] Even though these complex debates about what *can*, and what *should* go for further medical research and training today can seem to be so fast moving that the past is another country, they still merit more historical attention. Consequently, the historical work that Richardson pioneered was a catalyst, stimulating a burgeoning field of medical humanities study, and one with considerable relevance for contemporary social policy trends now.

How then do the hidden histories of this book relate to what is happening today in a biotech age? The answer lies in the immediate aftermath of WWII when medical schools started to reform how they acquired bodies for dissection and what they intended to do with them. Seldom do those procedures and precedents feature in the historical literature. This author studied in-depth older legislation like the Murder Act (running from 1752 to 1832) and the first Anatomy Act (covering 1832–1929) in two previous books. Even so, few studies move forward in time by maintaining those links to the past that continue to have meaning in the post-1945 era in the way that this study does.[34] That anomaly is important because it limits our historical appreciation of medical ethics. It likewise adds to the problem of how science relates its current standards to the recent past. Kwame Anthony Appiah (philosopher, cultural theorist and novelist) conducting the Reith Lectures for the BBC thus reminds us: 'Although our ancestors are powerful in shaping our attitudes to the past' – and we need to always be mindful of this – we equally 'should always be in active dialogue with the past' – to stay engaged with what we have done – and why.[35] Indeed, as academic research has shown in the past decade, the policing of the boundaries of medical ethics that involve the sorts of body disputes which are fundamental to us as a society also involves the maintenance of long-term confidence and public trust that have been placed in the medical sciences. This still requires vigilance, and in this sense the investigation and production of a seamless historical timeframe is vital. Such a process demands that we engage in an overview of the various threshold points that created – and create – hidden histories in the first place.

This is the subject of the next section, but since hidden histories of the body in the post-war period – stories like that of Randolph Turpin – are the product of, reflect and embody the powerful reach of intricate networks of power, influence and control, it is first necessary to engage briefly with the field of actor-network studies. Helpfully, Bruno Latour wrote in the 1980s that every-thing in the world exists in a constantly shifting network of relationships.[36] The human actors involved operate together with varying degrees of agency and autonomy. Retracing and reconstructing these actor networks therefore involves engaged research and engagement with research, argue Michel Callow, John Law and Arne Rip.[37] This approach to historical studies can enhance our collective understanding of how confidence and public trust change over time, as well as illuminate mistrust in the medical sciences. Latour argues we thus first need to 'describe' the network of actors involved in a given situation. Only then can we investigate the 'social forces acting' that shape the matrix of those involved. Latour along with Michel Callow hence prioritised the need to map the dynamic interactions of science and technology since these disciplines have come to such prominence in Western society. How the sociology of science operates in the modern world was likewise an extension of their work. Actor network theory and its study are therefore essentially 'science in action' and are one of the foundational premises of the case studies in Part II of this book.

Latour pioneered this novel approach because he recognised that science needed help to rebuild its reputation and regain its authority in the modern period, at a time when the ethical basis of so much medical research and claims to be in the public good became controversial in the global community. In 1999, John Law and John Hassard outlined a further development of actor network theory, arguing that if it was to become a genuine framework for transdisciplinary studies then it had to have five basic characteristics:

- It does not explore why or how a network takes the form its does.
- It does explore the relational ties of the network – its methods and how to do something within its world.
- It is interested in how common activities, habits and procedures sustain themselves.
- It is adamantly empirical – the focus is how the network of relationships performed – because without performance the network dissolves.
- It is concerned with what conflicts are in the network, as well as consensus, since this is part of the performative social elements.[38]

Michael Lee Scott's 2006 work further refined this model.[39] He pointed out that those who defend the achievements of science and its research cultures too often treat its performance like a car. As long as the car travels, they do not question the performance of the results, the function of its individual components or its destination. Only when science stumbles or breaks down, is its research apparatus investigated. When society treats science like a well-performing car, 'the effect is known as punctualisation'. We need medical mistakes and/or a breakdown of public confidence, argues Scott, to 'punctuate' our apathy about the human costs of the medical sciences to society as a whole. In other words, belief in science and rationalism is logical, but human beings are emotional and experiential too. If science has encapsulated our cultural imaginations for good healthcare reasons, we still need to keep checking that its medical performance delivers for everybody and is ethical. This notion of 'encapsulation', Scott explains, is important for understanding how the research cultures of the medical sciences really work. A useful analogy is computer programming. It is common for programmers to adopt a 'language of mechanism that restricts access to some of the object's component'. In other words, when a member of the general public then turns a computer on, most people are generally only concerned that the computer works today in the way that the car-owner does when they turn on the ignition key in the morning to go to work. Even so, those simple actions hand over a considerable part of human agency to new technology. On the computer, we do not see the language of algorithms (the mechanisms of the system) that have authority over us and conceal their real-time operation. Science operates in an equivalent way to computer programmes, according to Scott, because it has hidden and privileged research objectives, written into its code of conduct and a complex, interrelated and often hidden set of actors. This book takes its lead from this latest conceptual thinking in actor network studies, but it also takes those methods in a novel research direction too. We begin by remodelling the sorts of research threshold points created inside the system of so-called body bequests and what these 'donations' meant for the way that the medical sciences conducted itself, networked and performed its research expertise in post-war Britain.

Remapping Disputed Bodies – Missing Persons' Reports

The quotation 'volenti non fit iniuria' – no wrong is done to one who is willing – encapsulates modern attitudes towards ethical conduct in the dissection room, transplant operation theatre and more widely towards the use of human tissue and body parts for research purposes.[40] In practice, however, things are rarely this simple. Bronwyn Parry, a cultural geographer, has described this defensive position as follows:

New biotechnologies enable us, in other words, to extract genetic or biochemical material from living organisms, to process it in some way – by replicating, modifying, or transforming it – and in so doing, to produce from it further combinations of that information that might themselves prove to be commodifiable and marketable.[41]

In other words, the patient consents, is willing, and soon becomes the 'other', whether in life or death. A new cell-line, blood-product or genome sequence erases an original body identity. The 'donor' and 'donated human part' or 'tissue' are re-designated – 'Out there'.[42] As Margaret Lock explains – 'first a dead body must be recognised as alienable . . . legally available for transfer or sale. Current policies in North America and Europe treat cadavers and body-parts as "quasi-property", thus making them alienable, but their transfer may not involve payment' or at least not a direct payment.[43] Often there is (for instance) a refund of petty cash expenses to suppliers, as a way of working around regulations. The law of medical negligence on both sides of the Atlantic states in case law that the body is '*abandoned*' into these recycling schemes – known as bio-commons. If the person has consented to this, then it is a transparent process. Yet, often, and particularly under the Human Tissue Acts of 1961 and 1984, this was not the case (which Chapter 2 explains in greater detail). During the various government enquiries into NHS organ scandals, the conclusion was that all the original paperwork to reconstruct what really happened had been cursory, destroyed or never created in the first place. Generic figures covering the scale of organ retentions are thus often cited routinely in the historical literature, without checking their material pathways inside the research culture of the time. This book argues that the human material was traceable, provided we begin by reconstructing the threshold points of medical research. Thus, after 1945, the anatomical sciences, coroners and pathologists formed actor networks inside the research community of the medical sciences in Britain. They passed human material along a chain of human supply from operating theatre (amputated part or dead person) to hospital morgue or pathology laboratory, from the teaching lecture theatre or dissection room, to burial or cremation. Together they performed a series of research thresholds in disputed bodies and hidden histories of the dead. In remapping these, it is feasible to trace a whole series of what effectively became missing persons' reports, acknowledged by HTA2004. Conceptually, we need thus to start modelling a process that was hidden from public view.

The first research threshold point of the historical process for each individual 'body donation' was the need to put pressure on people to think more about giving. The second threshold point is usually then the approach made by a medical professional to obtain that tissue or organ when the time is right. The third threshold point normally comes with the medical decision to use that tissue or organ for a particular purpose. These threshold points go on being crossed until the human donor 'disappears' in terms of their whole body identity (see Chapter 4), but crucially their body part or human material does not. In point of fact, it is capable under certain circumstances of being recycled multiple times. A human heart transplanted from a young to an older person could (in theory) for instance be reutilised again, provided, that is, it remains healthy enough to be taken from one transplant recipient and given to another patient on a waiting list (see Chapter 5). Sometimes recipients need two hearts in their lifetime because each operation is time-limited by the effectiveness of immunosuppressant drugs. Mortality rates are much higher in such cases, but they are occasionally medically feasible. Tissue that is cultured or brain slices likewise could be recycled many times for different purposes under a myriad of medical research circumstances (see Chapter 6). This means that crossing these threshold points in modern science will always involve the potential for ambiguity, dispute, dilemma and resolution. Nothing is fixed, little is certain. Yet, medical science does two critical things with and around these threshold points which are in turn crucial for this book.

The first is that it treats each one of the threshold points described above as discrete. This is deliberate because such an approach distracts public attention from potential disputes about the fuzziness that surrounds medical ethics as each research threshold is crossed. The breaking up of a whole body history into parts across discrete moments on a research pathway is essential to disaggregate the

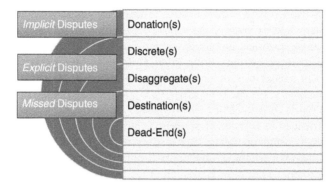

Figure 1.1 Re-modelling the threshold points in body bequests used for dissection and further research in the medical sciences, c. 1945–2015
Source: Author designed, themes embedded in Chapters 4–6, Part II, of this book.

human being from their 'body donation' point. In mapping, therefore, its historical process, we find – donation(s), discrete(s), disaggregate(s) and destination(s) – all to push past – dead-end(s) (see Figure 1.1). In other words, to become the 'other' you need a 'donation mechanism' that separates the 'gift' from its eventual destination, often called 'out there' or 'abandoned' as bio-commons in medical case law.

The second aspect is that medical science effectively treats each threshold point as *a*historical. The history of the person and the body or body part is there but it does not matter or is not central to the crossing of a threshold. To add to the confusion, the keeper of the record of what is happening at each threshold point is one step removed from the clinical bench of medical science itself. The regulator does not take an overview of the entire research recycling process but concentrates instead on monitoring each threshold point: essentially the modus operandi of the Human Tissue Authority and older legislation in the past (see Chapter 2). Regulators tend to wait until medical science reports to them the need for a license to use human material. This is a matter of professional trust, but it also distances that official oversight from the whole body of the donor from which in principle a wide variety of human material disappears from public view. Essentially, medical science's 'body donation mechanism' was (and is) given the capacity to act in a series of discrete steps in terms of its actor-network performance, and because its research professionals did just that, acts of bequest and donation move seamlessly into hidden histories of dead bodies and body parts. However, at each threshold point, relevant choices about its component activities and parts can become controversial – a drug development was judged worth the investment return – a specific treatment became commercialised – an experiment that was externally fundable was prioritised – and so on. In this sense, a set of related ethical questions arises that tends to remain unresolved in the historiography because few study them in-depth. What happens if these threshold points are not considered discrete in popular culture, and as a donor you regard them as *one whole* – as many people did around the time of the NHS scandals in 1999? What happens if this complete history does matter in certain cases, as it did in the case of Randolph Turpin at the start of this chapter? By way of further example, although there are rigorous screening protocols in place for cancer patients in full remission who donate, some recent transplant cases have been reported of a donor giving recipients undetected breast cancer at the point of transplantation.[44] Surgeons estimate the chances of this happening are 'between 1 in 10,000 and 5 in 10,000'; even so, the discrete history of each organ does matter to those living patients reliant on the dead for their healthy survival. Likewise, what happens when you have a whole set of body disputes that emerges in time to undermine public confidence and trust? These are complex issues, but ranging widely over the historiographical literature and primary materials, we can see that dealing in discrete thresholds generates three sorts of tensions (or disputes) between medical science broadly defined and 'ordinary' people and those (like the press) who represented them. These stress points are crucial to this volume.

First, they involve implicit disputes of the sort explored in Chapter 4. Here we encounter the stories of people who allowed use of their bodies by default rather than design, largely a reflection of the fact that nobody explained to them all the research steps properly. Second, we encounter explicit disputes of the sort explored in Chapter 5, where, for instance, coroners co-operating with transplant teams had the right to remove more than they declared officially after, say, road-traffic accidents, discovery of which brings them into direct conflict with families, the law or both. Finally, we can find missed disputes of the sort that underpin Chapter 6. Here, people were not able to dispute the use of dead bodies and their brain material because the discrete thresholds, layered onto complex actor-network relationships, kept them uninformed, such as at Alder Hey Children's Hospital when pituitary glands of dead children were taken as 'bio-extras'. In other words, it is true that 'no harm is done to *someone* that was willing' (as the Latin quotation stated at the start of this section). However, many people might have been unwilling to consent to the extent of what was about to be done to them or their deceased loved one, but they did not know this at the time, and these hidden histories matter to everybody. For, paradoxically, the medical profession prefers piecemeal methodologies that are untraceable, since these are not easily legally accountable. By pausing briefly to engage with a human story, this scenario can be poignantly and powerfully illustrated.

In the late 1950s, a distinguished and decorated hero of WWII died under tragic circumstances. For ethical reasons, this book does not identify this individual because they may still have living relatives. The 100-year rule has been applied to ensure that any distant kin who could not be consulted to give informed consent are still treated with the utmost dignity in this study, despite the fact that some of this information has been in the public domain for sixty years. Detailed record-linkage work reveals that the person in question had worked on mine sweepers in the Atlantic during WWII. Their career ladder was impressive. They were promoted after being 'Mentioned in Despatches' (MID) for bravery and eventually awarded the Distinguished Service Order (DSO). Once the war finished, like many service personnel, they were not discharged for some years after 1945. Even by the early 1950s, there was still a lot of cleaning up to do and de-militarisation of equipment to co-ordinate from the War Office in London. Thus, the war hero transferred to the regions, was allocated a new logistics job. Soon they were 'overworked', according to contemporary accounts. They had to process a large amount of paperwork in what became a busy semi-civilian job. As they were a diligent person, eventually the excessive workload triggered 'depression'. Since they had never had an experience of mental ill-health, they booked an appointment with a local doctor under the new NHS. That GP signed the person off work for a time, but then 'allowed [his patient] to return to work because he considered [the patient] was worrying so much about [the] paperwork piling up' that a leave of absence was counter-productive to the war hero's mental well-being.[45] By now, the individual was middle-aged, had a settled home life, was married in a stable relationship, but still they found it hard to cope at work. Eventually, they drove their family car one Sunday evening to a remote side-road near the coast in the South of England and attached a tube from the exhaust pipe into the passenger side, and then rolled up the window. At a subsequent Coronial hearing: 'the cause of death was stated as asphyxia due to the inhalation of carbon monoxide gas . . . while the balance of [name withheld by this book's author] mind was disturbed'. The individual in question did not donate their body to medical science in their will. Nonetheless, what happened next does indicate the research threshold points that this dead body was now about to cross in the hands of medical science.

The first threshold point was that by virtue of the physical fact of a suicide, the body in question became the responsibility of a coroner whose public duty it was to perform a post-mortem and report to an Inquest Jury. At this point, the coroner had two legal options: to extensively cut open the body and examine the lungs and heart and/or test the carbon monoxide levels in the tissue; or, examine the external appearance of the body and use his powers of discretion to declare a death by suicide. Historically, this latter option, a 'non-Jury' case, came under Coroners' Regulations. Since the early 1830s, when coroners started to be medically, not legally qualified, they had the discretion to save the costs of a post-mortem if a death was obvious, for example, in drowning cases. In other words, at this first threshold point, the body might be cut a little, some, or a lot. It all depended on the decision of the coroner, whether he was legally or medically qualified (or both) and the local political temperature, shaped by events surrounding an unexplained death. Today this practice continues with paper inquests, and it has always been part of Coronial discretionary justice.

The second threshold point that is then noteworthy is that despite a lack of bequest, this body went next to St Bartholomew's Hospital in London. The records indicate that the person died, there was a quick Coronial hearing and the body arrived at the dissection room within a total of two days. It is likely some testing had been done on its CO_2 levels and heart/lung tissue samples were removed for examination, but the body itself was substantially intact at this handover given the speed of delivery. It was now about to fall under the official jurisdiction of the dissection room because Coronial offices often had close working relationships with medical schools needing a steady supply of the dead to train students in anatomy in the 1950s. It had therefore travelled about 100 miles by van. In other words, the whole body had started to become the 'other' on that journey – literally and metaphorically moving by means of a medical bypass – but it was not, as yet, not 'out there' in parts – where its ultimate destination would be diverted to the cul-de-sac of history (as the Introduction outlined) until this book remapped it.

Crossing a third threshold point, the body of the dead person passed into the dissection room jurisdiction to underpin further teaching and research. It is evident from the original records that this phase took one and a half years in total, from entry to leaving the dissection room for the final time to be buried (cremation was not yet commonplace as it is today). In other words, this body was cut up extensively and no opportunity to learn missed. On entry, it was refrigerated and embalmed. This involved first washing the body. Then embalmers made initial small cuts at the neck in the carotid artery area and injected preservation chemicals into the inner thigh. The embalmer on duty pumped embalming fluid (a mixture of ethanol and formalin) into the arteries. About 25 to 40 litres was the normal level. Bodies were always refrigerated and checked regularly to see that the process was working. Additional fluid injected directly into areas of the body not responding to the chemical processes to fix the human material was likewise the usual procedure. Once preserved, cadavers, placed on a metal table in a temperature-controlled dissection room, were covered with a shroud until ready for teaching. The head was shaved for cleanliness too, akin to the sort of shorn-head appearance of all serving recruits in the armed forces. As the procedures for dissection were methodical on site, we can proceed to the fourth threshold point.

Allowing for the fact that the heart was still present (in some cases, coroners removed it as a precaution in suspected homicides, but this does not seem to have been so here), then medical students on site spent a concerted amount of time dissecting it. The lungs likewise were always the focus of intense interest, as would be the major organs like the liver and kidneys. The separated skin and each body part were prepared as prosthetics. The head generally was the focus of a month of teaching sessions too. Of importance here were the age, general condition of the body and its gender. The coroner's report said the deceased 'enjoyed reasonably good health' despite a recent episode of 'depression'. The person was middle-aged and had led an active life; therefore, the human remains were very good teaching aids. They were also useful for further research into mental ill-health in the brain, provided the pathologist had frozen below −20 degrees centigrade (rather than embalmed) that body part after a post-mortem. Consequently, the crossing of thresholds three and four technically represented a research opportunity to learn more about the potential physical manifestations of a suicide case and its neurology. Each threshold point was self-evidently a discrete step in which a whole body history was being dis-assembled into a series of hidden histories where the physical reality of completeness and the history of the person were eroded.

What happened then to each body part, organ, tissue or brain slice tends to fade from view into the jurisdiction of the pathologist and medical research community, as we shall see in the following chapters. After eighteen months, the body was buried with a Christian ceremony, complying with legislation. A family of undertakers in the employ of the dissection room at St Bartholomew's for almost 100 years did the internment (see Chapter 4). Consequently, here, as the ethnographer Marie Andree Jacob puts it: 'What deserves particular attention is the very creative ways actors [in this case, coroner, pathologist, dissector, student, medical researcher, lab technician and scientist] go around the law *while* going through the legal processes: for this is how legality is experienced.'[46] In other words, it is important not to be distracted by the medical sciences' insistence on the 'global' over the 'local'. Indeed, this reunification does require a lot more concerted effort in the archives. Nonetheless, what historical research has to do is 'privilege the microscope over the telescope' to trace each threshold point, engaging with its hidden histories of the dead and potential body disputes (explicit, implicit and missed).[47] That endeavour will provide a checking mechanism in respect of the success story of the 'body donation mechanism' of the medical sciences since WWII, testing in context the maintenance of public confidence and trust (or not) in actor networks and their achievements.

The material reality is that this suicide could have had many different types of threshold points. These would have shaped the sorts of disputes that could arise. The individual might have made a body bequest in a particular way that led to a medical breakthrough. If so, their bereaved family may have wanted to participate in its knowledge formation as a consolation after death but missed an opportunity to do so. On being opened up (even without this happening voluntarily), it is entirely feasible that a war hero would have a good physiology that a medical researcher was waiting on. Certainly, one cannot rule out the possibility that this body in the 1950s contributed to the development of crime scene forensic science. It could also have been used for new research into cancers caused by the presence of asbestos in the lungs, as the person had worked on mine sweepers in the war that would later prove to be of importance for the study of painful mesothelioma. As yet, Crick and Watson's discovery of DNA at Cambridge was just four years old. Had the war hero died ten years later, the potential was there in the cells for early genetic study. Even so, human tissue culture work took place at the Strangeways laboratory in Cambridge at the time of death and St Bartholomew's Hospital had shared training facilities and dissected cadavers with Oxbridge since the war. All of these possibilities and their potential thresholds could have created material afterlives. Speaking about them in this way is not about 'moral pronouncements' in which there have traditionally been 'two camps' – one defending science's achievements, the other doing the opposite – but instead focusses historical attention onto the nature, scope and meaning of body ethics in both a historical and modern sense.[48] And of course there is an irony here. Because the importance of discrete threshold points and their potential for generating dispute has rarely been acknowledged, medical science has gone about the Enlightenment project in a rather contradictory manner. Combating ignorance with reason, rationality and science has been dependent on the ignorance of donors about what was going on to achieve the ultimate goal called 'progress'. Should the combatting of medical ignorance rely on generating cultural ignorance to this extent, is a thought-provoking question and one with wide-ranging ethical implications. Soon it gave rise to public criticism and a demand that the human story must be restored to the relationship between medical researchers and teachers and the bodies that they relied upon. It is to this medical humanities issue that the chapter finally turns.

Everybody – *'Who Must Own the Organs of My Body?'*

I think it is self-centred of the public to feel they have a right to other people's organs without offering their own, and I think the present system, under which hundreds of kidney patients die each year while many more useful organs are destroyed is … inefficient. And yet, I cannot go along with the suggestion one's body, even after death, should be considered the property of the state. Perhaps this is a libertarian view, or perhaps it is simply the greatest irony of the transplant problem. The period of this great scientific advance has coincided with a decline in a sense of collective responsibility, and the advance itself, by making us think we can postpone death indefinitely, has discouraged us from making arrangements for our own demise.[49]

In many respects this short extract from a feature article in the *Independent on Sunday* in the early 1990s denoted the start of a public discussion about body disputes. It recognised controversial human harvesting issues that the general public may have wanted to raise about the regulation of organ donation, transplant surgery and 'body donation' bequests, but did not have the full information to do so. The rise of doctoring in British society as a profession over several hundred years had created a set of expectations for fee-paying patients that 'death's door' would be held shut for as long as possible by the medical sciences.[50] After 1948, NHS consumers became taxpayers with a stake in the best that medical science could share with everybody. It had once been the view that, as George Steiner, the moral philosopher, explains: 'Death has its history. The history is biological, social and mental. … Every historical era, every society and culture has had their own understanding, iconography and rites of mortality.'[51] In Western cultures, by the modern era, however, the way that people had traditionally edified 'the House of the Dead' (to use Steiner's analogy) was starting to change shape, and radically so. It no longer had in the popular imagination a clearly defined deadline – the metaphysical belief that this is your time, and date, and you must enter here after the traditional lifespan of three score years and ten – for that biblical timetable had eroded slowly with secularism and science. Patients now expected to push past the dead-end of life, and indeed, in many respects that so-called deadline seemed more alive than dead in emergency rooms that had lower mortality rates from improved resuscitation facilities. For Steiner this has created nonetheless what he calls 'the barbarism of specialisation' and with it the inability to see material things including the human body 'in its totality'. The real problem is that it has also tended, in his view, to misrepresent scientific invention as human creativity. It is important to reflect on this philosophical perspective because it has often been excluded from historical accounts of the 'success story' of the medical sciences in the modern era.

Steiner points out that science seldom looks back. Its mentality is to cancel a drug, medical procedure or surgical innovation and move on to the next big breakthrough.[52] Why study Newton when Einstein has taken a leap forward, was a rational position to take by the twentieth century; the new displaces the old. But this, Steiner believes, is contrary to the history of the creative arts over centuries. Creativity links the *whole* to each *part* – one artwork to another, one novel to a series of writings and so on. It is rare for new knowledge to cancel out old mind-sets and perspectives altogether. Knowledge is often compartmentalised for a time, retains the potential to re-join a creative conversation, may keep changing emphasis, and often productively so. What has tended to happen over a century of innovation in science that is worrying, for Steiner and philosophers of the body, is that the public have come to expect medical science to do the editing of information for them. This neglects the creative potential of knowledge formation, reinvention and retrieval in which everyone should be involved. Science instead will typically develop a new drug and work to lessen its side-effects because of the expense of clinical trials. Even if the drug is not really fit for purpose for some patients, the medical sciences will keep using it despite its downsides; until, that is, their lack of creative imagination to revisit their research agendas is held to public account. Occasionally we glimpse this sort of scenario, most notably in the case of thalidomide, which illustrates this key point succinctly.

Thalomid [*sic*] was the original name of the drug developed and sold in Germany in 1957 under the trade name Contergan.[53] It was marketed without proper clinical safeguards for nausea and morning sickness in pregnancy, then banned. Later, its chemical interaction that stunted human growth in the limbs persuaded some governments to issue it under special license for cancer and leprosy treatments to inhibit tumours. The 'dark remedy' had thus a 'one-track' scientific history, until a public outcry caused its creative potential to be unlocked. This is exactly the sort of predicament that troubled Rhoda Koenig (the journalist) in her 1990s short piece on organ donation that opened this section. The 'postponement of death', as she put it, makes everyone's eventual 'demise' not just difficult to talk about but there is an endemic cultural denial about difficult situations. 'Edit me down so that I survive longer' is all very well, as she explains, but it also disempowers the patient. Further complicating that situation was the reluctance of the medical profession to speak openly about the successes and failures of their clinical work, as the thalidomide controversy showed. Indeed, seldom was the legislative framework regulating laboratory practice, the development of drug rejection therapies or human tissue experiments, set out clearly in print in the immediate post-WWII era (see Chapter 2 for a more detailed discussion of the legalities). Innovations were publicised in the medical press like the *Lancet* and *British Medical Journal*, but almost never was the cohort of bodies or human tissue research activities acknowledged openly. It was not a legal requirement and thus omitted. Any publicity tended to be about promoting a new breakthrough and accrediting it to a doctor or scientist on their career path. A cultural fissure consequently started to open up after 1945 in Britain. The public thought they were being fully informed, when they were not; and the medical sciences assumed that the general public did not want to know what they did not know about!

Anatomists, clinicians and pathologists thus found themselves in a bad self-validating prophecy of their making: the public do not understand what we do, and we do not understand their attitude to us – ergo, we cannot work or co-create together. What exacerbated this situation was how talented doctors and scientists – ones genuinely working to improve the public good – made assumptions that laws in the past superseded present-day regulations. Soon it became clear that they were still working with outdated laws, broken down, tinkered with and rehashed, but never repealed. In stressing patient confidentiality (a legitimate legal concern), they seldom thought to look at the legal basis of their paperwork on bequests, post-mortems and so on. In other words, the methodologies of the medical sciences with their threshold points in human dissection and further research, done in discrete stages, ironically matched the way that the law itself had been revised in bits and pieces instead of in its entirety for the living and the dead. This cultural stand-off (for that is what it amounted to by the end of the 1990s) was further exacerbated by the medical sciences' scepticism about the value of human stories to their research endeavours. This scepticism is misplaced, argue moral philosophers and poets such as John Glenday; his poetic satire is biting about medical science's proverbial rubble from this recent past:

Rubble

> General term for a people who are harvested and reused
> Or broken. To be heaped randomly or roughly stored.
> That which is held for common use. Infill. Of little worth.
>
> Break them in different ways but they will always be the same.
> Hold them in the dark; remind yourself why they should stay forgotten.
> These days there is little interest in stones that bear names.
>
> May they be piled up and given this title in common.
> Let them take their place in the register of unspoken things
> May they never be acknowledged again.[54]

To disassemble might be a necessary and inevitable part of research, but to forget is not. This book thus builds on philosophies of the body and science since it challenges, resituates and rediscovers the human 'rubble' of a bio-commons.

Conclusion: *'No Decisions about Me, without Me'*

HTA2004 reflected a wide range of reactions to a recent (and not so recent) history of disputed bodies that has included – anger, blame, disappointment, frustration, regret and sadness. In many respects, it follows that the fallout of that history was always going to be far-reaching but not necessarily in the ways that the medical sciences would have anticipated. After 2005, body donations did not decline dramatically, and more people were willing to donate their organs in the first decade of the new legislation because of the work of the Organ Donation Task force set up by the government in 2008.[55] Rebuilding public trust can nonetheless be a complicated process. Often it is damaged far quicker than the long time it takes to be established. What continues to be at issue is the cultural fissure opened up by NHS scandals in 1999. These have been exemplified by the ongoing public stand-off over compulsory organ donation. On 17 July 2007 BBC News, for instance, reported that Sir Liam Donaldson (former Chief Medical Officer at the time of the NHS organ retention controversy) had done a *volte face*, despite his support for the principle of inclusiveness embedded into the new HTA2004 statute. He had embraced a system of 'presumed consent' because of long waiting lists for organs.[56] Yet, as the Shadow Health Secretary at the time, Andrew Lansley, replied: 'The state does not own our bodies, or have the right to take organs after death' – echoing the prescient journalism of Rhoda Koenig in the 1990s touched on early in this chapter. That concept of state ownership has been rejected in Scotland (for now), though adopted in Wales from 2015. In England, meantime, what remains the subject of lively debate is the ethical principle of '*No decisions about me, without me*', as it embraces in 2020 a new organ donation scheme based on the Welsh opt-out facility for the living and presumed consent for the dead. This proposal to change the law prompted lively discussion at a meeting of the Royal Society of Medicine (hereafter RSM) convened on 23 June 2016 to reflect on twelve years after 'the good, the bad and the ugly' of HTA2004.[57]

What remains palpable in bioethics is that if a person (alive or dead) gives (or has given) consent – whether for human tissue, cell-line, biopsy or organ – and if a medical researcher makes an invention or innovation that proves to be of commercial value from that human material – then that outcome distorts the 'goodwill' of the bequest. If we have moved from 'proprietorial' to 'consensual' medical ethics after HTA2004, then that legal emphasis has yet to become a medical reality in working practices. Moreover, there remains the difficult question of what happens when human tissue becomes recycled into computer data. Hugh Whittall, Director of the Nuffield Council on Bioethics, thus explained at the recent RSM conference in June 2016 that:

The long-term challenge is the issue of tissue banking. The value of a tissue sample, he says, is beginning to reside more 'in the huge amount of data it can deliver once you put it through any kind of biochemical or genetic analysis'.

'So to some extent, tissue banks could become redundant once you have got the data or information in the tissue. We then move from the framework of human tissue regulation into the framework of data and information regulation.' The interaction of regulatory control and legal and ethical frameworks is going to be very difficult, he thinks, because 'the two areas have not necessarily matched up completely'.

The current legislation … should be capable of working for 'another 10 or 15 years, because we quite deliberately introduced a degree of flexibility and discretion that could be exercised by the HTA'.[58]

The rising cost of regulation, the bureaucracy involved, the question of how far systems of medical research are streamlined enough to be inspected uniformly and, above all, the fast-moving e-globalisation of all our personal information, remain uncertain. 'Hack-work' was once pejorative slang for medical students cutting open corpses. Now to be 'hacked' involves breaches in data protection privacy laws and 'goodwill' needing a better firewall to protect the biomedical boundaries being broken down in medical science.

Looking back, leaping forward, it remains apparent that when the medical sciences had 'a degree of flexibility and discretion' in the past (to quote Hugh Whittall's phrasing above) they proved incapable of handling it. To build 'deliberately' therefore the same discretionary powers into HTA2004 to ensure it has longevity as a piece of legislation in terms of a Human Tissue Authority management culture, is dubious from a historical standpoint, however well intended its work. For it negates any historical sense of the research processes and their threshold points in the pieces of a medical mosaic. Indeed, it is striking that no historian of the body was (or is) invited to sit on the Human Tissue Authority. Such observations suggest that scientists, doctors, anatomists, coroners and pathologists continue to take a proprietorial view of the bodies and body parts in their professional hands. Few voluntarily adopted the mentalities of custodianship, and arguably this hidden history is still having important ramifications in scientific research circles today. As Sir Jeremy Farrar, Director of the Wellcome Trust, highlighted in his recent blog post on 10 September 2019:

The emphasis on excellence in the research system is stifling diverse thinking and positive behaviours. As a community we can rethink our approach to research culture to achieve excellence in all we do. The UK's research sector is powering ahead, with our world-leading universities generating knowledge and innovations that are improving lives around the world. But in the engine room of this great enterprise, warning lights are blinking on. The relentless drive for research excellence has created a culture in modern science that cares exclusively about what is achieved and not about how it is achieved. As I speak to people at every stage of a scientific career, although I hear stories of wonderful support and mentorship, I'm also hearing more and more about the troubling impact of prevailing culture. People tell me about instances of destructive hyper-competition, toxic power dynamics and poor leadership behaviour – leading to a corresponding deterioration in researchers' wellbeing. We need to cultivate, reward, and encourage the best while challenging what is wrong.[59]

Perhaps one of the greatest ironies is that the heritage sector may have better working practices in terms of the custodianship of our national assets than the medical sciences, which dominate public spending by government. Maybe because the heritage sector has always had a charitable status defined by trusteeship, its ethics were co-created in conversations with the entrance-fee-paying public. Yet, in medicine, people do pay their equivalent entrance fee in taxes to fund the NHS; its medical research base from patient case-histories is a national asset too: as the Covid-19 pandemic is highlighting. It is a point of view worth considering that whereas voters want politicians to protect the physical public ownership of the natural landscape of the environment, seldom are the insides of human nature seen as needing the same public property safeguards. One thing remains certain. This is a history not simply in our keeping, but in our collective making too. For, as Farrar emphasises, the medical sciences still need a more caring culture – 'not exclusively about what is achieved' but 'how it is achieved' too. The disputed bodies that have been missed and mislaid, exemplify the need for vigilance about the ethical basis of pushing back all our deadlines. We next therefore examine the legal framework of the messy business of these muddled research threshold points of the modern era.

Notes

1. 'English boxer Randolph Turpin has been elected to America's International Hall of Fame', *Daily Mail*, Sports news, 12 January 2001, issue 32350, p. 87.
2. 'Turpin: why were vital tests not made?', *Daily Mail*, News section, 22 July 1966, issue 21843, p. 1.
3. 'Turpin: why were vital tests not made?' *Daily Mail*, News section, 22 July 1966, issue 21843, p. 1.
4. 'Bankrupt Turpin takes a long, long count', *Daily Mail*, News section, 19 October 1962, issue 20679, p. 17.
5. 'Turpin: two questions must be answered', *Daily Mail*, News section, 19 May 1966, issue 21788, p. 10.
6. 'Turpin wrote farewell to his wife', *Daily Mail*, Lead article, 21 May 1966, issue 21790, p. 14.
7. 'Turpin: Girl, 4 "only witness"', *Daily Mail*, Lead article, 19 May 1966, issue 21788, p. 1.
8. 'Turpin "just burned up money"', *Daily Mail*, Feature article, 23 July 1966, issue 21844, p. 4, reconstructed his perilous finances and high-spending patterns.
9. 'The harder they get, the harder they fall', *Daily Mail*, Feature article, 18 May 1966, issue 21787, p. 7.
10. See, Ruth Richardson, *Death, Dissection and the Destitute* (London: Phoenix Press, 2001); Helen MacDonald, *Human Remains: Dissection and Its Histories* (New Haven: Yale University Press, 2005); Elizabeth T. Hurren, *Dying for Victorian Medicine: English Anatomy and Its Trade in the Dead Poor c. 1834–1929* (Basingstoke: Palgrave Macmillan, 2011); Tatiana Buklijas, 'Cultures of death and the politics of corpse supply: anatomy in Vienna, 1848–1914', *Bulletin of the History of Medicine*, 83 (2008), 3: 570–607; Michael Sappol, *A Traffic of Dead Bodies: Anatomy and Embodied Social Identity in Nineteenth-Century America* (Princeton: Princeton University Press, 2004).

11. Refer, for instance, William Bynum and Linda Kalof (eds.), *A Cultural History of the Body: Volumes 1–6* (London: Bloomsbury, 2010).

12. See, for instance, Erica Borgstrom, 'Planning for death? an ethnographic study of choice and English end-of-life care' (unpublished PhD dissertation, University of Cambridge, 2014), accessed 10/1/2017 at: www.repository.cam.ac.uk/handle/1810/245560

13. Notably featuring in the work of Michel Foucault, *Discipline and Punish: The Birth of the Prison*, translated by Alan Sheridan (London: Penguin, 1991); Foucault, *The Birth of the Clinic* (London: Routledge, 2003); Foucault, *Madness and Civilisation* (London: Vintage Books, 2006).

14. Refer, Arathi Prasad, *In the Bonesetter's Waiting Room: Travels through Indian Medicine – sponsored by the Wellcome Trust* (London & New Dehli: Profile Books, 2016).

15. See, for example, *Subaltern Studies Collective work, Subaltern Studies: Volumes 1–10 as a set: Writings on South Asian History and Society* (Oxford: Oxford University Press, 1999); Antoinette Burton and Tony Ballantyne, *World Histories from Below: Disruption and Dissent, 1750s to the Present* (London: Bloomsbury Academic Publishing, 2016).

16. A viewpoint highlighted in the admirable work of Julie-Marie Strange, *Death, Grief and Poverty in Britain, 1870–1914* (Cambridge: Cambridge University Press, 2005); Strange, 'Historical approaches to dying', in Allan Kellehear (ed.), *The Study of Dying: From Autonomy to Transformation* (Cambridge: Cambridge University Press, 2009), pp. 123–146.

17. Gerald Dworkin, 'The law relating to organ transplantation in England', *Modern Law Review*, 33 (1970), 4: 353–377, quote at p. 353.

18. Donald Longmore, *Spare-Part Surgery* (London: Aldus, 1968), p. 169.

19. E. Blythe Stason, 'The role of law in medical progress', *Law and Contemporary Problems*, 32 (1967), 4: 563–596, quote at p. 568.

20. Refer, Richardson, *Death, Dissection and the Destitute*.

21. See, context in, Hurren, *Dying for Victorian Medicine*.

22. Refer, notably, Naomi Pfeffer, *Insider Trading: How Mortuaries, Medicine, and Money Have Built a Global Market in Human Cadaver Parts* (New Haven: Yale University Press, 2017).

23. Scott Carney, *The Red Market: On the Trail of the World's Organ Brokers, Bone Thieves, Blood Farmers, and Child Traffickers* (New York: William Morrow, 2011).

24. Michiko Kukutani, 'Need a kidney? Need a skull? Just bring cash', *New York Times*, Book reviews, 16 June 2011. This trade was also satirised by Kazuo Ishiguro, *Never Let Me Go* (New York & London: Vintage Books, 2006), where in his dystopian novel children were 'cloned' specifically to 'donate' body parts.

25. Carney, *Red Market*, introduction, 'Man versus meat', p. 2.

26. Refer, key historiography in footnote 10 above.

27. Sally Satel, 'Generosity won't fix our shortage of organs for transplant', *Washington Post*, 28 December 2015, p. 1, argues that 'the tyranny of the gift' is an urgent ethics issue.

28. Refer, Richard M. Titmuss, *The Gift Relationship: From Human Blood to Social Policy*, 2nd ed. (London: London School of Economic Books, 1977). Titmuss first started these debates in 1970. Today academics have criticised his book extensively

because it tends to be an aspiration rather than a reality. Yet, today it is often still cited in official communiqués from government and the medical sciences on the merits of donation.

29. Margaret Lock, *Twice Dead: Organ Transplants and the Reinvention of Death* (Los Angeles: University of California Press, 2002), p. 5.

30. Ibid., p. 11.

31. Lock, *Twice Dead*, quotes at pp. 11, 13 & 38.

32. Donna Dickenson, *Body Shopping: The Economy Fuelled by Flesh and Blood* (Oxford: One World Books, 2008), pp. 42–43.

33. Ibid., p. 43.

34. Elizabeth T. Hurren, *Dissecting the Criminal Corpse: Staging Post-Execution Punishment in Early Modern England* (Basingstoke: Palgrave Macmillan, 2016), and Hurren, *Dying for Victorian Medicine*, cover both periods in detail.

35. See, Professor Kwame Anthony Appiah, Chair of Philosophy and Law at New York University, Lecture 1, 'Creed', *Mistaken Identities*, BBC Reith Lectures (2016), at: www.bbc.co.uk/programmes/articles/2sM4D6LTTVlFZhbMpmfYmx6/kwame-anthony-appiah; review by Gillian Reynolds, 'How this year's Reith lecturer broke new ground', *Daily Telegraph*, 19 October 2016, p. 32, column 1. The theme of Appiah's lecture series is how we can often be mistaken about the fixed boundaries of our identities, which can disappear in what he calls 'a blink of an historical eye'. In looking at how confusions have played out, he believes, that past mistakes mean admitting the positive and negative things we have done. This book is very much about navigating all of that landscape, not just the parts cleaned up for public consumption.

36. Bruno Latour, *We Have Never Been Modern* (Cambridge, Mass.: Harvard University Press: English translation, 1993); Bruno Latour, Steve Woolgar and Jonas Salk, *Laboratory Life: The Construction of Scientific Facts* (Princeton: Princeton University Press, 1986); Bruno Latour, *Science in Action: How to Follow Scientists and Engineers through Society* (Cambridge, Mass.: Harvard University Press, 1987); Bruno Latour, *Reassembling the Social: An Introduction to Actor Network Theory* (New York: Oxford University Press, 2005 & 2007 editions); Bruno Latour and Michel Callon, 'Don't throw the baby out with the Bath School! A reply to Collins and Yearly', in Andrew Pickering (ed.), *Science as Practice and Culture* (Chicago: Chicago University Press, 1992), pp. 343–368.

37. Michel Callon, John Law and Arie Rip, *Mapping the Dynamics of Science and Technology: Sociology of Science in the Real World* (Basingstoke: Macmillan, 1986); Andrew Feenberg, Michel Callon, Brian Wyne, et al., *Between Reason and Experience: Essays in Technology and Modernity* (Cambridge, Mass.: MIT Press, 2010).

38. John Law and John Hassard (eds.), *Actor Network Theory and After* (Oxford: Blackwell Books, 1999).

39. Michael L. Scott, *Programming Language Pragmatics* (New York: Morgan Kaufmann, 2006), quotes at p. 481.

40. *Nuffield Trust Official Report on Human Tissue: Ethical and Legal Issues* (April, 1995), with particular reference to Section III, entitled 'Ethical Principles: Respect for Human Lives and Human Bodies', produced by Bioethics Division, chapter 6, pp. 39–55, quotes at p. 44; to download a PDF copy, see, https://www.nuffieldbioethics.org/publications/human-tissue

41. Bronwyn Parry, *Trading the Genome: Investigating the Commodification of Bio-Information* (New York: Columbia University Press, 2004), p. 50; Dickenson, *Body Shopping*, p. 94.

42. Dickenson, *Body Shopping*, p. 95, raises the ethical issue of 'out there' and the ambiguities of Patent Law.

43. Lock, *Twice Dead*, p. 9.

44. See, for example, Rachel Rettner, 'Cancer spreads from organ donor to 4 people in "extraordinary" case', *Live Science*, 15 September 2018, accessed 5/8/2019 at: www .livescience.com/63596-organ-donation-transmitted-breast-cancer.html

45. The original name removed here from the Coroner's Report for ethical reasons. It can be located at St Bartholomew's Hospital Dissection register MS81/5-81/6.

46. Marie-Andree Jacob, *Contemporary Ethnography: Matching Organs to Donors, Legalising and Kinship in Transplants* (Philadelphia: University of Pennsylvania Press, 2012), p. 8.

47. Ibid., p. 10.

48. Jacob, *Contemporary Ethnography*, p. 10.

49. Rita Koenig, 'Who must own the organs of my body?' *Independent on Sunday*, Feature article, 13 May 1990, issue 16, p. 17.

50. Sandra M. Gilbert, *Death's Door: Modern Dying and the Way We Grieve* (London & New York: Norton, 2006).

51. George Steiner, *Grammars of Creation* (New Haven: Yale University Press, 2001), preface. Essentially, he acknowledges that technology and science may have replaced art and literature as the driving forces in our culture. Steiner warns that this has not happened without a significant cultural loss of public confidence and trust.

52. Ibid.

53. Trent Stephens and Rock Brynner, *Dark Remedy: The Impact of Thalidomide and Its Revival as a Vital Medicine* (New York & London: Perseus Publishing & Basic Books, 2001).

54. John Glenday, 'Rubble', in *The Golden Mean* (London & New York: Picador Poetry, 2015), p. 31.

55. It should be noted, it was the medical expansion of the Donation after Circulatory Death (DCDs) initiatives, rather than an improvement in family consent rates, which increased the number of donors since 2008, according to a report by NHS Blood and Transplant (2013).

56. See, www.news.bbc.co.uk/1/hi/health/6902519.stm, accessed 24/10/2016; refer also, Niall Frith, *Daily Mail*, 'Opt out scheme *only way to tackle organ donor shortage says Liam Donaldson'*, 17 July 2017, where he claimed that '70 per cent wanted to donate in death' but only '20 per cent carried organ donation cards'.

57. See, Royal Society of Medicine, 'The Human Tissue Act 12 years on, the good, the bad and the ugly', Pathology section, 23 June 2016, at: www.rsm.ac.uk/events/ptg03

58. Andrea McGauran, World Report section, 'Regulation of human tissue in the UK', *Lancet*, 388 (17–23 September 2016), 10050, e-4–e-5.

59. Sir Jeremy Farrar, 'We need to re-imagine how we do research', Wellcome Trust blog, 10 September 2019, accessed 01/10/2019 at: www.wellcome.ac.uk/news/wh y-we-need-reimagine-how-we-do-research. Note: the author has full academic freedom and was not obliged by funding to quote this viewpoint.

2   *Res Nullius* – Nobody's Thing

While the stories and hidden histories of the dead stand at the heart of this book, it is important to frame these narratives against the restrictions and permissions of the 'laws' that governed matters of consent, harvesting and research in modern British medical research. This seemingly simple endeavour is considerably complicated by the fact that as well as direct legislation on these matters, medical practice and the 'rights' of the dead and dying are shaped by legislation in other areas of criminal, civil and administrative law. Official and unofficial 'guidance' and long-established customs also have purchase on these matters. In turn, the fact that much 'law' merely clarified or amended previous legislation rather than repealing it, means that 'the law' becomes 'the laws'. Thus, there is often considerable scope for differential interpretations of legal permissions at any chronological point. In this sense, law matters very much for the interpretation of the stories that we will go on to encounter in the rest of this volume.

A starting point for this process is the long tradition in English Common Law that: 'A dead person cannot own the property of their body once deceased – the legal principle is *Res Nullius – Nobody's Thing.*'[1] In many respects, this lack of a human identity set the tone for how medical science represented its dissection and research work to government, as we have already begun to see in previous chapters. The importance of this basic principle becomes apparent in the eighteenth century, when many European states were threatened by revolution and the mob, and preventing criminal behaviour became a matter of urgency. In Britain, central government decided by 1750 that the forces of law and order should link heinous crimes like murder to a system of extra-physical punishments. Murder thus became punishable by death and dissection. The thinking was that this double deterrent would prevent ordinary people from seeking the radical political change threatened in Europe. These new regulations drew on ingrained body taboos in northern European cultures. Popular opinion held that any interference with the integrity of the human body in death was a moral shame. For the soul to go to heaven, the dead body had to be buried intact. As this author has argued extensively elsewhere, the culmination of these cultural mentalities was the passing of new capital legislation called the Murder Act (25

Geo. 2 c. 37: 1752) in England.[2] Based on the Common Law principle of *Lex Talionis* – that the punishment must match the degree of offensive committed – it had a biblical counterpart, 'an eye for an eye' of retributive justice, outlined in the book of Numbers, chapter 35. After 1752, if convicted of homicide in a court of law, the condemned faced a death sentence, was hanged on a public gallows, and then surgeons either dissected the criminal corpse or placed it on a gibbet to rot. The bodies thus released by the justice system became one significant strand of the supply that medical science required for its educational and research needs over the next eighty years. It relied on 'Nobody's Thing'.

It was not to be enough. There was meantime a corporate ambition amongst practitioners to gain full professional status from an expansion of European medical education. At Bologna, Padua and Paris, training doctors in human anatomy had been a national priority since the Renaissance. Now others, particularly in northern European countries and cities where Enlightenment values gained a strong intellectual foothold, like Edinburgh, followed suit. Yet, those in Britain faced a logistical problem. The murder rate lagged behind the expansion of human anatomy training. Not enough people were convicted of homicide to supply dissection tables, and medical students thus lacked enough corpses to dissect. Grave robbing soon became commonplace, and newspapers reflected public concern that the unscrupulous were indiscriminately digging up the dead for anatomical profit. Resurrection men sold the dead of the rich, middling-sort and labouring poor, disinterred for dissection. This class question of who owned the dead body and who should be charged legally for stealing human remains became a highly emotive one in contemporary British culture, until, that is, the controversial Anatomy Act (2 & 3 Will. 4 c. 75: 1832 (hereafter AA1832) changed the medical status quo. Two catalysts changed public debates about the need for more legal supply lines in human anatomy by the 1830s. First, the famous 'Burke and Hare' murders in Edinburgh revealed how the destitute who were killed for medical profit entered the supply chain of anatomists in Scotland. Second, the simultaneous death of an 'Italian boy' in London, murdered and traded for a similar dissection sale, caused public outrage. These scandals would result in the medical profession successfully lobbying for a better and more plentiful legal mechanism of supply but crucially one still based on class inequalities. AA1832 permitted the poorest in society to become the staple of dissection tables, supplied by asylums, infirmaries, workhouses and street deaths, amongst the homeless, friendless and nameless of society. In turn, key aspects of AA1832 were to remain in force until HTA2004, a remarkable 172 years. Officially, AA1832 was supposed to end when the New Poor Law closed in 1929.[3] In reality, as we shall see, its class ethos, tinkered with and rehashed a number of times, did not alter that much. This was because, as Richard Smith and Peregrine Horden have observed, early Welfare State council care homes were really just workhouse infirmaries renamed. They still supplied the dispossessed for dissection.[4] In other words, in terms of body supply-mechanisms there was a great deal more continuity than discontinuity inside the healthcare system, a theme that runs throughout this book. Starting from this point, Table 2.1 summarises key statutes and important regulatory changes in British law on matters of consent, biomedical research regulation and the rights of the dead.

A full description of the technicalities of this legislative canvas is neither possible nor desirable in the context of this book. Broad trends are, however, important. Thus, prior to WWI a raft of intersecting changes influenced fundamentally public and legislative attitudes to the supply of the dead for dissection and research. The passing of the Third Reform Act (48 & 49 Vict. c. 3: 1884), the creation of County Councils (51 & 52 Vict. ch. 41: 1888), democratisation of the New Poor Law under the Local Government Act (56 & 57 Vict. c. 73: 1894) and the Liberal Welfare Reform Programme (1906–1911) encapsulated a growing sense that poverty and pauperism were not the fault of individuals.[5] Having the vote without the citizenship rights of healthcare and welfare provision was thus regarded as an empty political promise by the labouring poor, and no longer tenable in a modern society. The progressive extension of the franchise to women, the structural and cultural effects of the war, increasing political and economic assertiveness by the working class and the final demise of the New Poor Law in 1929, all signalled the increasing fragility of public support for the legislative base that underpinned the use of bodies for medical research and teaching. During the 1930s, however, the modus operandi of the medical sciences did not really alter that much. It was resistant to the direction of wider cultural shifts happening in British life, and continued to rely on Victorian legislation.[6]

Change when it came was from an ostensibly unusual angle. The growth of the Victorian information state had been a boon for the medical sciences by the early twentieth century.[7] In particular, the expansion of the Coronial Office proved to be an important stepping stone in the piecemeal regulation of dissection and its further research agendas by the 1930s. This was the culmination of fifty years or more of a strategic realignment of the professional classes inside the expanding Information State in which coroners sought to be pivotal to the development of forensic medicine and crime-scene evidence, working closely with the anatomical sciences, as well as pathologists. As this author has shown elsewhere, some coroners were so successful at expanding their official jurisdiction that by the turn of the century a medical school which did not co-operate with the Coronial Office risked losing an important source of supply in the dead.[8] It came therefore as less of a surprise to the medical profession as a whole that coroners were the first to lobby about the need for 'special examinations' (not just post-mortems) under the Coroners (Amendment) Act

Table 2.1 *The official boundaries of bio-security in modern Britain and Europe*

Timeline	Legislation/regulations	Main features of its remit
Ancient Times	English Common Law – *Res Nullius – Nobody's Thing*	A dead person cannot own the property of their body once deceased
1832	Anatomy Act	The dead must repay any welfare debt to society. Welfare costs paid from public taxation merit post-mortem. The individual dissected and dismembered for the purposes of anatomy teaching and medical research
1926	Coroners (Amendment) Act	Extended retention powers over post-mortems
1926	Registration of Stillbirths Act	Stillborn children now constitute a potential 'living' person in law and as such their death and burial must be registered officially
1950s	Pituitary Gland Programme	Extraction of Human Growth Hormone post-mortem by anatomists, coroners, pathologists
1952	Corneal Grafting Act	Regulates the removal of eye material taken from cadavers post-mortem
1960/1	Declaration of Helsinki	World Medical Association's new ethical framework for medical research
1961	Human Tissue Act	Human tissue from a dead patient considered in law to be an *unconditional gift*. In the case of material derived from fatal operations (organ, body part, tissue) provided the patient when living gave consent for the surgical procedure that led to that removal, once removed in law is *abandoned*. It hence becomes the legal property of the medical establishment, removed for the therapeutic benefit of the consenting patient before their death. Doctors need '*only make reasonable enquiries*' where human material originates
1962/3	Medical Research Council (MRC) Annual Report	Seen as a cornerstone of medical ethics in Britain. Future funding of research studies dependent on adhering to a new Ethical Code of Conduct. Has been revised many times, especially in 1979 (see below)
1977	National Health Service Act	Section 25 – *where the Secretary of State has acquired: (a) supplies of human blood . . . or (b) any part of a human body . . . s/he may arrange to make such supplies or that part available* (on such terms, including terms as to charges, as he thinks fit) to any person
1979	Medical Research Council (MRC) Ethical Code	Compulsory for scientific and medical research studies based in Britain
1984	Coroners' Rules	Clarified post-mortems by coroners and the Preservation of Material. Rule 12 stated that: *A person making a special examination shall make provision, as far as possible, for the preservation of the material submitted to him for such period as the coroner thinks fit*

Year	Legislation	Description
1984	Anatomy Act	Passed to repeal aspects of 1961 legislation but did not clarify adequately use of tissue and organs, and their ownership
1986	Corneal Tissue Act	Permitted the removal of eyes or parts of eyes for therapeutic purposes, medical education and research by persons who are not medically qualified, subject to appropriate safeguards. Amended parts of the HTA1961 so responsibility for medical death resided with doctor(s) who had cared for the patient
1989	Human Organ Transplant Act	Passed to prevent the illegal trade in organs globally and to protect the vulnerable from becoming victims of organ harvesting
1988	Anatomy Regulations	A written record kept of all bodies and body parts retained by medical schools for human anatomy teaching and medical research
1989	Human Fertilisation and Embryology Act	Specifically regulates research into fertility and embryology research due to international concern about the future of designer babies
1998	European Directive on the Legal Protection of Biotechnological Inventions	Directive 98/44/EC of the European Parliament and of the Council of 6 July 1998 and ratified under the Treaty of Rome – Harmonises the laws of Member States on patentability of biotechnological inventions, plant varieties (as legally defined) and human genes – under BREXIT review in the UK
2004	Human Tissue Act	It is a criminal offence to use or store human bodies or body parts without explicit consent. Human tissue can, however, be subsequently used in medical research under presumed consent provided it has been first removed for the benefit of a living patient being treated and they have not sought to object in person
2008	Health and Social Care Act (Regulated Activities)	Saying Sorry campaign of NHS Litigation Authority
2009	*Jonathan Yearworth and others v. North Bristol NHS Trust* (known as the Yearworth Judgment)	Court of Appeal Judge warned that patients were entitled to compensation if their bodies generated sperm before undergoing chemotherapy and these a hospital mistakenly destroyed. It was not a defence in law that the hospital now owned that sperm and was not liable for its mistake. The case was an admission that Common Law may be no longer reliable, with regards to, the development of medical technologies and body/parts/products ownership
2014	Care Act (NHS)	Duty of Candour – admission of errors is now a clinical responsibility to NHS patients

(16 & 17 Geo. 5 c. 59: 1926). For the purposes this chapter's legislative review, the part of the Bill ratified that mattered most to anatomists was *Sections 21–24*, which gave the coroner special powers for:

Post-Mortem and Special Examination

21. Post-Mortem examination without an Inquest.
22. Power of Coroner to request specifically qualified person to make a Post-Mortem and Special Examination.
23. Fees to Medical Witnesses.
24. Power of Removal of body for Post-Mortem Examination.[9]

All of these slippery legal terms, notably 'Special Examination', created material ambiguities that were eventually repealed by HTA2004. Meantime, what the legal framework did was to extend the already extensive powers of the coroner and the nature of discretionary justice in their hands. This they made, and remade, during the modern era, and often to the benefit of their professional contacts in dissection rooms and pathology labs, as we shall see in Part II.

At the same time, central government passed the Registration of Stillbirths Act (16 & 17 Geo. 5 c. 48: 1926), alarming anatomists. They worried that their natural allies at the Coronial Office in sponsoring this new legislation might cut off dissectors from parts of their historic supply-lines. Previously a stillbirth – defined by the Victorians as the death of a fetus after the twentieth week of pregnancy – went unrecorded as an 'official' death. In English law, spontaneously aborted fetuses (accidental and unnatural) physically had to breathe independently when separated from their mothers or they did not exist legally as a human being. To save money, normally such grieving parents buried their dead offspring without paying a sexton's fee or covering a doctor's death certificate expenses.[10] Often when a mother and child died together, burying both in the same coffin was commonplace; families registered just the dead parent in the parish burial records of a local church. Anatomists could therefore ask coroners for their stillbirth cases without any official oversight and the promise of a small supply fee to those struggling to make ends meet in relative or absolute poverty. But after 1927, acquired human material now had to be recorded officially: '*"still-born" and "still-birth" shall apply to any child which has issued forth from its mother after the twenty fourth week of pregnancy and which did not at any time after being completely expelled from its mother, breathe or show any other signs of life*'.[11] Then the Births and Deaths Registration Act (1 & 2 Eliz. 2 c. 20: 1953) altered this stipulation again. The qualifying time span of official notification increased to '*within 42 days of the birth*'. This regulatory change meant that anatomists who acquired (or were supplied) with dead fetuses for the purposes of teaching and research could no longer do so unofficially, and without a time limit, as they had done for 200 years.[12] The outcome of the legislation was that it convinced the medical sciences of the vital importance of co-ordinating with coroners more closely by the 1950s. The professional tensions that arose in this process are explored in Part II of this book.

By the early 1950s, a series of new laws and regulations about the use of the dead by the medical sciences became even more piecemeal. These generally reflected concerted public health campaigns that again had their roots in the late-Victorian era. Two in particular stand out because they were to have long-term consequences for disputed bodies, and issues surrounding them were to feature in public debates around the time of the NHS scandal at Alder Hey Children's Hospital. The first was the Pituitary Gland Programme (hereafter PGP) that began in the USA in 1958, extended to the UK under the auspices of the Medical Research Council (hereafter MRC). The aim of the initiative was to investigate whether children born with a shorter stature needed growth hormone treatment. The medical facts were that Growth Hormone Deficiency (GHD) appears on the pituitary gland, a pea-size gland at the base of the brain. Its function in the body is to be the 'master controller' to 'make hormones and control the function of other glands' efficiently.[13] Once it starts to malfunction, it 'slows down or stops from the age of two or three years onwards. It is often first detected through routine monitoring using growth charts although it can become more obvious when a child starts nursery or school and is much shorter than other children in the class.' Children characteristically display GHD by 'growing slowly' but crucially they do so 'in proportion', that is, 'the length of their arms and legs stay at the same ratio to their chest and abdomen'. Thus, 'their face may look younger than their actual age. They may also seem chubbier, more than other children, due to the effect of growth hormone on fat storage in the body. Puberty may occur later than usual or not at all.' By early adulthood, typical symptoms will have started to manifest, as:

- Increase in fatty tissue, especially around the waist
- Decrease in lean body mass (muscle)
- Decrease in strength and stamina, reduction in exercise capacity
- Decrease in bone density, increase in rate of fracture in middle age and beyond
- Changes in blood cholesterol concentrations
- Increased sensitivity to cold or heat
- Excessive tiredness, anxiety or depression
- Reduction in quality of life[14]

Medical science in Britain was therefore from the 1950s concerned to do new research on whether GHD had links to poor diet, a lack of sanitation or substandard housing: all social problems once familiar to the late-Victorians, exacerbated by the Wall Street Crash (1929) and the food rationing privations of WWII. The main diagnostic tool was to extract GH post-mortem in order to see 'if it could be manufactured in the laboratory and used to treat patients with hypopituitarism'.[15] This PGP initiative would expand exponentially in the 1960s, and by the 1980s it had grown into a commercial enterprise in northern

Europe, but one still reliant (in Britain) on the relatively cheap extraction of GH by anatomists, coroners and pathologists. The standard MRC payment for each post-mortem extraction was 1s 6d in the 1950s, increasing to £0.20p by 1985. As the amount of GH extracted each time was very small, multiple extractions happened until official approval for a more profitable, synthetic replacement for NHS use occurred in the 1990s. It was this hidden history that Professor Van Velzen exploited at Alder Hey Children's Hospital when he removed organs, including pituitary glands, as so-called 'bio-extras'. The standard means of harvesting GH was thus a classic case of 'going *around* the law while going *through* legal processes' overseen by the MRC and then supposedly the NHS.[16] And, it proved to be a pivotal catalyst for HTA2004.

Meantime a second post-war initiative involved the passing of the Corneal Grafting Act (15 & 16 George 6 & 1 Eliz. 2: 1952). This too had its roots in late-Victorian public health concerns about the welfare of the poorest children in England. Many suffered from common eye diseases and eye defects due to vitamin deficiencies and birthing problems associated with substandard medical practices before the establishment of the NHS. Professor Arthur Thomson, for instance, who ran the dissection program at Oxford University medical school from 1885, pioneered eye research and was funded by the MRC to do ophthalmology and its neurology from WWI. The new legislation in 1952 was hence the culmination of fifty years of research work, which seemed to justify expanding regulation of the removal of eye material from cadavers, post-mortem. As the *British Medical Journal* announced:

The use of cadaver material for medical purposes [has been] ... governed by the Anatomy Act of 1832 (2nd and 3rd William 4, cap 75.), which put a stop to the practices of the 'resurrectionists', and aimed at ensuring a legal supply of subjects for anatomical dissections from the bodies of unclaimed persons dying in public institutions. That Act did not help the provision of material for corneal graft surgery, since a complicated legal procedure has to be carried out before the body is available, and does not permit the removal of a fresh organ from the body since this is permissible only on a Coroner's order. Nor did the Act allow any person to bequeath his or her own eyes for graft purposes, as in law the dead body has no property. Legal opinion was that the removal of cadaver eyes for graft purposes, even with the consent of relations was, therefore, illegal. In addition, a large number of enlightened people in Great Britain who wished to bequeath their eyes for corneal grafts were, by law, prevented from doing so. It seemed, therefore, that if these obstacles could be removed the supply of donor material would be legally increased; surgeons would not run the risk of legal actions and the voluntary bequest of eyes would probably be sufficient for anticipated needs.[17]

Importantly, this legislation created two further initiatives that should have opened up a medico-legal space for donors and their families to enquire more about bodies and their body parts in their material afterlives. All the eye grafts were sent to a new eye-bank and cornea plastic units based at prominent hospital-based eye units such as that at the Queen Victoria Hospital in East Grinstead Suffolk. Aware also of the sensitivities surrounding the gift of eyes, with many people feeling squeamish about donating them even after death, government launched a major publicity campaign. The BBC contributed, the press (both quality and tabloid newspapers) withheld sensational cases and emphasised instead the positive outcomes for NHS patients, and together the Women's Voluntary Service and the Royal College of Surgeons approached bereaved families in hospital emergency rooms for donations. In other words, in this specific context at the start of Queen Elizabeth II's new reign there seemed to be a concerted effort to be more engaging and open-handed. The confusion therefore about material afterlives came about after the passing of three amendments to AA1832: namely the Human Tissue Act (9 & 10 Eliz. 2 c. 54: 1961), Human Organ Transplant Act (Eliz. 2 c. 31: 1989) and Anatomy Act (Eliz. 2 c. 14: 1984).

In what follows in the rest of this chapter, these are styled HTA1961, HOTA1989 and AA1984 to avoid confusion. Before summarising their key features and explaining why they gave rise to disputed bodies by the late 1990s, it is important to set these cumulative legislative initiatives in the context of the history of international law. This is because what was happening in Britain did not occur in political isolation. Thus, as P. Sohl and H. A. Bassford explain: 'During the 1900s with the growth of complexity in both scientific knowledge and the organization of health services, the medical ethical codes addressed themselves to elaborate rules of conduct to be followed by the members of the newly emerging national medical associations.'[18] Then 'after World War II the World Medical Association was established as an international forum where national medical associations could debate the ethical problems presented by modern medicine'. Against this backdrop nonetheless concern was also being expressed that there was danger of seeing international consensus as 'progress' whilst ignoring its 'cultural relativism'. In reality, everyone welcomed the international framework of medical ethics, but it had to be applied in countries with 'different methods of financing medical services' and therefore differential socio-economic forces shaped doctoring and medical research cultures that were constantly evolving during the post-war era. In other words, we need to briefly engage with what the Hippocratic principle to 'first do no harm' meant in principle (the international foundation of medical ethics) before considering how it got applied in practice in modern Britain (the national imprint of HTA1961, HOTA1989 and AA1984).

Primum Non Nocere – First Do No Harm – International Medical Ethics

Once the Nuremberg Trials in 1945 exposed the atrocities of Nazi medical experimentation in the death camps of Auschwitz-Birkenau, there was an international effort co-ordinated by the Security Council members of the United

Nations to protect individuals from future exploitation.[19] The Nuremberg Code (1947) hence outlawed human experimentation of all descriptions that involved doing harm to the patient. Linked to the Declaration of Geneva (1948), this reflected widespread condemnation of war crimes in medicine, as well as a global commitment to monitor medical ethics to an international standard. The subsequent Declaration of Helsinki (hereafter DofH) in 1960/1, however, did not become international law. Instead, the UN ratified it as a code of practice, and monitored its uptake. One influential organisation to adopt its framework voluntarily in June 1964 was the World Medical Association (hereafter WMA). WMA consisted of a collection of voluntary national associations containing some eight million doctors worldwide, who signed up to self-regulate their commitment to medical ethics, education and the highest professional standards in patient-practitioner relationships. A crucial part of their commitment was that the WMA promised to remain politically neutral of the UN. At its 50th anniversary celebration in 2014, what was celebrated by WMA was the fact that their original DofH was now regarded as the cornerstone of human rights, a code of medical ethics that seeks to protect individuals against human experimentation in a global medical marketplace. It has unquestionably become *the* standard by which all ethical codes in individual nation states are judged in the human rights arena. It is not a code fixed in aspic: quite the opposite. Seven revisions happened since 1964, and that evolution is a creative process that keeps medical ethics valid in biomedicine today. In summary an overview remains:

The fundamental principle is respect for the individual (Article 8), their right to self-determination and the right to make informed decisions (Articles 20, 21 and 22) regarding participation in research, both initially and during the course of the research. The investigator's duty is solely to the patient (Articles 2, 3 and 10) or volunteer (Articles 16, 18), and while there is always a need for research (Article 6), the subject's welfare must always take precedence over the interests of science and society (Article 5), and ethical considerations must always take precedence over laws and regulations (Article 9).

   The recognition of the increased vulnerability of individuals and groups calls for special vigilance (Article 8). It is recognised that when the research participant is incompetent, physically or mentally incapable of giving consent, or is a minor (Articles 23, 24), then allowance should be considered for surrogate consent by an individual acting in the subject's best interest. In which case their consent, should still be obtained, if at all possible (Article 25).[20]

The principal issue nonetheless with this important DofH codification is not its best intentions but, rather, its flaws. Few countries have queried the dignity of the human research subject. Most agree that an ethics committee should oversee scientific research that involves people (whether alive or dead). There is likewise consensus that good practice is what medicine is all about. Nation states do, however, differ on the degree of legal emphasis contained in the original DofH and its seven revisions. For the purposes of this book, there has been a great deal of contention about the meaning of 'informed decisions' (Articles 20, 21 and 22) and what system of consent (opt-in versus opt-out) should be adopted on location. In some countries like England, patients have to make a positive choice to enter a clinical study or donate their human remains to medical research in writing prior to death. Whereas, in the Welsh National Assembly, for instance, from 1 January 2015, an opt-out system of organ donation has been officially ratified because of organ donation shortages; that is, if you die it will be presumed in law that you intended to donate unless you took steps when living to state otherwise.[21] Recently, the Conservative government under Theresa May ratified new legislation in Parliament that followed the Welsh example in organ donation – though not without controversy. Thus, the fundamentals are the same but their resource management does differ, and this matters if historians are to trace their research threshold points and actor networks (discussed in Chapter 1), as well as their body disputes that have taken place in different places, at different times and for different reasons using donated bodies.

There has been, therefore, an increasing recognition in legal circles that translational medical ethics require good communication, an ongoing dialogue to reflect cultural change, and that in the modern world this has been a very complicated process since WWII. Some legislation succeeded, other bills did not. This was because in the recent past, civil servants who drafted government business in Britain were tasked with reconciling 'medical ethics, business ethics, professional ethics, and human rights considerations' as well as taking into account a doctor's 'fundamental fiduciary responsibility to the patient in the context of a growing secular, libertarian tradition'.[22] That complex and fast-moving bioethical backdrop started to expose the need for 'a fundamental reorientation' of issues of informed consent. Slowly, as legislation did not have the impact intended, patient groups began to argue that legal and ethical guarantees were not as robust as the medical sciences claimed. However, this often only became the focus of public attention after a number of body disputes came to press attention. This was because unless you can measure something, it is often difficult to manage it properly. Much modern medical research contained body parts, brain slices and tissue samples. It was consequently easier for those inside the system to evaluate international ethical policies translated to national contexts, rather than actual practices that were piecemeal locally. Approved policies also took time to be adopted, refined and applied by their intended users; continually these had the potential to result in multiple variables. It is therefore necessary to return to a discussion of keynote legislation and core medico-legal issues in the UK, since these ambiguities frame the research cultures in the rest of this book.

A Toothless Tiger[23]

On 6 November 1967, the Right Hon. Julian Snow MP, Minster for Health in Harold Wilson's first Labour government (1964–1970), was asked by Cranley Onslow, MP for Woking, in the House of Commons: 'if he is satisfied that general practitioners are sufficiently aware of the provisions of the Human Tissue Act 1961; and if he will make a statement'.[24] The Minister replied that: 'My Department gave general practitioners guidance on the provisions of this Act in a memorandum issued in September, 1961 and I have no reason to believe that this has been generally overlooked. I am, however, glad to take this opportunity of again drawing attention to this guidance.' The matter, though, did not rest there. Over the next four years, there were numerous debates and discussions in Parliament about the efficacy of HTA1961. At issue was its implications for organ transplantation, and the degree to which it had placed more, not less, discretion in the hands of coroners, doctors, pathologists and transplant surgeons to decide on the material fate of donations from the dead and living donors in hospital care. So much so, that during a heated Prime Minister's question time in the House of Commons on 15 June 1971, Edward Heath (leader of the Conservative party) in reply to a question about the need to repeal HTA1961 and replace it with a new HTA statute at a forthcoming Queen's Bill, announced:

I realise that it is not only a question of opinion in the medical profession but that many hon. and right hon. Members have expressed the view that there should be legislation on this subject. Nevertheless, I think that if the hon. Gentleman studies the matter closely he will recognise that it is extremely controversial. What is required is a clear indication that legislation will improve the situation, and at the moment I think that that clear and convincing proof is lacking.[25]

At issue was that HTA1961 was supposed to have sorted out the class injustices of AA1832, but instead it had led to more ambiguity, confusion and misinformation. For the general public, what the legislation was supposed to have done was to set out what exactly informed consent meant in plain English, but it was flawed by the slippery civil-service speak of Parliamentary parlance. As Professor Margaret Brazier, Chair of Law at the University of Manchester, noted in the *Journal of Medical Ethics*:

The Human Tissue Act 1961 is a toothless tiger imposing fuzzy rules with no provision for sanctions or redress. Absent directions from the deceased . . . the act provides that the person lawfully in possession of the body (often the hospital where the body lies) may authorize removal of body parts for the purposes of medical education or research providing that having 'made such reasonable inquiry as may be practicable' [even though there is] . . . no reason to believe that the deceased had expressed objections to such a process or that 'the surviving spouse or any surviving relative of the deceased objects to the body being so dealt with'. Under the Human Tissue Act it may appear that the requisite authorization, consent if you like, comes from the hospital. Hospitals permit themselves to remove organs and tissue which they desire to put to scientific or medical uses.[26]

Hindsight, she conceded, is a wonderful thing. Nonetheless, those who drafted HTA1961 should have been aware that although 'consent is such a simple word' it was also self-evident that a lack of clarity had resulted in many disputed cases. Helpfully, Brazier also elaborated on the legal position of the medical sciences:

A previous Master of the Rolls, Lord Donaldson, took a straightforward view of consent to medical treatment by living patients. He likened consent to a flak jacket. Once consent is obtained, the doctor is protected from legal gunfire. Consent protects his back. He cannot be sued. Academic lawyers, those rather precious creatures, dislike the analogy, ignoring as it does any analysis of the interests consent protects, avoiding even any mention of autonomy. Moreover, whether you like flak jackets or not, the crucial question remains of who has the requisite authority to provide the flak jacket to the doctor.[27]

There were essentially two medico-legal issues: 'Whose consent *should* have been obtained for organ retention? And whose consent *ought* to be obtained for organ return?' In other words, the main flaw in HTA1961 was exactly what the ethnographer Marie-Andree Jacobs identifies as a central problem with 'the law: how was everyone involved absorbing and using legal frameworks', and in what ways were those 'actors' going '*around* the law while going *through* legal processes?'[28] In many respects, these key ethical questions were not resolved by the raft of new legislation in the 1970s and set out in Table 2.1. This despite how widely the medical profession welcomed the Medical Research Council's new Ethical Code in 1979, which made MRC funding dependent on following new EC guidance. By the opening of the 1980s, there seemed to be an urgent need for yet more piecemeal legislation, tackling but never resolving discrete aspects of the consent issue.

The enterprise culture of Margaret Thatcher's Conservative government (1979–1990) saw the start of an unprecedented expansion of biotechnology in Britain.[29] In part, this reflected just how much early transplant surgery had benefitted from improved surgical training techniques, as well as the development of the next generation of drug-rejection therapies by the pharmaceutical industry. There were public health campaigns organised by the Department of Health to get more of the general public to carry organ donation cards, but still sociological studies found that half of those bereaved were prepared to give and half were not. As transplant lists grew longer, and patients' expectations rose, wanting to push past the dead-end of life, more and more parliamentary questions reflected on the need to deal separately with human organ transplantation. The result was the passing of HOTA1989. It had been preceded by

AA1984, and the Anatomy Regulations Act (1988) (hereafter ARA1988). HOTA and ARA were in principle about better accountability. The first prevented the illegal trade in organs and protected the vulnerable from becoming victims of organ harvesting. The latter made it compulsory for a written record to be kept of all bodies and body parts retained by medical schools for human anatomy teaching and medical research in Britain. This second medico-legal guarantee was heralded as a major ethical step forward, but it was nothing of the sort because the original AA1832 had a very robust system of tagging bodies to paperwork at each stage the corpse was moved on or changed hands.[30] It was, therefore, reintroducing an old law that HTA1961 had watered down, reviving it again to mask that HTA1961 was flawed. Because no official body had oversight of the entire process of medical research and its various hidden histories of the dead, older standards could be recycled in the belief that this was progress. It was clumsy and careless to reverse AA1832 legislation that was not fit for purpose in its HTA1961 form.

Focussing on the central aims of the various pieces of legislation passed in the 1980s to protect patients and facilitate further medical research, one aspect of AA1984 stands out. Amendments to statutes dealing with the legal use of organs and human tissue did not clarify who owned human material removed from its source. Moreover, it was clear that the issue of informed consent in a whole variety of contexts was very complex indeed. This was because it involved a balancing act of four sorts of agency: the patient, scientific research, medical doctors and public scrutiny. Thus, in letters to the *British Medical Journal* (hereafter *BMJ*) at the time the new AA1984 became law, some clinicians were asking uncomfortable ethical questions. What would happen to vulnerable patients with mental ill-health, manipulated into clinical trials by virtue of their vulnerability, and would those that committed suicide be automatically handed over by coroners for medical research post-mortem? Of concern were those patients who helped test new psychiatric drugs or 'electroconvulsive therapy' that aimed to alleviate severe depression. Is it possible, enquired Dr Neville-Smith in a letter to the *BMJ*, that fully informed consent is never achievable because the person in mental ill-health has an unbalanced mind? Others were likewise questioning what happens in organ donation to those so bereaved after a fatality that they cannot think straight. In response, a member of the psychiatric department at Leicester Royal Infirmary claimed that:

SIR,- Dr Neville-Smith raises an important ethical issue when he questions the nature of informed consent. It is, however, impossible to offer a simple solution. The protection of the individual patient, the need for research to improve both fundamental knowledge and patient care, and the need to maintain a humane and scientific profession must all be secured by policies acceptable to doctors and open to public scrutiny.[31]

It was the emphasis in this letter of reply on matters of consent being 'acceptable to doctors' (first – paternalism) and open to 'public scrutiny' (second – accountability) in that running order of priority that would prove to be contentious by the end of the 1980s. Eventually, the *Isaacs Report* (2003) would set out how and why the various statutes had proven to be inadequate by the end of the 1990s, even without the various NHS scandals that were to be catalysts for HTA2004:

9.3 No claim by statute is available to the person from whom tissue is removed. Indeed, the implication of the Human Tissue Act 1961, the Human Organ Transplants Act 1989 and the Anatomy Act 1984, though it is not expressly stated, is that the tissue removed pursuant to these Acts is given free of all claims, that is an unconditional gift. The Human Fertilisation and Embryology Act 1990, is less straightforward. Donors of gametes or embryos may impose conditions on use and may vary or withdraw any consent given. By adopting a scheme of consents, however, the Act avoids vesting any property claim in the donor [*sic*].[32]

The ethical issue was that the piecemeal nature of legislation was matching the piecemeal climate of actual research on the body – disassembled into parts – opened up for transplant harvesting of organs – and disaggregated to facilitate tissue, cellular and DNA modification. As Ronald Munson in his thought-provoking study of organ transplantation, ethics and society observes: 'Here is the "body that will not die" or at least not until the medical sciences is "done with it".'[33] Thus, the ethical question remains, why was (and is) the public not sharing in the profitable outcomes of this enterprise? For, Munson insists, to describe the reach of scientific research as a simple 'gift exchange' in a biomedical era is misleading, especially when 'transplantation ... is a second-rate technology. ... It's a crude, stop-gap measure to keep people from dying.'[34] It is a viewpoint shared with many others in the wider scientific community. Sir Robert Lechler, Chair of Immunology at King's College London, thus explained in an interview with the *Times* on 14 July 2018 that soon: 'organ regeneration could end "barbaric" transplants'.[35] His latest regenerative medical research aims to allow patients to 'regrow their own diseased tissue ... through stem cell changes to their genetic machinery'. The leading journal *Nature* likewise featured the latest laboratory discovery that there is a 'latent capacity of some organs to grow back when they are damaged' without the sort of debilitating side-effects that can blight the lives of transplantation patients on permanent immune-suppressants drugs. Science now recognises that transplantation does extend life expectancy but it also has opportunity costs for patients too, and ones seldom elaborated honestly in public health campaigns. As Jacobs reflects in a similar refrain: 'what emerges from documentation practices [in patient case notes] is agency in abeyance, a form of submissive self'.[36] It was this lived experience that would culminate in HTA2004, but not before the question of brain research was resolved.

Brain Banking

The final catalyst that would contribute to a very public set of debates about the need for a repeal of old legislation in its entirety was the publication of the *Isaacs Report* in 2003. Jeremy Metters, HM Inspectorate of Anatomy, conducted a public enquiry into the retention of brains at Manchester University for post-mortem investigation and further medical research. As he explained:

It is important to remember that this investigation followed the chance discovery by Mrs Elaine Isaacs in April 2000 that the brain of her late husband had been retained for research in February 1987.

Had Mrs Isaacs not come across the letter sent to Mr Isaacs' general practitioner by the joint research team, she would never have known that her husband's brain had been retained, and the widespread retention of brains, and other organs, from Coroners' post mortems might have remained undisclosed.

Most of the brains from Coroners' cases in the 1980s and 1990s were initially held for entirely proper diagnostic investigation into the cause of death. A very much smaller number were retained specifically for research or teaching. The feature that unifies both these categories is that very few relatives were aware of the practice and I found no evidence that any were asked for their consent for later research or teaching use.

In this way the requirements of the Human Tissue Act [1984] were consistently disregarded.[37]

Metters undertook an audit and discovered that '21,000 brains collected between 1970 and 1990 were still held' for medical research. It was unclear how and under what circumstances Coronial cases generated human material from hospital mortuaries, or asylums, in England and Wales. He concluded that: 'Among the limited number of consent forms that I have examined, few specifically mention organ retention.' He thus reflected that: 'It appears the assumption was made that a signed post mortem consent form also indicated agreement to organ and tissue retention. It will never be known how many relatives were aware that organs might be retained from hospital post mortems without their knowledge.'[38] There was hence a need for an explicit and transparent form of informed consent keeping relatives fully and transparently engaged. This required new legislation to restore public confidence in post-mortems. His view was that there were 'serious weaknesses in the Human Tissue Act (1984)'. Perhaps the most obvious human one was that the statute made little allowance for the fact that:

The sudden death of a relative is among the most stressful of life's experiences and the closer the relative the greater the distress. The same usually holds true for the relatives of those whose deaths are reported to the Coroner for other reasons.

Many who are suddenly bereaved are 'in shock' in the days that immediately follow. More ready access is needed to the advice, support and counselling that is available for the relatives of those who die in NHS hospitals. . . .

When for the Coroner's purposes a formal statement is needed, there should be no pressure on a relative for its urgent completion or duress over the contents. While 'in shock', erroneous information may too easily be included.

As many relatives do not, at first, take in details of what is explained to them a written summary should be provided.[39]

It was imperative that those bereaved had a process of informed consent explained to them, a notion that echoed what some correspondents had been saying in the letter page of the *BMJ* since 1984. In the case of Mr Isaacs whose brain had been retained, allegedly used for medical research, but in reality 'destroyed' (according to the official report) without the knowledge of his Orthodox Jewish family, an apology was sent by Professor Deaking, head of the brain research unit at Manchester University, on 28 July 2000, that read:

I do fully understand and sympathise with the additional distress this discovery has caused you. I very much regret that current standards and safeguards about post-mortem tissue that would have prevented this occurrence today, were not in place 13 years ago. At that time there was little awareness that a relative might have strong views or legitimate rights concerning the removal of tissue and this was overshadowed by a strong desire to assist research. While not in any way condoning these attitudes, it is worth reflecting that this UK research led directly to understanding the causes of Alzheimer's disease and to entirely new treatments for this incurable condition [sic].[40]

There were two key misleading elements in this well-intentioned statement. The first is that Jeremy Metters, HM Inspectorate of Anatomy, concluded that: 'My enquiries have subsequently confirmed that no research had been undertaken on Mr Isaacs' brain, which had probably been disposed of in 1993.'[41] So the apology and its justification based on a medical research defence – namely the contribution that brain retention in this case may have made to a future cure for Alzheimer's – was a false one.[42] It was in fact very rare for a medical researcher at the time to be able to explicitly identity from their flimsy paperwork what they were hoping to achieve with specific human material at the point of so-called 'donation' or subsequently because the culture of record-keeping was to keep it sparse. This therefore looked and read like an officious excuse for an apology to those who read it. There was then the question of the culture of medical research and a lack of knowledge about wider cultural and religious sensitivities at the time that formed the basis of the second statement of apology in the letter to the Isaacs family. Again, this was incorrect.

Mrs Isaacs had repeatedly told the police, coroner and attending doctor on the night of her husband's suicide that he was an Orthodox Jew and that she needed therefore to bury the body intact within twenty-four hours according to her family's religious traditions, but she was ignored. This failure of oversight is striking. Given the publication of Ruth Richardson's renowned book, *Death, Dissection and the Destitute*, in 1987, there was ample information in the public domain about the cultural and religious meaning of death and dissection since the original AA1832. Richardson's study received a lot of publicity in the medical press, and it was well known in the media that criticisms were being made about the cultural conduct of the medical research community per se. Indeed, so respected was her work that the Chief Medical Officer, Sir Liam Donaldson at the time of the various public enquiries into the NHS organ retention scandals at Liverpool and Bristol, had asked Richardson to assist with the cultural dimensions of his findings. It would therefore have been more honest to say in the Isaacs letter of apology that the medical profession did not choose to inform itself, rather than trying to use a weak ethical defence that *'current standards and safeguards were not in place'* and there was *'little awareness'* of the impact on grieving relatives. Indeed, it would be the scale of retention both at Manchester ('5,000 organs and tissues held at 4 locations'[43]) and elsewhere (some 50,000 organs[44] rising to 105,000 in the subsequent Redfern report[45]) that prompted a public backlash. It was no longer tenable to say that the medical sciences were sincere, but sincerely wrong.[46]

Today there is now an international recognition that bioethics is a very significant but also a somewhat complex and confusing legal framework which individual clinicians apply in their cultural settings in the global community. One key criticism of bioethicists that endures is how 'in terms of the classic triad of thought, emotion and action' – they have 'focused almost exclusively on thought – ethical thinking *per se* – and given inadequate attention to emotion and action'.[47] Thus, 'what has been lost in the academic processes' of evaluating the evolution of international and national ethical frameworks are 'concrete human dimensions … the connection between ethical discourse and the full dimensions' of clinical decision-makers in a biomedical research facility between actors, particularly as technology advanced after WWII. To advance clinical ethics thus requires more careful historical consideration of rhetoric (ethical codes internationally) and reality (muddled national legislation), and its ambiguities. Moreover, as George Belkin wrote, we need medico-legal perspectives that are:

less concerned with generating rules of conduct than with deepening and enriching the self-understanding and perspective brought to bear when people confront choices and each other. And a humanist ongoing engagement and routine reflection can make medicine more deeply ethical than can duels over methodologies or ethics per se. Bioethics has narrowed how reflection in medicine about medicine takes place and has inhibited rather than rescued a medical humanism by an overrated focus on restrictive reduction to 'the ethical'.[48]

This book sits at this intersection – between rules and practicalities – between laws and choices in research spaces – between human stories and medical ethics that really happened.

Conclusion

A raft of legislation in Britain, stretching from the Murder Act in 1752 to the Human Tissue Act in 2004, had sought to regulate the use of human material from the dead and the living for teaching and research purposes. Largely, however, regulations were piecemeal, and Parliament never took a robust over-sight of all the stipulations to check that they still made sense in a fast-changing biomedical world. Those working inside laboratories (pathologists and neurolo-gists), dissection rooms (anatomists), medical schools (clinicians and doctors), as well as specialists attached to cancer study centres, all assumed that the particular law they were following was correct. Few stopped to think about, much less check on, the robustness of their medical ethics and governance criteria. Everyone assumed that methods and training were correct, standard practice within the medical science community. It was the cultural changes taking place in modern British society which would lead to their investigation properly by the Chief Medical Officer around the Millennium. Meantime, the network of actors involved – in which the Coronial Office would prove to be a linchpin – followed fundamentally flawed statutes. The legal framework turned out to be akin to standing on ethical quicksand. Thus, to engage with the sort of 'medical human-ism' that Belkin called for recently, we end Part I of this book by navigating a selection of human stories in Chapter 3 that reflect the main research themes to come in Chapters 4–6 in Part II. In this way, instead of dissecting bodies and mislaying their material histories, we begin to reconstruct, trace and analyse what it meant to conduct medical research behind closed doors, to sign up to train in human anatomy and to experience medically what soon became known collo-quially in popular culture as the *Ministry of Offal*.

Notes

1. Randall Lesaffer, 'Argument from Roman law in current international law: occupa-tion and acquisitive prescription', *European Journal of International Law*, 16 (2005), 1: 25–58.
2. Refer, Elizabeth T. Hurren, *Dissecting the Criminal Corpse: Staging Post-Execution Punishment in Early Modern England* (Basingstoke: Palgrave Macmillan, 2016).
3. See Elizabeth T. Hurren, *Protesting about Pauperism: Poverty, Politics and Poor Relief in Late-Victorian England, c. 1870–1900*, Royal Historical Society Series (Woodbridge, Suffolk: Boydell & Brewer 2015 paperback edition).

4. Peregrine Horden and Richard Smith (eds.), *The Locus of Care: Families, Communities, Institutions and the Provision of Welfare since Antiquity*, Routledge Studies in the Social History of Medicine (New York & London: Routledge, 1988).

5. See, Hurren, *Protesting about Pauperism*, provides key historical context for trends.

6. See Elizabeth T. Hurren, *Dying for Victorian Medicine: English Anatomy and Its Trade in the Dead Poor c. 1834–1929* (Basingstoke: Palgrave Macmillan, 2011), chapters 5 and 6.

7. Edward Higgs, *The Information State in England: The Central Collection of Information on Citizens since 1500* (Basingstoke: Palgrave Macmillan, 2003).

8. See, Elizabeth T. Hurren, 'Remaking the medico-legal scene: a social history of the late-Victorian coroner in Oxford', *Journal of the History of Medicine and Allied Sciences*, 65 (April 2010): 207–252.

9. A complete PDF copy of *British Parliamentary Papers, Coroners (Amendment) Act* (16 & 17 Geo. 5 c. 59: 1926), was consulted on 20/10/2016 and can be accessed online at: http://www.legislation.gov.uk/ukpga/1926/59/pdfs/ukpga_19260059_en.pdf

10. Refer, for instance, Elizabeth T. Hurren and S. A King, 'Begging for a burial: form, function and meaning of nineteenth century pauper funeral provision', *Social History*, 20 (2005), 3: 1–41.

11. Hurren, *Dying for Victorian Medicine*, pp. 308–309 on stillbirth official changes.

12. Ibid., discusses this backdrop in chapters 4, 5 and 6; see, also, Elizabeth T. Hurren, 'The pauper dead-house: the expansion of Cambridge anatomical teaching school under the late-Victorian Poor Law, 1870–1914', *Medical History*, 48 (2004), 1: 19–30, which identifies research on children and stillbirths.

13. Refer, *US Library of Medicine*, Medline Information Resource, 'Pituitary disorders', accessed 20/10/2016 at: https://medlineplus.gov/pituitarydisorders.html

14. Ibid.

15. In those who needed urgent treatment, there were four main types of deficiency that they suffered from, including a lack of: 'growth hormone, puberty hormones (or gonadotrophins), thyroid stimulating hormone (TSH, which stimulates the thyroid gland to make Thyroxine), and Prolactin and Adrenocorticotrophic Hormone (ACTH, which stimulates the adrenal stress hormone, cortisol). The posterior pituitary makes the fluid balance hormone called anti-diuretic hormone (ADH)' – Refer, *The Pituitary Foundation*, for accurate medical information about the range of conditions and current treatments available at: www.pituitary.org.uk/information/what-is-the-pituitary-gland/

16. Marie-Andree Jacob, *Contemporary Ethnography: Matching Organs to Donors, Legalising and Kinship in Transplants* (Philadelphia: University of Pennsylvania Press, 2012), p. 8.

17. B. W. Rycroft, 'The Corneal Grafting Act', *British Medical Journal*, 37 (1953): 349.

18. P. Sohl and H. A. Basford, 'Codes of medical ethics: traditional foundations and contemporary practice', *Journal of Social Science Medicine* 22 (1986), 11: 1175–1179.

19. Notably, Paul J. Weindling, *Nazi Medicine and the Nuremburg Trials: From Medical War Crimes to Informed Consent* (Basingstoke: Palgrave Macmillan, 2006); Weindling, *Victims and Survivors of Nazi Human Experiments: Science and Suffering in the Holocaust* (London: Bloomsbury, 2014); Weindling, *From Clinic to*

Concentration Camp: Reassessing Nazi Medicine and Racial Research, 1933–1945, The History of Medicine in Context (New York & London: Routledge, 2017); and importantly, Michael Marrus, *The Nuremberg War Crimes Trial of 1945–6: A Brief History with Documents* (Basingstoke: Palgrave Macmillan, 1997).

20. See, World Medical Association Declaration of Helsinki, 'Ethical principles for medical research involving human subjects', *Journal of the American Medical Association*, 20 (27 November 2013), 10: 2191–2194, DOI: 10.1001/jama.2013.281053, retrieved 21/10/2016.

21. 'Organ donation opt-out system given go-ahead in Wales', BBC News, 2 July 2013, accessed 21/10/2016 at: http://www.bbc.co.uk/news/uk-wales-politics-23143236

22. Mary Jane Kagarise and George F. Sheldon, 'Translational ethics: a perspective for the new millennium', *Archives of Surgery, Journal of the American Medical Association* (2000), 135: 39–45.

23. Margaret Brazier, 'Organ retention and return: problems of consent – symposium on consent and confidentiality', *Journal of Medical Ethics*, 29 (2003): 30–33. Professor Margaret Brazier, Chair in Law at Manchester University, had been asked to address the proposals of the Independent Review Group in Scotland on the Retention of Organs at Post Mortem to speak of authorisation rather than consent, and its attendant ethical issues when she spoke out about the flaws in HTA1961.

24. *Hansard*, HC, vol. 753, cols. 334W, 6 November 1967, 'Prime Minister's Question Time answer on proposal to amend Human Tissue Act 1961 in the forthcoming Queen's Bill', reply by Prime Minister, Right Hon. Edward Heath, Leader of the Conservative Party.

25. Ibid., 15 June 1971, vol. 819, cols. 229–30.

26. Brazier, 'Organ retention and return', p. 31.

27. Ibid., p. 32.

28. Jacob, *Contemporary Ethnography*, p. 8.

29. A historical connection made, persuasively, in Darrell M. West, *Biotechnology across National Boundaries: The Science-Industrial Complex* (Basingstoke: Palgrave, 2007).

30. Hurren, *Dying for Victorian Medicine*, explains this context in chapter 1, pp. 16–17.

31. Sydney Brandon (Department of Psychiatry, Leicester Royal Infirmary), Letters to the Editor, *British Medical Journal*, 289 (1 September 1984): 558.

32. See, http://image.guardian.co.uk/sys-files/Society/documents/2003/05/12/isaacs_report.pdf, accessed 24/10/2016, *Isaacs Report* (2003), Section 9.3. We will be returning to this report below since it dealt with the question of brain retention primarily.

33. Ronald Munson, *Raising the Dead: Organ Transplants, Ethics and Society* (Oxford: Oxford University Press, 2002), preface.

34. Ibid., p. 22

35. Oliver Moody, 'Organ regeneration could end "barbaric" transplants', *Times*, 24 July 2018, News section, p. 4, and leading article, p. 9, on *Nature*-published discoveries.

36. Jacobs, *Contemporary Ethnography*, p. 42.

37. *Isaacs Report*, Recommendations section, p. 11. See Chapter 6 later in this book on how Mr Isaacs died on 26 February 1987 aged 54. His family were of Orthodox Jewish descent and their belief was that the body should be buried whole, within 48

hours of death according to Jewish law. However, because Mr Isaacs had been treated for mental ill-health and he committed suicide at home, his body entered the post-mortem process of the Manchester Coronial Office. His body was taken to Prestwich mortuary where his brain was removed during post-mortem and kept for further research purposes at Manchester University.

38. Ibid., Recommendations section, p. 11.
39. *Isaacs Report*, Recommendations 14 and 15, p. 24.
40. Ibid., pp. 49–50, quoted in italics as per the original report.
41. *Isaacs Report*, p. 50.
42. Brains were likewise taken for research at Cambridge Addenbrookes Hospital for research into Huntingdon's disease and sometimes a 'control' brain was needed on which no research was done. This will be again discussed in Chapter 6.
43. *Isaacs Report*, p. 52, stated: 'The inventory had identified over 5000 organs and tissues held at four locations. These were: (i) the University Medical School in Oxford Road; (ii) the Central Manchester Hospital site (including the Children's Hospital); (iii) the Salford (Hope) Hospital site; (iv) the South Manchester Hospital (Wythenshawe/Withington) sites. A full list of specimens is held at each site, with a copy held centrally. Among these specimens were 473 brains in brain collections that had been reported to the Chief Medical Officer's Census.'
44. See for instance, Professors Ian Kennedy and Liam Donaldson's census estimates as reported in '50, 000 organs secretly stored in hospitals', *Guardian*, 11 January 2001.
45. See, Elizabeth T. Hurren, 'Patients' rights: from Alder Hey to the Nuremberg Code', *History and Policy Papers* (6 May 2002), accessed 3/11/2016 at: http://he alth-equity.pitt.edu/4042/1/policy-paper-03.html
46. A split infinitive; and yet, an apt expression of the situation at the time.
47. See, Stephen Scher and Kasia Kozlowska, *Rethinking Health Care Ethics* (Basingstoke: Palgrave Pivot, 2018), p. 4.
48. George S. Belkin, 'Moving beyond bioethics: history and the search for medical humanism', *Perspectives in Biology and Medicine*, 47 (2004), 3: 372–385, quote at p. 378.

3   *The Ministry of Offal*

Introduction

Francis Partridge, diarist and writer, attended a Christmas wedding in central London on 23 December 1962.[1] Recently widowed, her financial affairs were precarious. She would shortly take the difficult decision to sell her Wiltshire home, Ham Spray House, it being too expensive to maintain on a small widow's pension. Francis looked forward, even so, to her only son's yuletide marriage.[2] He had been a great comfort to her in the dark days of early bereavement. Bleak times seemed to be behind them both because there was now the promise of a future grandchild. Her son's fiancée was pregnant and would shortly give birth to a baby girl. Little did Francis know, however, that her hopes of enlarging her family circle would soon be dashed, and cruelly so. Her beloved son, an up-and-coming talented writer, was to die of a heart attack just nine months after his wedding and only three weeks after the birth of his new daughter.[3] On 7 September 1963, the day of her son's death, Francis's grief as recorded in her diary was raw: she wrote – 'I have utterly lost *my* heart: I want no more of this cruel life'.[4]

On her son Burgo's wedding day, Francis's heart had in fact been full of hope.[5] She invited a wide circle of friends to the celebration, many from amongst the famous Bloomsbury set of artists, painters and writers, her relatives by marriage. Her new daughter-in-law, 17-year-old Henrietta, was the offspring of David 'Bunny' Garnett.[6] He was a former bi-sexual lover of Duncan Grant the painter and the ex-husband of Francis's sister.[7] As Bunny lived in France, it was a gathering from across Europe and England that promised to closer entwine the bonds of friends and family. Francis wrote an affectionate and amusing account of those assembled in her diary:

Notes on the wedding: the absolute charm of Duncan, arriving with a button-hole in a white paper bag, beaming at everyone. The geniality of Bunny who suddenly began talking about the necessity of leaving one's body to the doctors with a look of great jollity on his face (more suitable to the occasion, than the subject). His father's mistress, old Nellie someone-or-other, has just died and when Bunny went to arrange the funeral he found to his relief that the body-snatchers had been already, and all the trouble and expense were spared him: '*You just ring up the Ministry of Offal, Sackville Street*' is what I remember his saying, but I suppose he can't have.[8]

Having lost a husband and 28-year-old son to heart failure over a three-year period, Francis had every reason to revisit her diary entry on the *Ministry of Offal*. New medical research might have prevented the early deaths of those she loved. Yet, even this dispassionate, highly intelligent woman could not bear to donate her husband's or son's body to medical science. Here was someone so shockingly bereaved, in such emotional turmoil, that the physical pain she experienced was almost impossible to bear. The amusing quip at her son's wedding had foreshadowed a tragic end to her intimate family life, akin to a Grimms' fairy tale. As Burgo's publisher, Antony Blond, wrote years later:

One afternoon whilst talking on the phone to Charlotte [Blond's wife], Burgo died. He was suffering from von Falkenhausen's disease [an aortic aneurysm discovered at the post-mortem] and part of his aorta had flaked off and choked him. I am told that when his mother was informed she telephoned Harrod's and asked them to collect her son's body, cremate him, and send her the bill.[9]

For a woman who did not believe in an afterlife, there was no solace gained from a sense of spirituality. Nor could she bear to contemplate the bodies of her loved ones displayed for public consumption in any respect. Indeed, in accordance with her rationalist and atheist beliefs, Francis refused to hold a formal funeral for Burgo – a decision that his publisher said he 'never forgave her' for taking.[10] The alternative consolation of the gift to humanity of her son's body was unconscionable as she sank into depression, unable to write her diary for the next two years. The gap came to symbolise the gulf that death left in her life.

Even so, Francis was a writer and what she could constructively do was to chronicle the human condition of trying to live with the pain of a double bereavement. As Anne Boston remarked of her diaries covering this sad period: 'The stages of grief stand out almost like a clinical case history. At first she feels eerily like an amputee, at the same time fearing her sense of loss still lies in wait.' Francis hence remarked in 1962 that grief is like a 'ghastly elephant trap. . . . I have buried and suffocated some part of it and one day I shall wake and find I've been falsely bearing the unbearable and either kill myself or go mad.'[11] It is precisely this sort of scenario that has often resulted in disputed bodies in modern biomedicine. For Francis could afford a cremation, she had legal control of the body and she never had to resort to voluntary donation out of poverty. A doctor did not compel her to think about when exactly the dead-end of life happens in a laboratory or dissection-room setting. Everyone respected her wish to cremate her son with dignity and in the way that she and her daughter-in-law envisaged. And without the proverbial *Ministry of Offal* this would also have been the ending story in all cases of untimely or tragic death. In practice, however, most 'ordinary' people did not know that at

Coronial Inquests parts of their loved ones were used to establish a cause of death and for further medical study under one of the Human Tissue Acts outlined in Chapter 2. The *Ministry of Offal* had a fleeting presence in a doctor's interaction with patients or in written guidance and advice. This is not necessarily a criticism of medical science. Many researchers and other professionals acted within current guidance at the time, and the story above clearly shows the dilemmas involved in reconciling research ethics with painful personal sensibilities. In later life, Francis thus still recalled 'the sharpness of the death of her husband and son' even after forty years of bereavement.[12] Yet this was also the sort of person expected to be open to body donation. Francis never espoused religious beliefs that constructed medical research as some-thing taboo: quite the opposite. Even so, like many of her contemporaries, it was the physical shock of grief that out-weighed the call of medical science. In this case, her wishes were respected. In others, the wishes of families were either ignored or never canvassed or undue pressure was applied for consent. The rest of this chapter unpicks some of the competing influences that shape how disputes about bodies (the focus of Part II of this book) might originate. Running from the early twentieth century to the present, it will concentrate on five core sets of life writing.

The first, letters by Mrs Pearl Craigie, explores how negative public senti-ment about the use of bodies and the harvesting of organs could develop and the defensive attitudes in the medical establishment that could thus develop. The second, third and fourth sets of life writing – respectively, Richard Harrison, Jonathan Miller and Michael Crichton – illustrate the complex ethical, moral and personal standpoints of those who benefitted from or con-ducted anatomical research and its teaching activities. A final set of life writing – the author's own reflections on visits to modern anatomical spaces and dissections – focusses on the sentimental and experiential aspect of ana-tomical practices, in effect showing how the three types of body disputes that underpin the agenda for Part II of this book can sometimes (but not always) be generated by complex feelings when involved in medical research cultures rather than an intent to deceive. Here then, we encounter the human flow of medical research and the tides of public opinion in the serpentine river of life and death of a biomedical age.

Mrs Craigie's Complaint

At the turn of the twentieth century, female novelists who came to prominence in the press often did so with strong political convictions, and many went on to become journalists. One leading columnist was 'John Oliver Hobbes', the pseudonym of Mrs Pearl Mary Teresa Craigie. She used her writing talents and feeling for a good story, not just to entertain, but to tackle social inequalities in British society. Thus, the *London Review* observed how Mrs Craigie 'with an unfailing finger pointed out the sores of modern life' and did so in the belief that she should be 'a woman who faithfully served her contemporaries to her utmost ability' in popular print culture.[13] During the Edwardian era, she focussed public attention on hidden histories of the dead, to the embarrassment of those dissecting at leading London medical schools.

In the late spring of 1906, a series of letters appeared in the *Daily Mail*, which caused considerable consternation in medico-legal circles. They were penned by Craigie (see Illustration 3.1), a former president of the *Society for Women Journalists* in London.[14] One controversial letter asked 'Mr Sydney Holland ... Chairman of the London Hospital' to reveal 'how a post-mortem examination may be performed with the act of dissection'. Craigie queried the standard methods of cutting up a dead body according to the various definitions set out

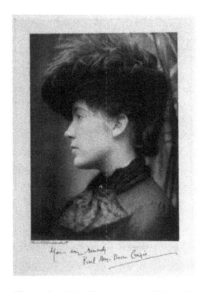

Illustration 3.1 Photograph of '*Mrs Craigie*' for an article by Margaret Maison, 'The Brilliant Mrs Craigie', *The Listener Magazine*, 28 August 1969, Issue 2109, p. 272. The photograph originally appeared in the flyleaf of John Morgan Richards, *The Life of John Oliver Hobbes told in her correspondence with numerous friends* (John Murray, Albermarle Street, 1911). As this publication is now out of the copyright clearance restrictions and this author owns a copy of that original book, the image is being reproduced here under creative commons Attribution Non-Commercial Share Alike 4.0 International (CC BY-NC-SA, 4.0), authorised here for open access, and non-profit making for academic purposes only.

in a medical dictionary, pointing out that it was self-evident that there was a great deal of difference between:

Dissection: The operation of cutting-open a dead body.
Post-Mortem: An examination of the body after death: autopsy.
Autopsy: Dissection and inspection of a dead body.[15]

She wanted to know explicitly: 'Mr Holland speaks of the "small disfigure-ment" caused by a post-mortem examination. With all respect, I must ask him whether he has personally seen many bodies after the operation in question, or bodies not especially prepared for his inspection?' Mrs Craigie also queried whether relatives could dispute the use of their loved ones' remains for post-mortem and subsequent medical research, or whether medical science ignored their intimate feelings. She challenged the prevailing medico-legal viewpoint that post-mortem protected patients from future medical negligence and was always a positive experience that the bereaved had consented to. Surely, she queried, this was dependent on the number of material cuts to the body of a loved one:

Again: is it always made clear to every patient (or to his or her relative), on entering other hospitals, that, in the event of his or her death, the body may be subjected to the 'small disfigurement' in question?[16]

She was sceptical that a relative would be told of deaths caused by the 'hospital's own negligence', or indeed from 'carelessness, or ignorance or bad nursing'. The common situation was surely that hospital doctors would instead close ranks to protect their reputations. Thus, she enquired, if the bereaved objected to a post-mortem and further medical research, 'in the event of a refusal' are the 'relatives reminded that they have received free treatment'? This question of financial obligation was to have remarkable longevity in Britain, and indeed often shapes media debates today about the need to open up patient data for research in the NHS (as we shall see throughout this book). Meantime, Mrs Craigie's questions about the ethical basis of medico-legal research and its actual working practices were to prove to be remarkably forward-thinking. In many respects, a lack of informed consent – her central complaint – was not resolved until the Human Tissue Act (Eliz. 2 c. 30: 2004), as we saw in Chapters 1 and 2. And so, in 1906 her letters caused an outcry at the start of a century of controversy. To appreciate her impact in the media and how defensive the medical science became at the time, we need to briefly reflect on her social origins and the reach of her social policy journalism in popular culture.

One of the reasons that *Mrs Craigie's Complaint* (as it was styled in the national press) received such widespread publicity was that not only was she a successful novelist but also a well-known playwright and contemporary of Oscar Wilde on the London stage.[17] Craigie was an American by birth, born in

Massachusetts, but brought up in London by wealthy Anglo-American parents. As the *Listener* magazine explained:

Her father, John Morgan Richards, was a successful businessman of Non-Conformist stock. At the time, there were only about a dozen American families living in London. Mr Richards became founder and chairman of the American Society in England. He introduced the sale of American cigarettes into this country and became a leading light in the brave new world of advertising. His interests were literary, as well as commercial, and at one time he was proprietor of the *Academy Magazine* and *Carter's Little Liver Pills*. His pioneering spirit made him a large fortune and he realised a cherished dream by buying a castle on the Isle of Wight.[18]

Richards thus had the financial wherewithal to fund his eldest child's expensive education. Pearl enrolled at Misses Godwin's boarding school at Newbury in Berkshire (1876–1877) before entering a number of private day schools in London. By 1885, she had grown into a confident young teenager and spent a year in Paris, where she became an accomplished pianist. Mrs Craigie was renowned, however, for having made an ill-fated marriage aged 19 to Reginald (known as Robert) Walpole Craigie, seven years her senior, and a banker.[19] On her honeymoon Pearl realised that she had made a serious mistake, as her husband proved to be an alcoholic and a philanderer. Her marital problems were, she told friends, akin to 'being strangled by a boa constrictor'. Nevertheless, she did her marital duty by giving birth to a son, John Churchill Craigie, in 1890. Soon, though, a legal separation and divorce followed in August 1895. In between, to avoid her husband's excessive drinking and womanising, Pearl enrolled as a student of classics and philosophy at University College London. She also started to do some serious creative writing and developed intimate friendships with gentlemen in her social circle. In part, these inspired Henry James's famous novel, *The Wings of a Dove* (1902). Consequently, according to commentators in the media, Pearl espoused the 'new woman' of the 1890s. For she was determined to speak her mind, earn an independent living and thus break free from the marital restraints of her bitterly unhappy home life. To become financially independent, and secure the sole custody of her only child in the divorce court, she published a novel, *Some Emotion and a Moral*, in 1891. The storyline concerned the trials of infidelity and a bad marriage.

It soon became an instant best-seller. Pearl was delighted when it sold '80,000 copies' in the first year. The publicity surrounding her publishing success and the notoriety of her divorce case reflected her wide social circle of not just political but bohemian friends too. Many were up-and-coming artists, poets and dramatists of the fin-de-siècle. They included the first contributors to the famous *Yellow Book*, a magazine devoted to the decadent arts, featuring Oscar Wilde, George Tyrell, Aubrey Beardsley and George Moore.

She likewise was befriended by the elderly William Gladstone (former Prime Minister) and a young Winston Churchill. Yet, her closest friendships were from amongst a wave of wealthy young American women who migrated to England during the annual social season. Many went on to marry into the top ranks of the British aristocracy. Most bought their title but soon found the marriage bargain to be disillusioning. One such was Consuelo Vanderbilt, who resented, but had to comply with, an arranged marriage to the 9th Duke of Marlborough in exchange for her dowry of $2.5 million. Consuelo by 1906 (the date of Pearl Craigie's letter to the *Daily Mail*) had separated too and was to divorce in 1921. In many respects, then, Pearl espoused a new form of female liberation, and it was on this basis that medico-legal figures of the Gilded Age on both sides of the Atlantic derided *Mrs Craigie's Complaint*.[20]

In all the articles and letters written to counter *Mrs Craigie's Complaint* by those associated with the London Hospital and the medical research culture of the time in England, three things stand out. First, the responses all had an aggressive, affronted tone. To paraphrase their male sentiments, most said: Who is this woman with the effrontery to question what we as a medical profession do with the dead body? They next all sought to reassure the public that the dead were treated with the utmost respect. Again, a précis in the media often ran something like this: Why does this over-sensitive female writer, who is divorced and has converted to the Roman Catholic Church to assuage her guilt, think she has the right to interfere in our work of national importance? A third trend was that all responders to her letters stated categorically that only the poorest were dissected and a post-mortem for the rich and middle classes did not in any respect resemble what happened to the 'unclaimed' from amongst the lower classes who could not afford a pauper funeral. The line of argument stressed was 'that there was never a time when the hospitals of this country were so much endeared to all classes of the community'.[21] Yet, this trinity of stock responses was disingenuous and thus Mrs Craigie kept pressing for better public accountability.

Not one single medical correspondent was prepared to elaborate on the reasonable questions Mrs Craigie posed in print. Nobody defined what the material differences were between an autopsy, post-mortem and dissection. One angrily said: 'I think Mrs Craigie should have taken the trouble to understand the differences between dissection and post-mortem' before going into print.[22] Of course, this only made readers of the *Daily Mail* more suspicious as to why the medical profession was not prepared to do so in the first place. Even a family acquaintance, Edwin Howard MRCS, did not explain explicitly that dissection meant dismemberment in his letters to the editors of several national newspapers in which he defended his profession. Nor did he concede how little materially was left at the end to bury. For, as this author has shown elsewhere, at best it was only about one third of the body at the end of an average dissection done during the Edwardian era.[23] In other words, what Mrs Craigie had done was to ask some inconvenient questions.

The timing of Mrs Craigie's letter was particularly unwelcome for the London Hospital. Mr Sydney Holland, to whom her letters were addressed, was the 2nd Viscount Knutsford, a barrister and hereditary peer, who chaired the London Hospital House Committee from 1896 to 1931. He had just completed a major fund-raising drive, and would clearly have been embarrassed socially by the allegations of medical impropriety.[24] The press dubbed Holland *The Prince of Beggars* for the sheer number of financial activities he had personally undertaken to raise money to rebuild the rundown infrastructure of the London Hospital.[25] By 1906, he had generated enough capital donations to rebuild the premises in their entirety, and this gave the hospital doctors a new opportunity to increase their involvement in medical research. It was likely therefore that in the future they would want to acquire more, not fewer, bodies to dissect. In private, Holland conceded that the hospital focussed on '*B.I.D.*' patients – '*Brought-In-Dead*' – the initials doctors used in their medical case-notes to indicate that a body might be suitable for medical research after post-mortem.[26] The irony was not lost on those like Mrs Craigie that they would be 'bid for' in an expanding supply system that was becoming very competitive. In Part II we will be examining how these networks of actors acquired human material, their common activities, habits and procedures, building on and extending in new directions the conceptual approach of Bruno Latour, Michel Callon and John Law in actor-network theory, outlined in Chapter 1.[27] For whilst historians and sociologists have considered in general terms how actor networks were fashioned by the science and technology of the twentieth century, there is a much less refined sense of how and for what purpose anatomists, coroners and pathologists generated and regenerated complex chains of human material to sustain new research cultures. In this book, we will be describing this actor network by mapping it out. From 1945 to 2000, its acquired human material created notable research agendas, attracting external funding, building professional status and making careers. This had performative elements that were intended and unintended, orthodox and unorthodox, seen and unseen. In other words, we are going to take our research lead from Mrs Craigie and her searching enquiries about '*B.I.D.*' Her opponent Holland meantime was also a keen advocate of vivisection, believing that animal research was justified for the public good. So much so, that in 1908 he would become the president of the *Research Defence Society*, a position he held until 1931.[28] He was therefore a committed and vocal exponent of human and animal research: passions that set in context *Mrs Craigie's Complaint* and the press coverage it generated.

What Sydney Holland chiefly objected to was the accusation by Mrs Craigie in a letter to the *Daily Mail* of 28 April 1906 that said: 'it is known that the hospitals are not under any Government inspection'. This was despite the Anatomy Act (2 & 3 Will. 4 c. 75: 1832) setting up an Anatomy Inspectorate to oversee dissection and its supply lines from infirmaries, large teaching hospitals and workhouse premises.[29] As Pearl pointed out, 'Some are well managed; some are less well managed.' The fact that inspection was seriously underfunded meant it lacked rigour. She then used emotive language to describe bodies handed back after post-mortem: 'I leave your readers to imagine the feelings of parents and others on receiving the bodies of their dead brutally disfigured and coarsely sewn up as though they were carcasses from Smithfield' livestock market. There is no doubt that this was a controversial way to question contemporary medical ethics, and many thought that she should have used more measured language. Today, she would be criticised by some historians of science and medicine for her 'neo-liberal' values in a pre-liberal era (ironically), whereas she defended that what she espoused was a 'basic humanism'.[30] Pearl Craigie was a plain-speaking American who liked to take risks, and she thought that people of education in the public sphere of the arts should be radical. Thomas Hardy, the novelist, was praiseworthy of this character trait in her, often quoting the definition she espoused about the role of an artist in society. They should be a person, she said: 'who thinks more than there is to think, feels more than there is to feel, and sees more than there is to see'.[31] Even so, she had only a partial picture of reality, as subsequent letters to the press revealed.

Most dead patients underwent a post-mortem, but it was not their whole body that was taken for further research but rather their body parts, organs, tissues and cells that could and were often removed, supposedly to establish a cause of death, as we have already seen in earlier chapters. Coroners and the medical men they employed to do post-mortem work had a lot of discretion to remove human material as they saw fit. Mrs Craigie could not have known this in 1906, but she had potentially hinted at a trade shrouded in secrecy. There were in fact many unseen aspects to the business of anatomy and its supply lines.[32] For instance, an amputation of a leg or arm sold after operative surgery often entered the chain of anatomical supply in London. The poorest, used exten-sively for teaching and research purposes, were divided up before burial. Bodies were broken for sale because a body in parts was more profitable than whole. Generally, the anatomist on duty did their best to make sure the body contained enough human material sewn up inside the skin for burial. The dead body thus weighed enough to meet grieving relatives' expectations at the graveside (a theme we return to below). Meanwhile, the reference to Smithfield market in *Mrs Craigie's Complaint* was ironic, because across the road from the famous meat market stood St Bartholomew's Hospital, which always competed with the London Hospital to buy the dead and destitute of the East End for medical research and teaching purposes (see Chapter 4 for the modern period). In other words, the comments by Mrs Craigie were ill informed on the essential details, but they did hint that larger ethical problems existed. Predictably, perhaps, Sidney Holland picked on the inaccuracy of the finer details. He chose to ignore the bigger ethical dilemmas that the medical profession faced: there was a trade in the dead, it was active in 1906, and it would continue to be so at least up to the 1960s and often until very recently in most medical schools in Britain.

Sydney Holland admitted to the *Daily Mail* that the London Hospital undertook some '1,100 post-mortems every year'.[33] He did not, though, reveal how many actual full-scale dissections this involved. Instead, he stressed that in the case of post-mortems generated on the hospital wards, when he received a complaint from a relative about medico-legal impropriety, he always investigated them personally. Holland appreciated that 'the horror of post-mortem being made on anyone one loves is shared by the poor as well as the rich' but reiterated that only a 'small disfigurement' occurred, disguised by being covered over when relatives came to view the body. This was misleading: the poorest cut 'on the extremities and to the extremities' could not accurately be described as having a 'small disfigurement'.[34] Class played a central role in cutting a little, or a lot. Holland, by concentrating on what happened at a post-mortem *before* a body went for dissection, was being deliberately evasive. Instead, he defended that Mrs Craigie was not in a position to verify her statements, and that in his opinion 'she has permitted her tender feelings, stimulated perhaps by a complaint she has not tested, to tempt her to publish one more work of fiction, which, unlike her others, will give pain to many, and pleasure to none'. In a follow-up letter, he did reveal when pressed that there had been some 'one hundred and ten thousand' post-mortems in the 'last ten years' but stressed 'we have had only three complaints'.[35] He also emphasised that 'very special and loving care is shown to the dead in the London Hospital'. There was a mortuary chapel, built from the bequest of William Evans Gordon, a major benefactor. Yet, this still did not elaborate on the fate of those sent for a full-scale dissection and dismemberment. Instead, Mrs Craigie faced accusations of being an interfering female of a sensitive disposition, given to storytelling, who was not in command of the material facts. It was difficult to see how she could be so, when the dead-end of life seldom featured in public. Searching questions often created this sort of medical backlash, and it could be biting to protect the fact of many missed body disputes of the sort analysed in later chapters.

There was to be one final twist in this storyline about disputing the dead-end of those used for medical research. Pearl Craigie died within just three months of penning her robust exchanges with Sydney Holland in the *Daily Mail*. On 13 August 1906 she was staying at her father's house in London, excited about a touring holiday she was about to embark on to Scotland. Retiring to bed, she said she felt tired, but ill-health was not suspected. In the morning, a maid tried to rouse her in her bedroom, but to no avail. She had died of a heart attack in the night. Her shocked parents and her 16-year-old son were grieved to discover that, as her sudden death was unexplained, she would have to undergo an autopsy followed by a post-mortem. At a Coronial Inquest conducted in Paddington by Dr George Danford Thomas, the GP called to the death-bed scene (Dr Leslie Meredith) recalled that he 'found Mrs Craigie lying on her back in bed, dead'.[36] He thought that she had expired 'painlessly' and been dead 'three or four hours, probably more' sometime the previous evening. His post-mortem examination concluded with an informative summary: 'One division of the heart was dilated and the muscle was thin and degenerated. Death was due to cardiac failure, and entirely due to natural causes.' The jury heard the medical circumstances in full:

CORONER: Her death might have occurred anywhere suddenly?
DR LESLIE: Oh yes
CORONER: She must have fallen right back on her bed, dead?
DR. LESLIE: Yes.
CORONER: And that would be a painless death?
DR. LESLIE: Yes, quite . . .
CORONER: The case seemed a perfectly simple one. The deceased had probably been exerting herself. She was an active woman, and the heart not being able to stand the strain had given way, causing her death, which was quite painless. The deceased was a married lady. The marriage had been an unhappy one, and she took proceedings and obtained a divorce.[37]

Despite having been divorced for eleven years, this legal status, her gender and financial plight determined the courtroom's attitude to Pearl Craigie's unexpected death. The Inquest Jury was very concerned to make sure she had not committed suicide in despair at her failed marriage, or due to the exertion of having to work to earn a living. The fact that she would have strongly objected to a post-mortem of any description never featured in court. Yet until cause of death was confirmed, Craigie and her body did not belong in mainstream society. The need to establish why she died required that her family engage with a medico-legal process she had opposed determinedly and in recent memory. They understandably wanted to bury her but had to wait until the body was returned to them by the Coronial Court, and without her heart (a recurrent theme in such cases to which we return in Chapter 5). And when it was given back, at the reading of the will they discovered that Pearl wanted a cremation, which created yet more controversy. She had converted to Roman Catholicism in 1892 and the parish priest felt strongly that a burial would be more appropriate under the circumstances. Cremation was still a contentious and novel request in 1906. A requiem mass was thus held at Farm Street in Mayfair, and Pearl Mary Teresa Craigie was buried at St Mary's Cemetery, Kensal Green in London. Despite her best efforts to prevent it, her cut-open heart, major dissected organs and tissue samples did not join her cadaver sewed back up for internment in the ground, superseding in death all the things she objected to in life. The press did not disclose, moreover, tissue retention for long-term heart research goals. Yet, as we shall see, heart failure and research to prevent it was one of commonest entries in the dissection registers of leading medical schools like St Bartholomew's in London (see Chapter 4). It was incontrovertible that a 38-year-old woman in the prime of her life would have been a valuable research commodity and that, if not retained for further research, class had protected her from a fate the poorest could seldom hope to avoid. In many respects then *Mrs Craigie's Complaint* personified a dead-end that medical science denied and in which the *Ministry of Offal* did have a basis in reality. The material reality of what went on behind the closed door of this ministry – in effect the substance of the answer that Mrs Craigie was searching for when she penned her first letter to the press – can be garnered from another, later, representative set of life stories.

KEEP OUT – Private!

On the eve of WWII, Richard Harrison aged 17 was a grammar school boy living in London, where he was a diligent student.[38] Studying hard was essential if he was to realise his ambition of becoming a qualified doctor. He needed to obtain his Higher National Certificate in the sciences because entrance to a good medical school was very competitive. Like most young people of his wartime generation, Richard wanted to get ahead in his career plans. It was likely that he might have to enlist in the armed forces as war threatened across Europe. As a prospective medical student, he was eager to win a place at a prestigious London teaching hospital. He hoped to train somewhere with an excellent reputation. Before the National Health Service (hereafter NHS) in 1948, junior doctors needed a good reference from their medical school to be able to buy into a solvent general practice to start earning back the cost of their expensive, privately funded education.

Richard's father encouraged his son to engage with the recruitment brochures of medical schools that he sent for in the post. Together they made a decision to apply to St Bartholomew's Hospital, central London, and for three key reasons: first, it was where his mother had been treated successfully for laryngeal carcinoma; second, the medical staff had treated her with courtesy and professionalism which augured well; and third, the hospital was within travelling distance of the family home in Mill Hill, north-west London. Richard could commute daily, live at home to save costs, and do extra work in the holidays to earn his keep. As there was no tradition of a career in medicine in the Harrison family, Richard was nervous about his chances of securing a place at medical school. Yet, he impressed the interview committee by telling them that he never forgot his childhood inspiration, the medical novel *The Elephant*

Man and Other Reminiscences written by Sir Frederick Treves, which he had read aged 13. It was, he believed, 'the best volume of surgical memoirs ever published'.[39] This was a curious coincidence because Mr Sydney Holland, 2nd Viscount Knutsford, had been responsible for the dissected body of the 'Elephant Man' in the collection of the London Hospital. Without knowing it, Richard Harrison had a strong connection to a hidden history of medical research that *Mrs Craigie's Complaint* had hinted at some thirty-three years before he became a new medical student. For now, Richard was convinced that by training at St Bartholomew's he would be at the centre of an exciting medical world.

Richard obtained a training place in the Indian summer of 1939. He remembered: '*the huge poster covering the wall of the building nearest to the Old Bailey which proclaimed Barts was the Mother Hospital of the Empire. It convinced me that I had made a sensible choice* [*sic*].[40] Soon, however, the German Blitz on London would affect the training of all medical students. The *Daily Mail* announced on 29 September 1939 that some '6,000 medical students' were about to 'study amongst the sandbags'.[41] Central government then asked Oxford and Cambridge universities to prepare for a threefold increase in evacuated students from the capital. New medical students, like Richard Harrison, arrived at either Queens' College, Cambridge from St Bartholomew's Hospital or St Catharine's College, Cambridge from the London Hospital Medical School, sent there for the duration of the war. On his arrival, Richard found that 'Cambridge in wartime was a sombre, not very sociable, place. Barts was *at* the university, but not truly *of* it [*sic*]'. He needed to find a way to make his mark, and he did so in the dissection room. The sign on the door read *KEEP OUT – Private!* Even so, Richard gained permission to enter this exclusive and privileged medical space. In doing so, he provides us with insights into the material substance of *Mrs Craigie's Complaint* and the medical profession's appellation *The Ministry of Offal*.

Like most medical students, Richard reflected that he was nervous about dissecting his first corpse:

We were required to dissect, and in considerable detail, the whole of the body. From time to time I had wondered, in desultory fashion, whether that might prove an emotional, even a fearful experience.[42]

He soon discovered that 'I need not have worried'. For 'our subjects were unclaimed corpses from the workhouse which had been steeped in preservation for so many weeks before reaching us that they would have been quite unrecognisable to anyone who might have known them in life'. Later he recalled what the bodies preserved with formaldehyde looked like: 'They were, indeed, so shrunk and wizened, with such tough and leathery skins, as not to be instantly identifiable as human at all.'[43] A relieved Richard explained that this inhuman appearance helped him to develop a clinical mentality of medical research in the dissection room: 'As we teased them apart we gave little thought to the existence each had led.' The priority was to compare each corpse according to *Cunningham's Manual on Practical Anatomy*, the set textbook. Yet, Richard was troubled too: 'I suppose we had become conditioned to the fact that we would have to dissect a human body.' It may have been mundane and routine after a while, but from time to time he was reminded that others might dispute his dispassionate demeanour. One incident he called to mind:

Visitors to the dissecting room were not encouraged, but one weekend, when it was deserted, I took my father. He was not a squeamish man, and had seen much service on the Western Front but I heard not long after that, for 24 hours, he felt unwell and could eat nothing.[44]

Richard was close to his father and it disturbed him that a man familiar with the horrors of trench warfare in WWI could still react in the way he did to death, and its dead-end.

The main reason that medical students like Richard developed a detached attitude was, of course, that the corpse they dissected was not a complete body shell for long. It soon became a fragmented human being in the dissection room. Seldom did medical students and those training them in anatomy discuss the material reality of dismemberment, and so Richard's recollections are strikingly honest:

Though we each dissected the whole body, it was not a single particular body. Six teams, each of three students, were assigned to every cadaver – one team to each limb, and two others to the torso and the head. This caused arguments at the start of each term, since those working on the arm began by approaching the shoulder from behind, whilst the 'leg' men commenced on the front of the hip. So a notice was hung from the subject's toes during the first fortnight, saying: '*Body will be turned at 2pm*'.[45]

Here we can trace the development of a medical discourse in anatomical action. The person on the dissection table without a name was a 'corpse' – then a 'cadaver' – the 'subject' – a 'body' to be 'turned over' – facedown. As Richard conceded, 'Gradual disintegration thereafter resolved the problem' of how to divide up the dead on a daily basis. There was also a further practicable problem to overcome – generally offensive to public sensibilities. Richard elaborated that

Each corpse was weighed when it came into the department. It had to weigh, when eventually buried in consecrated ground, about the same as it had done originally. So, at the end of each day, Arthur, the attendant, transferred the fragments, from each cadaver back to its specific coffin. At least he did in theory. In practice, he moved down the long, brightly lit, and spotlessly clean room, sweeping the pieces of tissue from each glass-topped table into one bucket. He divided its contents between all the coffins, tipping into each as much as he calculated would satisfy HM Inspectors [of Anatomy]. If that seems like an arbitrary or irreverent procedure I always understood Arthur had arranged when the time came, he too would be dissected.[46]

In many respects, this first-hand testimony is not only representative of what happened inside many medical schools in Britain; it also provides confirmation of *Mrs Craigie's Complaint*.

To use Richard Harrison's precise phrase, anatomists buried 'fragments' of corpses in pieces that were 'calculated' to be concealed. The macabre may have made medical history but it remained in the scientific shadowlands. There was no public engagement effort, and communication was clumsy. Seldom did a newspaper feature an article that led with: We did this with your dead-end to push past the deadline of life. Nor was that status quo debated or reformed as cultural tastes changed – effectively it did not exist in the public domain. Richard Harrison made clear that in his medical training he was taught 'punctilious history taking' at the bedside, but never at the dissection table for the obvious reason that his patient cohort was dead. Few thought to ask whether the dead should have a post-mortem passport, in which their material journey could be mapped and précised for relatives to connect them to the gift of donation and its medical legacy. The attitude was that it took too much time, effort and resources to design and maintain identity links, and without public pressure to do so, the practical option was to follow 'proprietorial' rather than 'custodial' medical ethics.[47] Ever since, this has essentially been the medical sciences' default position, enshrined in law, until, that is, HTA2004. Thus, the profession kept disputed bodies and bodies in dispute with modern medical research behind the *KEEP OUT – Private!* sign. A similar representative life story takes us forward in time to trace how this set of training attitudes endured after the 1950s into the 1970s.

'Say Ah!'

One key question that historians examining these sorts of personal accounts always need to ask themselves is how reliable and representative this recollection is of what happened. Did it reflect what occurred elsewhere? The answer is often straightforward – many medical students experienced dissection as a dehumanising encounter and they were relieved to do so. Jonathan Miller, writing for *Vogue* magazine in 1968, for instance, recounted his training as a doctor in the 1950s, which was in many ways similar to the sort of human anatomy sessions experienced by Richard Harrison in the 1940s:

That anatomy course stands out for another reason, too. As with most students, it was my first encounter with the dead. On the first day of term we were assembled in a lecture theatre and told what to expect. Afterwards we all trooped down to the tiled vestibule outside the dissection rooms and dared each other to be first inside. I cannot remember now just what macabre fantasies I had before going in the first time, but I remember quite clearly the vapid sense of anti-climax when we finally pushed through the frosted glass doors and stood facing our subjects.[48]

Once inside he was surprised how mundane the furniture, equipment and room looked. Again, the dead were called 'subjects', a professional language that Miller adopted easily. He recalled, 'In our ignorance we had expected some ghastly parody of our living selves' but instead 'what we saw bore so little relationship to life that it didn't seem to have anything to do with death either'. This was the grey zone of the dead-end of life, in which paradoxically the deceased would help the living push past a deadline. Soon he echoed Harrison's impressions, but here the scale was greater. Miller trained at University College Hospital London (hereafter UCHL). The anatomy department had a policy of obtaining bodies of the homeless found dead in the streets around the back of Euston, King's Cross and St Pancras stations. These were in plentiful supply during the cold winters of the early 1950s:

The bodies were laid out on fifty or sixty glass-topped tables, arranged in rows right down the length of an enormous shed lit from the windows in the roof. Most of them had been aged paupers. The pickle had turned them grey and stiff, and they lay in odd unfinished postures, like those pumice corpses fixed in headlong flight from the hot ash at Pompeii. Even their organs were dry and leathery, blood vessels filled with red lead, and hearts chocked with the ochre of brick dust. It was only much later, when we came to autopsies – dissection, that is, performed on the recent dead – that we finally experienced the ordeal of which we had been so mysteriously cheated.[49]

Miller then went on to describe what it was like to dissect a fresh cadaver. He soon came to appreciate the clinical importance of those aged paupers he encountered. Unbeknownst to him at that time, they were either destitute street deaths or passed on from old infirmaries and workhouse premises now run by the new NHS:

The body is opened from the chin to pubis and the organs are taken out and examined one by one and laid on a side table like a windfall of rotten exotic fruit. When it's all been cleared, the carcass lies open to the sky with the ribs and spine showing like the hull of a wet canoe. It's always a shock to see how much we hold inside us and the florid variety of it all. Heart, liver, spleen, bladder, lungs and guts, we know them all by name but we don't feel them and know them directly as we do our limbs and torso. This bloody cargo of tripes [sic] is carried from day to day more or less without being felt.[50]

Unlike Harrison, Miller explains why this sort of clinical intimacy is essential for general practice. He elaborates on his belief that it may always be necessary for the dead with hidden histories to continue to inform the case histories of living patients, regardless of medicine's technological prowess:

The doctor is not just a critical spectator, he is a participant . . . licensed by law to go right up close to the actors [patients] and poke the suffering innards. He can feel the physical vibrato of the patient's pain and overhear the otherwise silent complaints of the injured heart. There is no job on earth that brings one into such close and such refined contact with the physical substance of human feeling.[51]

Every time a junior doctor asks a new patient to 'Say Ah' to be able to hear properly the heart and lungs functioning, it is ironically from holding the hearts of the dead that they owe their dexterity.

What is thought-provoking about this personal memoir is its candour and emotional engagement. At UCHL, remaining *unfeeling about* the autopsies of dead aged paupers was essential for a future doctor's ability to *feel for* his patients (literally). Indeed, Miller concludes that before he dissected 'it was almost as if one were deaf before going onto the wards'. For he says that taking his transferable skills from the dissection table to the bedside, meant that: 'The scales suddenly drop from one's sense and for the first time one can hear the complex eloquence of the tissues.' He observed often that: 'The muffled gibberish of the cells and organs suddenly makes sense, becomes grammatical, and makes itself heard in verses and paragraphs of distress.' Yet, he never knew the names of his aged paupers nor how they arrived at their autopsy. Even so, he was sensitive to his situation, more attuned perhaps than many others. For it is one of the greatest ironies of this type of medical education that students soon discover how the shapes of organs 'like the kidneys also provide a perfect illustration of the old-age anatomical truth: the body is designed to protect itself, *not* to be easy to dissect'.[52] Barriers have to be broken when going under the lancet, just as the doctor trained in human anatomy will later have to cut through the sensibilities of patients who might dispute her or his actions. Cutting-edge reach is paradoxically always about cutting into and up the deadline of life. That process can be strikingly personal, something that goes a little way to explaining why in the past and present some researchers suggest that too much knowledge about its unsavoury material side can be incompatible with the competing 'public good' of giving consent for the use of bodies in death. The final section of this chapter thus tries to show through personal experiences – notably by other medical students in the 1970s and this author's visits to current dissection spaces – just how complex the issues explored through the stories that underpin Part II of the book actually are.

'Cut!'

How candid would you want your dissector to be? Would you ask in advance to know everything, a bit or not that much? The usual riposte to this unsettling question is: Well why worry? After all, you will be dead! This is a material fact of life. All bodies are abandoned, you might reasonably reply. You cannot change decay. Yet, what about the question of dignity in death? Donors and their relatives need reassurance that loved ones are handled decently because there has been a long history of disrespect for those dying in destitution. And since that hidden history is inextricably bound up with ongoing questions of public trust in the medical sciences, it is not something that can be simply argued away by holding that it does not matter for the dead because it is the living who celebrate, commemorate, cremate and bury. So what was it like to experience dissection in the more recent past? Here is how Michael Crichton describes his first encounter with a dissected body at medical school by the 1970s:

NOBODY moved. Everybody looked at one another. The instructor said that we would have to work quickly and steadily if we hoped to keep on schedule and finish the dissection in three months. Then, finally, we began to cut. The skin was cold, grey-yellow, slightly damp. I made my first cut with a scalpel. . . . I didn't cut deeply enough the first time. I barely nicked the skin. '*No, no,*' said my instructor. '*Cut!*'[53]

Crichton soon lost his appetite for this dead work. He was not supposed to find this difficult. It was a rite of passage – something all medical students did with dark humour. So why could he not simply grin and bear it like his fellow students? If laughter is the best medicine, he still found it difficult to see the funny side: 'The second-year students regarded us with amusement, but we weren't making many jokes in the early days.' In fact, he observed that most trainees 'were all struggling too hard to handle the feelings, to do it all'.[54] A lack of life experience created emotional hurdles not found with instructions in dissection manuals.

Then the atmosphere in the dissection room intensified as each body was broken up. Dissection soon gave way to dismemberment and the realisation that: 'There were certain jobs in the dissection [room] that nobody wanted to do.' Soon, he explains, the medical students 'portioned out these jobs, argued over them'. His recollection is that: 'I managed to avoid each of these jobs' until, that is, the demonstrator in anatomy said, '*OK, Crichton, but then you have to section the head* [sic].' He kept thinking, do not panic – 'The head was in the future. I'd worry about it when I got there. But the day finally came':

They handed me the hacksaw. I realized I had made a terrible bargain. I was stuck with the most overt mutilation of all. . . . I had to go through with it, try to do it correctly. Somewhere inside me, there was a kind of click, a shutting off; a refusal to acknowledge, in ordinary human terms, what I was doing. After that click, I was all right. I cut well. Mine was the best section in the class. People came round to admire the job I had done.[55]

To test the integrity and reliability of memories like this, there are two options. Either analyse yet more autobiographies published in the past twenty years or so for comparable reasons, or leap forward in time to find out in person exactly what dissection has been like since the 1980s. Several logistical issues are the deciding factor.

Medical students' memories are a mixture of feelings, general recollections and post hoc rationalisations – in other words, bias needs balancing out. Entering hence a selection of dissection spaces today to check credentials seems sensible, but it also does present its own contemporary challenges. There is the need for a strong stomach. Just because, for instance, this author has written extensively about the history of dissection does not mean that they would relish the thought of cutting up a body personally, any more than Richard Harrison, Jonathan Miller or Michael Crichton once did in the 1950s to 1980s. Then there is the question of how to judge what is happening inside the dissection space when your perception is going to be coloured by the vast amount of academic reading that you have done on this subject for fifteen years. Seeing the present with fresh historical eyes will take a great deal of reflection and self-control. Indeed, as E. H. Carr always reminded his undergraduate students at Cambridge, find out about your historian and you will then understand the sort of history they write.[56] Another thing to keep in mind is that medical schools have regulations about dignity standards and you generally need an invitation to enter the dissection room. This is an ethical requirement that is admirable, but it can also compromise the degree of physical freedom visitors can have once inside a dissection space. A uniform of a white laboratory coat is standard, talking loudly is discouraged and engaging with the reactions of students must be about participant observation. Nonetheless, on balance it is necessary to have a checking mechanism, because otherwise the unarticulated parts of this rite of passage – the feelings, sentiments and beliefs of those behind the closed doors of the *Ministry of Offal* – could be missed, or misconstrued. All good historians know that what is not said can be as important as what is – indeed, as Marianne Barouch, the dissection room poet, reminds us:

> *People say a lot of things.*
> *And think three times that many.*
> *Nothing like this place ever crossed my mind.*[57]

Three features of contemporary dissection spaces which this author visited as preparation for this book are an important addendum to the medical experiences we have already encountered in this chapter.[58]

The first is that they are seldom what you expect. Of course, they look clinical because they must be kept clean (refer to Illustration 3.2).[59] The furniture and basic equipment are much the same as they have been for a hundred years or more. And the layout of the tables in rows feels familiar from old photographs (compare to Illustration 3.3). But the air of anticipation, the sense that this room might be a bit smaller, lit slightly differently or run by individuals you have never met before, creates a first-time feeling on entering each new dissection venue. Indeed, the architectural variety and pragmatic use

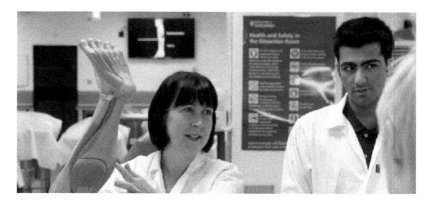

Illustration 3.2 Publicity photograph of 'Students Dissecting at the New Medical Centre' ©University of Leicester – see, https://www2.le.ac.uk/depa rtments/medicine/resources-for-staff/clinical-teaching/images/students-in-dissecting-room/view, accessed 10 January 2017, authorised for open access, and non-profit making, reproduced here under (CC BY-NC-SA, 4.0), for academic purposes only. Authorised by the University of Leicester where the author works.

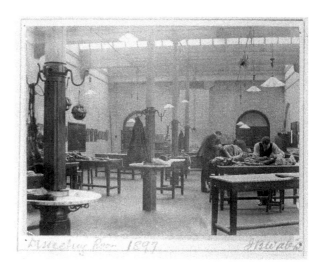

Illustration 3.3 ©Wellcome Image, L0014980, 'Photograph of Newcastle Dissection Room 1897', by J. B. Walters, copyright cleared under creative commons Attribution Non-Commercial Share Alike 4.0, reproduced here under (CC BY-NC-SA, 4.0), authorised for open access, and non-profit making for academic purposes only.

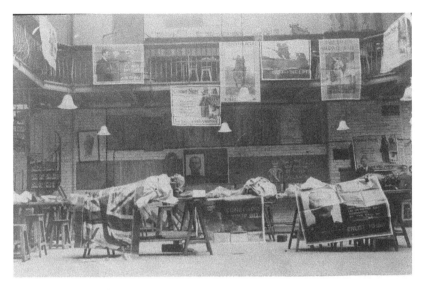

Illustration 3.4 ©St Bartholomew's Hospital Archives, Photographic Collection, 'Dissection Room, 1915', copyright cleared under creative commons Attribution Non-Commercial Share Alike 4.0, reproduced here under (CC BY-NC-SA, 4.0), authorised for open access, and non-profit making for academic purposes only.

in the past of these medico-legal spaces is surprising for the uninitiated. We can see this, by way of example, in archive images of St Bartholomew's Hospital dissection room in London. It was once hung with military recruitment posters from the WWI. These were also used to cover the cadavers being dissected each night (Illustration 3.4). Later teaching facilities were streamlined by building a separate new lecture theatre for the anatomy department to ensure clean sight lines: dissections were selected for special lectures and body parts placed on the lectern at the front of the room for students to observe (Illustration 3.5).[60]

Then once inside modern premises, a second experience starts to be stimulated naturally. The five senses recalibrate their normal running order. On entering the room, it is a place for smelling and listening, and then looking. Even a visual learner generally sniffs the air on entry, because the olfactory imprint of chemicals onto your skin, clothes and hair is what most people worry about. Being led by the nose into the room is commonplace. Quickly, though, the head turns to the side, because to most visitors' surprise there is the low hum of air-conditioning units. These reduce any lingering chemical smells and keep the atmosphere crisp and fresh on entry. The eyes soon start to adjust to the lights overhead too, before modifying their lenses from a portrait view (seeing

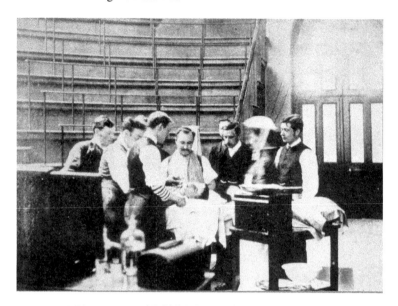

Illustration 3.5 ©Wellcome Images, s3_L0018000_L0018253, 'The New Operating Theatre at St Bartholomew's Hospital around 1910', looking recognisably modern with its stacked lecture theatre seats, Wellcome Trust Collection, digital download image reference, https://wellcomecollection.org /works/mtgyyb5w, reproduced under (CC BY-NC-SA, 4.0), authorised for open access, and non-profit making for academic purposes only.

the upright students and demonstrators in the foreground) to a landscape scan (glimpsing the actual corpses and dissection tables in the background). The brain is now processing information fast in the first few minutes to make the visitor feel safe and circumvent the hyper-arousal mechanism of fight or flight that deals with fear in the body. An unnerving feeling can be trigged on entry: the sense that someone is standing just behind you. Some nervous visitors shudder and then realise that there is no reason to be spooked. A member of staff assigned to stand behind the visitor's back makes sure they do not faint after a few seconds. The third feature of this experience is that most people generally want to look across the room, not down immediately to an actual corpse. It is the equivalent of having a fear of heights where you want to look out at a view but not down from a sharp precipice at what is below. This is so the mind has time to adjust to seeing a dead body with a human face. Generally, therefore, the new visitor is guided to an area of the room where the demonstrator in anatomy has pre-prepared a dissection of a limb called a prosthetic. First-time students are learning how to handle the human material with dignity, and touch the preserved tissues that will be the basis of their working life from now on. The ancient philosophy 'healer, know thyself' starts here. There is a human connectedness is this room even for those who have less interest in the anatomical sciences per se as a discipline-defining pursuit in their future careers.

One of the most common unforeseen experiences is the quality of human expressions still preserved in human body parts. Even an experienced visitor to these sorts of spaces can still be drawn to the touching beauty of the shape of a hand; the fingers that look female or male; the expressive quality of digits in an open greeting; all placed on the table for inspection. It is not difficult to spot a former farmer whose hands have toiled the soil for half a century – callouses, stodgy fingers, a big firm grasp; or the hairdresser who once chatted busily to her customers will have the telltale indentation of scissors marks on her forefinger. Again, all echoing what the poet Marianne Boruch recounts in her dissection-room visitor's book *Cadaver, Speak*:

> *The hand in cadaver lab – the first fully human thing*
> *we did. I thought. No hands alike, raging*
> *small vessels run through them – you'd never*
> *believe how many ribbons. The arm*
> *kept springing up, no*
> *not to volunteer. We tied it down with the ordinary rope*
> *you'd get at the hardware store, and even then –*[61]

Wrists too are surprisingly evocative. The thinner they are, the more elegant is the mental impression of the absent person. A ring mark on a third finger's paler skin likewise signifies a love token, taken perhaps in consolation by the bereaved before body donation. Slowly the fragmentary clues start to build a picture of the dead. Painted nails are redolent of a wartime generation for whom make-up was part of a person's glamour. Tattoos too 'are a reminder that this not just a body, but *some*body'.[62] It is striking how very few hands point the finger when preserved; all the moral judgements have evaporated. These are open hands that you can slip your hand into in a greeting and they can stimulate a student to respond in kind. Some stroke the hand and arm – *intuitively* (they often say later) – *impulsively* (most tend to claim) – *calmly* (say those whose interest in the science of dissection takes over quickly). There is a concentrated honesty in those present and it is a refreshing experience, because in the dead all pretence is stripped away.

Perhaps the most unanticipated aspect of visiting dissection rooms is the reaction of some of the staff on duty to the corpses and body parts. Those who work part-time to prepare the prosthetics generally tend to do shift work in local NHS general hospitals. Some are skilled in emergency medicine or intensive care nursing, and so this space can be challenging. For to them, it is a room full of failure. *Every-body* was a life that medical science could not save from death. The demonstrators in anatomy are dissecting their let-downs. Often, one of the most difficult emotional experiences involves unwrapping a cold storage body and recognising them as a patient who died in the care of the demonstrator; death can intrude uninvited into even the most impartial medic's memory. There is then a lot of subjectivity surrounding the research subjects; just as there is a lot of emotional anticipation in what will become an emotive scientific endeavour. One thing, though, from all the visits is obvious. Whether at Harvard Medical School (where Michael Crichton trained in the 1970s) or at a British medical school since then, most students find that they have 'that click' deep somewhere inside themselves. The switch can be flicked to shut off their emotions, or not. It really does depend on the person. Crichton discovered that he had a talent for dissection, but he still looked for his emotional exit strategy, eventually becoming a successful film-maker and novelist. Johnathan Miller also left medicine. He became a renowned literary polymath and playwright, with a deep respect for his former general practice. Richard Harrison meantime worked tirelessly for patients with cancer and gynaecological problems until his retirement. He had few plaudits in the press, but it was, he thought on reflection, a life lived well. All nevertheless depended on hidden histories from the corpses in dissection rooms, secretly dreaded and silently taken for granted in their youth.

Janus-Like Hidden Histories of the Dead

In Paul Thompson's seminal book about the value of oral history, *The Voice of the Past* (2000), he wrote that it is a combination of the written and spoken historical record that 'can give back to the people who made and experienced history, through their own words, a central place'.[63] Yet, in rediscovering threshold points, their research pathways and paperwork processes by actors who created hidden histories of the dead inside modern medical research cultures, it is evident that much more archival record linkage work is necessary to arrive at a revisionist perspective. Many closed conversations were never collected either on paper or recorded. In the official evidence base, there were gaps, silences, incomplete and shredded files. Private conversations were evasive in public. Even so, these were peopled with honesty, integrity and a sincerity too. Professional standards of behaviour continued to exude both medical altruism and clinical mentalities. Equally, medical staff and their students were trained not to speak openly outside their rank and file, or give only a partial account of their working lives about what really happened behind the dissection room door, pathology laboratory or hospital morgue because of wider cultural sensitivities about death, dying and the re-use of the dead in society. Part II thus sits at this complex cultural intersection where so much was consigned for filing but did not necessarily get forgotten. Often it was pared down, but could later be at least partially recalled, and thus, although considered lost forever, in fact endured in living memory to a remarkable degree. Chapters 4–6 nonetheless guard against the justifiable criticism of oral history that it could result in 'the collection of trivia' or 'become little more than the study of myths'. For as Julianne Nyhan and Andrew Flinn alert us:

> If oral history aimed to recover 'the past as it was', questions [from the 1970s] were asked as to whether the testimonies based upon retrospective memories of events (as opposed to documentary records produced contemporaneously and then authenticated and analysed through a professionally recognised method of 'objective' historical scholarship) could be relied on to be accurate. It was asked whether oral histories were not fatally compromised by the biases and uncertainties introduced by the interview process; and in the case of collective, community-focussed projects whether the selection of interviewees would introduce an unrepresentative or overly homogeneous data collection sample into the studies.[64]

Thus, the new case-material generated in this book essentially symbolises how the above historical debate moved on, and, recently so, with the advent of the digital humanities. Now historians of science and medicine test the validity of oral histories 'by subjecting them to rigorous cross-checking with other sources, arguing for the general accuracy of memory and its suitability as a source of historical evidence, importing methodologies from sociology and the other social sciences', particularly with regard to the representativeness of selected testimony.[65] Historians today concur that every piece of historical evidence – whether written and spoken – is partial, and through rigorous archival checking it is feasible to arrive at a new 'critical consciousness'.[66] To achieve this, finding and fusing new source material, according to Alessandro Portelli, will mean that we arrive at a new consensus in which: 'The peculiarities of oral history are not just about what people did, but what they wanted to do, what they believed they were doing, and what they now think they did.'[67] The *Oral History of British Science* (2009–2013) is one example, deposited at the British Library, of this fascinating and necessary research journey. Admittedly, the *ORHBS* has been criticised for being innovative yet inward-looking, seminal yet celebratory, significant yet not self-reflective enough, for some scholars. Concern has been expressed that some scientists are too quick to praise the past because of a club culture mentality. Even so, new digital oral history collections like this do mark a break with the more fragmented past on paper. Speaking up about the hidden past of the dead will always be about human paradoxes that sit today at the 'intersection and interaction with society, culture and ideology':[68] and this is where this book's novel contribution is located too.

Part II thus builds on Thompson's view that 'the richest possibilities for oral history lie within the development of a more socially conscious and democratic history'.[69] It does not seek to explore that historical record out of context, to apply 'neo-liberal' values to a time when the thinking was very different in the immediate aftermath of WWII. Instead, it is framed by a Janus-like approach, looking back to better understand a hidden past, and forward to engage with the long-term lessons of its lived experiences. As its focus is implicit, explicit and missed body disputes; at times there may be more of an emphasis on case-histories where things went wrong with medical ethics and inside research cultures in Chapters 4–6. This is balanced with a holistic sense that human beings can only learn from past mistakes when they get to know what those were in the first place to make future improvements. In other words, this is not a book about covering up, blame or pointing the finger – instead, its central focus is about joining in and renewing recent conversations about cultural change – from the proprietorial ethics of the past – to a custodial ethics of the future – from an ethics of conviction that framed the professionalisation of medical training – to an ethics of responsibility in a global community of precision medicine. For at the dead-end of life, as we shall see, there were many different sorts of hidden histories of the dead, and these created body disputes with stories that did not have to be buried or cremated without acknowledgement. Its bio-commons had medical dimensions and ethical implications not just in our keeping, but in our making too. In modern Britain from 1945 to 2000, we return to it, by looking forward to its past.

Notes

1. Anne Chisholm, *Frances Partridge: The Biography* (London: Weidenfeld & Nicolson, 2009).
2. 'Ralph Partridge died 30 November 1960 at Ham Spray House Wiltshire', *Times*, Death Notices, Friday, 2 December 1960, issue 54944, p. 1.
3. Burgo Partridge, *A History of Orgies* (London: Sevenoaks Publishers, 1958); this first book was published to acclaim.
4. Francis Partridge and Rebecca Wilson (eds.), *Francis Partridge, Diaries, 1939–1972* (London: Phoenix Press, paperback edition, 2001), p. 387, entry 7 September 1963. Ralph, her husband, died 30 November 1960 aged 66.
5. Named Lytton Burgo Partridge, he was known as Burgo in the Bloomsbury family circle.
6. Sarah Knights, *Bloomsbury's Outsider: A Life of David Garnett* (London: Bloomsbury Reader, 2015). His first wife (and Francis's sister) died of cancer and he then married Angelica Garnett.
7. Frances Catherine Partridge CBE (1900–2004) was a long-lived member of the Bloomsbury Group. She married Ralph Partridge (1894–1960) in March 1933. The couple had one son, (Lytton) Burgo Partridge (1935–1963). Ralph had previously been married to Dora Carrington, who committed suicide in 1932.

8. *Francis Partridge, Diaries*, p. 367, entry 23 December 1962. See also, *Garnett Family Papers*, acquired by Northwestern University Library, USA in 2008, and deposited in the Charles Deering McCormick Library of Special Collections with an online catalogue at: http://findingaids.library.northwestern.edu/catalog/inu-ead-spec-archon-1489.
They reveal that a few weeks after Bunny's mother gave birth to him she suffered severe gynaecological complications (probably a prolapse of the uterus), which meant that she no longer enjoyed full sexual relations with her husband, as she had to wear a surgical support for the rest of her life. She took the decision to release him from the moral bonds of marriage and encouraged him to take a mistress – a painter named Ellen Maurice Heath aka 'Nellie Heath' (1873–1962). She was the daughter of Richard Heath, an engraver, and brought up in France. Her father was a devout Christian Socialist and multi-lingual. He wrote *The Captive City of God* about the alienation of the working classes from middle-class materialism. He returned to live in England in 1899, where he set up in Rugby a Christian community called *The Brotherhood of the Kingdom*. For a time, Ellen's brother, Carl Heath, was tutor to the Garrett family before he converted to Quakerism. Ellen was thus intimately involved in Bunny's upbringing through her brother and status as mistress in the family.
David Garnett in his youth won a place at the Royal College of Science to study botany, and this may account for the contacts he had in his wider social circle with the so-called *Ministry of Offal*. He was happy to take responsibility for the donation of Nellie's body to medical science since she had loved him as a child, and he wanted to fulfil the last wishes in her will. At http://www.npg.org.uk/collections/search/portraitLarge/mw185159/Ellen-Maurice-Nellie-Heath   a   contemporary portrait of 'Nellie' is available at the National Portrait Gallery in London, from a black and white photograph in the Bauhaus archives taken in 1937 and donated in 1995. 'Nellie Heath' worked predominately in Hampstead, London, where she had a studio. She was also the former lover and muse of two renowned men: first, her patron Walter Sickert, the artist, with whom she had studied painting in Paris, and then D. H. Lawrence, the novelist. She had an affair with the latter just before WWI. Lawrence first admired her paintings around 1913 according to his private letters, and the brief affair developed with the full knowledge of Lawrence's wife, see, Mark Kinkead-Weekes, *D. H. Lawrence: Triumph to Exile 1912–1922*, volume 2 of *The Cambridge Biography of D. H. Lawrence* (Cambridge: Cambridge University Press, 1996), p. 80.
9. A. Blond, *Jew Made in England* (London: Timewell Press, 2004), p. 128.
10. Burgo's literary agent, Antony Blond, was very critical of this decision but only voiced it after Francis's death in his autobiography, *Jew Made in England*, p. 128.
11. Anne Boston, review of Francis Partridge, *Hanging On: Diaries 1960–62* (London: Collins, 1990), *Guardian*, 1 November 1990, p. 22.
12. 'Bloomsbury groupie: she loved Ralph, who loved Lytton, who loved …', *Guardian*, 11 January 1999, p. B4.
13. Desmond Mountjoy Raleigh, 'Character sketches: Part II, in memoriam: Pearl Mary-Teresa Craigie', *The Reviews of Reviews London*, 34 (September 1906): 251–254, quote at p. 251.

14. She was also a regular contributor to *The Women's Penny Paper* and *Woman's Herald*, 1888–1893.

15. 4 May 1906, '*Mrs Craigie's Complaint*', letter to the Editor of the *Daily Mail* by Pearl Mary-Teresa Craigie, 56 Lancaster Gate, Hyde Park London W 1. This address was her father's main residence in the capital where Pearl lived with her son after her divorce.

16. 4 May 1906, '*Mrs Craigie's Complaint*', letter to the Editor of the *Daily Mail*.

17. Hugh Chisholm (ed.), 'Craigie, Pearl Mary-Teresa', *Encyclopaedia Britannica*, 11th ed. (Cambridge: Cambridge University Press, 1911).

18. Margaret Maison, 'The brilliant Mrs Craigie', *The Listener*, 28 August 1969, issue 2109, p. 272.

19. See, John Oliver Hobbes and John Morgan Richards, *Life of John Oliver Hobbes Told in her Correspondence with Numerous Friends* (New York: Ulan Press, 1911).

20. Refer, Mildred Davis Harding, *Air-Bird in the Water: The Life and Works of Pearl Craigie (John Oliver Hobbes)* (Madison, N.J.: Fairleigh Dickinson University Press, 1996).

21. 30 April 1906, *Daily Mail*, reply by Richard Kershaw 'hospital official' [living at Wrexham Lodge West Hampstead] to *Mrs Craigie's Complaint*.

22. 1 May 1906, *Daily Mail*, reply by Edwin Howard MRCS, Shanklin, Isle of Wight to *Mrs Craigie's Complaint*. Craigie Lodge, St Lawrence, Isle of Wight was the family home of Pearl Craigie and her parents. Built as their holiday villa, it was where Pearl often wrote. Her father later retired from business and took up permanent residence until his death. There is a plaque to commemorate Pearl Craigie's life still at the villa today.

23. Refer, E. T. Hurren, *Dying for Victorian Medicine: English Anatomy and Its Trade in the Dead Poor, c. 1834–1929* (Basingstoke: Palgrave Macmillan, 2012).

24. Neville Langton [private secretary to Sydney Holland] *The Prince of Beggars: Being Some Account of the Beggings of Sydney Holland, 2nd Viscount Knutsford, During his 25 Years as Chairman of the London Hospital* (London: Hutchinson and Co, 1921).

25. See notably the caricature sketch by Spy [Leslie Ward] '*How Much*', depicting Holland with another begging letter in his hand published in *Vanity Fair*, August 1904 edition, p. 1.

26. See, Royal London Hospital Records, GB 0387 PP/KNU, Holland, Sydney, 2nd Viscount Knutsford (1855–1931), PP/KNU/1 – Speeches and notes, 1897 – 1931; PP/KNU/2 – Correspondence, 1898 – 1929; PP/KNU/3 – Publications, 1910 – 1925; PP/KNU/5 – Photographs, [c. 1904] – 1931; PP/KNU/6 – Miscellaneous Items, 1897 – [c. 1931]. Refer also, his comments on how to define '*B.I.D.*' patients to Lavinia L. Dock published in *The American Journal of Nursing*, 1906 edition.

27. Selectively, refer: Bruno Latour, *Science in Action: How to Follow Scientists and Engineers through Society* (Cambridge, Mass.: Harvard University Press, 1987) and *Reassembling the Social: An Introduction to Actor Network Theory* (New York: Oxford University Press, 2005); Michel Callon, John Law and Arn Rip, *Mapping the Dynamics of Science and Ethnology: Sociology of Science in the Real World* (Basingstoke: Macmillan, 1986); John Law and John Hassard (eds.), *Actor Network Theory and After* (Oxford: Blackwell Books, 1999); Bruno Latour and

Michel Callon, 'Don't throw the baby out with the Bath School! A reply to Collins and Yearly', in Andrew Pickering (ed.), *Science as Practice and Culture* (Chicago: Chicago University Press, 1992), pp. 343–368 – conceptual themes that will be developed and discussed in subsequent chapters, notably Chapter 4, where their specifics are applicable.

28. See, the recent bequest of the *Research Defence Society papers,* Wellcome Library, London. I am grateful to the archivist for permitting me to access those from 1908–1931.
29. Mrs Craigie, Letter to the Editor of the *Daily Mail*, 28 April 1906.
30. See by way of example, Duncan Wilson, *Tissue Culture in Science and Society: The Public Life of Biological Technique in Twentieth Century Britain* (Basingstoke: Palgrave Macmillan, 2011); and Wilson, *The Making of British Bioethics* (Manchester: Manchester University Press, 2014). Michael Brown also made similar claims in 'Book review section', *History*, 98 (2013), 330: 302–304. There are regrettably many academics working today in the history of science who tend to excuse a lack of forward thinking in medical ethics, whilst exclusively praising medico-scientific achievements. This book argues that the medical sciences cannot on the one hand defend their obligation to be progressive for society, but then on the other hand ignore its fixed medical ethics. We will be returning to this important theme in Chapter 7.
31. Margaret Maison 'The brilliant Mrs Craigie', *The Listener*, 28 August 1969, issue 2109, p. 272.
32. See, Hurren, *Dying for Victorian Medicine*, chapter 4 and conclusion.
33. Sydney Holland, Letter to the Editor of the *Daily Mail*, 3 May 1906.
34. Hurren, *Dying for Victorian Medicine*, chapter 3, explains the material realities of an anatomical education.
35. Sydney Holland, Letter to Mrs Craigie and the Editor of the *Daily Mail*, 7 May 1906.
36. 'Mrs Craigie's death: the victim of a weak heart', *Daily Mail*, 16 August 1906.
37. Ibid.
38. Richard Harrison recounted his medical training in 2009 before his death in 'A student at Barts: seventy years ago – feature article', *Barts and the London Chronicle* (Autumn/Winter issue, 2009), pp. 1–6.
39. Ibid., p. 1.
40. Harrison, 'A student at Barts', pp. 1–2.
41. *Daily Mail*, Friday, 29 September 1939, issue 13551, p. 3.
42. Harrison, 'A student at Barts', pp. 1–6.
43. Formaldehyde preserves or fixes tissue or cells in a person or animal that is dead. Today it is used in DNA and RNA sequencing too. A solution of 4 per cent formaldehyde fixes pathology tissue specimens at about 1 mm per hour at room temperature. It is also used as a fixative for microscopy and histology. For embalming purposes, it will disinfect and temporarily preserve human and animal remains. It is the ability of formaldehyde to fix the tissue that produces the telltale firmness of flesh in an embalmed body.
44. Harrison, 'A student at Barts', p. 3.
45. Ibid.
46. Harrison, 'A student at Barts', p. 3.

47. Again a point explored convincingly in, Prue Vines, 'The sacred and the profane: the role of property concepts in disputes about post-mortem examination', *Sydney Law Review*, 29 (2007): 235–261: a research theme introduced in the Introduction and more fully developed with new case material in Part II.

48. Jonathan Miller, 'Saying ah', *Vogue*, 1 January 1967, p. 40 and article continued on p. 46.

49. Ibid.

50. Jonathan Miller, 'Saying ah', p. 46.

51. Ibid.

52. Bill Hayes, *The Anatomist: A True Story of Gray's Anatomy* (New York: Bellevue Literary Press, 2009), p. 27.

53. 'Hack work' reprinted in the *Guardian*, 9 August 1995, column 11, taken from Michael Crichton, *Travels* (New York & London: Vintage Books, 2014 paperback edition), and also reprinted in 'Travelling with Michael Crichton', *Esquire*, Book Review section, 8 November 2008, p. 1.

54. Ibid.

55. Crichton, *Travels*, in which the early chapters cover his turgid time at medical school and desire to escape its confines.

56. E. H. Carr, *What Is History?* (Cambridge: Cambridge University Press, 1961).

57. Marrianne Boruch, *Cadaver, Speak* (Port Townsend, Wash.: Copper Canyon Press, 2014). She said this about the subtleties of her working experiences with medical students in dissection spaces during her tenure as a Visiting Fellow and poet in Scotland and the USA over the course of 2009.

58. I am grateful to those anatomists in London, Cambridge, Oxford and Leicester who talked to me about and facilitated my entry to dissection rooms and who are at all times concerned with the dignity of the gift to humanity.

59. This typical layout is taken from a publicity photograph of the new Medical Centre ©University of Leicester.

60. The same architectural design was used for the new lecture theatre for dissection after WWII – see ©Royal Institute of British Architects Archive, 'Photographic Image of St. Bartholomew's Medical School, lecture room of the anatomy department'. It has not been possible to reproduce the second image because of copyright costs.

61. Boruch, 'Hands', in *Cadaver, Speak*, p. 55.

62. Hayes, *The Anatomist*, p. 51.

63. Paul Thompson, *The Voice of the Past, Oral History*, 3rd ed. (Oxford: Oxford University Press, 2000), p. 3.

64. Julianne Nyhan and Andrew Flinn, introduction, 'Why oral history?', in *Computation and the Humanities: Towards an Oral History of the Digital Humanities* (Basingstoke: Palgrave, 2016), pp. 21–36, quote at p. 26.

65. Ibid., p. 27.

66. A conceptual approach first pioneered by Luisa Passerini, 'Work, ideology and consensus under Italian fascism', *History Workshop Journal*, 8 (1979): 82–108, quote at p. 104.

67. Alessandro Portelli, 'The peculiarities of oral history', *History Workshop Journal*, 12 (1981): 96–107, quote at pp. 99–100.

68. Nyhan and Flinn, *Computation and the Humanities*, p. 28.

69. Thompson, *Voice of the Past, Oral History*, p. iv.

Part II

Disputing Deadlines

Because the body really
is Mars, is Earth, or Venus, or the saddest downsized
Pluto. Can be booked, bound, mapped then. . .
                    Complete: because
            the whole body ends, remember?
                But each ending
                goes on and on. . .
                                Tell me.
            Then tell me, who that
                '*me is*', or the
            '*you understand*', the any of us, our
        precious everything we ever, layer upon
                bright layer.

Marianne Boruch, 'Human Atlas', *Cadaver, Speak*
(Port Townsend, Wash.: Copper Canyon Press, 2014, p. 43)

4   Implicit Disputes

Mapping Systems of Implied Consent

Overview

Chapter 1 argued that the way in which bodies and body parts have been obtained for medical research and teaching creates three core forms of dispute. These have incrementally (and sometimes sharply, as for instance with the NHS Alder Hey organ retention controversy) shaped public understandings of the ethics and practices of medical science and thus the possibilities of, and constraints on, medical research. This chapter analyses the first of our categories: the implicit dispute. An implicit dispute is what happens when a person dies, their body enters a medical research and teaching culture, but informed consent is implied, never documented in full for the bereaved. A lot is therefore left unsaid, and deliberately so. It is normal for these sorts of bureaucratic processes to be very light touch, and to have audit procedures that look robust, but are the opposite. The aim being to make it a difficult logistical task to track at the time, or retrace later, exactly what is happening, or has happened, to human material once it enters a system of body supply. Even an insider might not know who exactly had shared a body and body parts, and what scientific studies these relate to. Those grieving thus never got an opportunity to make an informed choice. They are given the impression at the time of a loved one's death that informed consent existed, when it did not. Instead, it was often implied, particularly by those staffing large teaching hospitals. In modern Britain, a proper system of consent was an aspiration, not a uniform working practice. As we shall see, implicit disputes thus constituted what modern research scientists would term 'bio-commons', and reconstructing their human stories is the central focus of this fourth chapter.

There are many ways in which such disputes can be analysed, but in this chapter we focus (detailing the 1950s and 1960s in particular) on disputes over bodies that became available because of bad weather. A first section explores the connection between foggy weather patterns, the deaths of the poorest members of society and the consequent supply of bodies and body parts for medical research and teaching.[1] While everyone may have disliked fog, it was a boon for a medical community needing more research material.[2] The chapter then moves on to develop this theme across a number of sections, focussing on the case study of a young boy who died in the 'Great Fog' of 1952 and was dissected for teaching and research purposes. Remapping the material journey of his brief life-story and body reveals the extra time of the dead created by the actor network of hospital staff, anatomists, coroners, and scientists. Subsequently, the chapter generalises this individual experience, reconstructing the body supply network for St Bartholomew's Hospital in London from 1930 (when the New Poor Law ended) until 1965 (when a 'mechanism of body donation' was put in place that other medical schools in the capital subsequently copied). The next step in this critical analysis is to expand upon the new data, focussing on a number of representative stories of those taken for dissection and who did not consent to the 'donation' process. They ended up being dissected by virtue of being alone, friendless, socially isolated, or they died inside NHS premises where medical research was a priority. The penultimate section compares St Bartholomew's data to national statistics on 'body donation' figures for the whole of England during the 1990s, arguing amongst other things that women come to be the mainstay of the body bequest process, and that current practices for encouraging organ and body donation do not reflect that material fact. The final section thus asks how the implicit disputes that arise out of the covert (if at the time perfectly legal) supply of bodies and body parts for medical research and teaching have shaped trust in medicine and the development of professional boundaries, a theme taken up again at length in Chapter 5. In this way, this fourth chapter builds on some of the core themes of this book, as outlined in Chapter 1, including: notions of expertise, the ambiguities of consent, the rise of the information state, deferential power relations and the particular authority of individual actors in the wider medical science and research community. We begin our engagement with these themes by exploring the medical hazard of fog; in a hidden history of disputed bodies, few could escape the old English weather lore –

> *Whether the weather be fine*
> *Whether the weather be not*
> *Whether the weather be cold*
> *Whether the weather be hot*
> *We'll weather the weather*
> *Whatever the weather,*
> *Whether we like it or not.*

Fog – Weather Warning!

In December 1952, *The Times* newspaper featured a severe weather warning about the harmful effects of a deepening winter fog across the capital:

A 'LONDON PARTICULAR'

Of all the afflictions which visit the inhabitants of this temperate climate, fog is the most exasperating. There are some who think well of frost or snow, and rain is an undoubted necessity. It refreshes the earth and the air, and at one time was the only decent scavenging system London knew. But there is no decent use for fog. It cripples business and brings even winter sports to a standstill. Fog is a dirty and stifling cloud without any silver lining at all. We could do well without fog. . . . Fog is altogether too big a job for Science to handle.[3]

By the 1950s, air-pollution trapped in fog attracted considerable column inches in the British medical press.[4] Smog from the constant burning of coal fires in houses, shops and factories across the capital was blighting Britain's major cityscapes. Newspapers described the daily distress of commuting under a 'green-yellow miasma' lingering on London's streets.[5] The toxic haze eventually led to a concerted public health campaign around the time of this 'Great Fog', known as the 'pea-souper', of 1952.[6] Scientists could not, as *The Times* observed, disperse fog, but it had boons for medical research and teaching. Weather crises such as that in 1952 increased emergency admissions to hospitals and more people died of heart and lung complaints, prompting a synchronicity of greater body supply on the one hand and calls for better medical research on the other hand. Moreover, there was also a deeper history.[7] Trading dead bodies in fog, moving them under the cover of darkness, buying and selling at the back of Poor Law infirmaries and workhouses or on the streets of London had been commonplace for centuries. After the NHS was created in 1948, the old welfare institutions of the New Poor Law had become County Council care-homes, and they continued their supply-lines. Still the anatomical sciences waited in wintertime for the Grim Reaper to stalk British cities in the fog. Yet seldom did the scientific community speak openly about this fact of life because of public sensitivities surrounding dissection.

There is no doubt that the dense smog that hung over London at the start of December 1952 was an exceptional weather event, even for the damp British climate. A low, dank cloud covered the capital. It sat stubbornly on top of impenetrable smoke pollution. Out-of-doors everywhere was wet with a cold miasma. Foggy rain dripped from trees and formed a drizzly haze under lamp-posts. Along the packed streets, passers-by coughed, spluttered and wheezed, to and from work. *The Times* ran a daily health feature on how to combat colds, sneezes and asthma. They did so because of widespread concern about the high number of extra emergency admissions to large teaching hospitals that had stretched medical services to almost their breaking point. In North West London, *Times* journalists reported on how Harrow public school pupils experienced a cacophony of illness even though they lived on top of a steep hill, 406 feet above the rest of the capital. Most had contracted sore throats, chest cackles, and high temperatures. Cancelling sports in the foggy conditions meant that everyone stayed indoors in their boarding houses to manage the spread of infection. Tragically, however, the Headmaster of Harrow, Dr R. W. Moore, died aged just 46 during the foggy pall of 1952. His obituary explained that 'early in 1951 he had an attack of bronchial pneumonia' and despite being X-rayed and operated on to alleviate his condition, the symptoms returned with renewed vigour in the winter fog of 1952.[8] All the pupils at Harrow 'underwent X-ray examination', but Moore died of the latest outbreak. The *Times* health correspondent highlighted that many London residents were experiencing the same severe symptoms of bronchial pneumonia. It was the worst outbreak since 'the influenza pandemic of 1918'. Civil servants at the Ministry of Health meantime emphasised the virulence of the 1952 pneumonia strain. They warned central government that the peak in mortality rates from fatal lung diseases was akin to the sort of death statistics of 'the last great cholera epidemic of 1866'.[9] A public health report was thus urgently prepared for the London County Council. It revealed that some '2,484' residents in the capital died from a 'tenfold increase in bronchitis' in the reporting period from 5 November to 5 December 1952.[10] Within days, however, the foggy conditions worsened. Medical science was on hand to treat patients but also to benefit from higher fatalities in its dissection spaces.

During early to mid-December 1952, all of the daily newspapers devoted their front pages to the deepening winter fog that descended over London and would not shift.[11] A combination of high pressure, near-freezing temperatures, light winds and thickening smog had intensified the hazardous public health crisis. The Automobile Association told *The Times* on 8 December 1952 that 'it is the worst fog they had ever known'. The *Daily Telegraph* reported on how the dense smog had 'blacked out central London and a band 40 miles across. . . . All buses had stopped by 10 p.m. Hundreds of cars were abandoned. . . . Thousands of people did not get milk.'[12] Nightly there was a shutdown of all the capital's transport systems because bus and train drivers could not see more than 100 yards ahead on the roads or railway networks. Only the underground stayed open, but even underneath London the fog seeped into the drainage system tunnels. Airport traffic-control staff took the unprecedented decision to divert '500 planes' from London Heathrow to Hurn aerodrome in Bournemouth. Few planes could land safely in the capital because they did not have the radar capabilities to guide them blind onto the ground. The ambulance service faced a crisis it could not cope with as well: 'It took five or six times as long as usual to get cases to hospital', according to the *Daily Telegraph*; so bad was it that: '. . . women gave birth to babies in fog-bound ambulances'. Yet, it was the rising daily death toll, disproportionate amongst children and their grandparents, which caused the greatest public concern. In two weeks, 'some 4,000 died'. The death toll then rose to '10,000' in total by the close of the Christmas holidays of 1952.[13] A single case-history from this tragic period – a young boy aged 7 living in the Harrow area and dying in December 1952 – symbolises the central themes of this chapter because we can trace what happened next to his human remains. Out of the medical miasma of fog emerges the material journey, reconstructed from detailed record linkage work on the mechanisms of body donation.

TAB – A Hidden History Remapped

TAB was born in North London at the end of the WWII to parents (Mr WAB and Mrs HAB) who had married in their twenties sometime in 1938.[14] They spent their savings on a small deposit to mortgage a three-bedroom house in Hendon. Having rented a property during the first year of their marriage, they wanted stability at home to start a family. Like many of their wartime generation, the ABs did not want to waste time. Their philosophical attitude was that if Mr WAB died at the front, then Mrs HAB would have the consolation of children. In Hendon during WWII, Mrs HAB gave birth to two boys – one in 1941, the other in 1945. She conceived each sibling during Mr WAB's leave of absences from the armed forces. Detailed record linkage work reveals that whilst the eldest child (RAB) was to survive the 'Great Fog' of 1952, his younger sibling (TAB) did not. On 5 November 1952, TAB 'died from pneumonia' aged 7 in hospital. Under normal circumstances, once the funeral had been staged at a local church, his short life story would have ended but for the fact that he had died from prevalent pneumonia and his small body was thus a very valuable research and teaching tool for a medical profession facing a deepening epidemic of this deadly disease. Remapping its material journey from emergency admission to dissection and burial reveals the multilayered, hidden histories of a hospital coroner's case. For the first time, we can trace a series of discrete research steps that were never officially recorded (Figure 4.1) but which go to the heart of attitudes towards body ethics in the immediate post-WWII era.

On the night TAB died, an ambulance transported him from Hendon to Harperbury Hospital near St Albans in Hertfordshire.[15] Bonfire Night was a busy time for the emergency services in North London. Yet, this does not explain why a small boy breathing poorly went on a thirty-minute road journey about fifteen miles from home to hospital. There were four logistical issues shaping the local GPs decision-making. These helped to create research threshold points, stage-managed by an actor network of hospital staff, anatomists, a coroner and his pathologist. The first consideration was that out-of-doors most local people walked to and from work with a handkerchief over their face, often covered in a layer of coal dust from London's dirty air. The 'Great Fog' of 1952 would culminate in politicians on all sides of the House of Commons passing the Clean Air Act (4 & 5 Eliz. 2 c. 52: 1956) as a national priority.[16] The GP thus judged it prudent to move TAB out of the immediate area of the

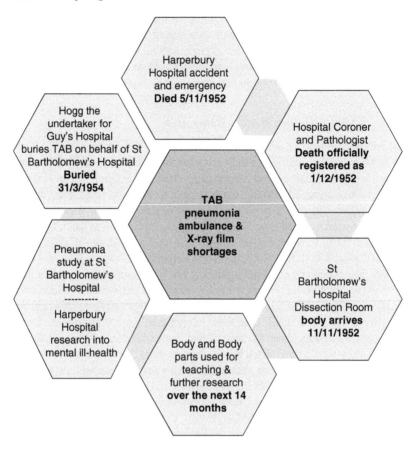

Figure 4.1 Remapping the threshold points of the dissected body and body parts of TAB, 5 November 1952–31 March 1954
Source: Reconstructed from St Bartholomew's Hospital Dissection register MS81/5–81/6 and associated detailed record linkage work in the archives.
Ethical note: case details de-identified and anonymised.

contagious pollution in Hendon. If air pollution was foul at the top of Harrow hill, 406 feet above London, then it was self-evidently best to remove the patient out of the capital altogether. Even so, a second practical factor shaped the decision-making too.

During WWII, St Bartholomew's Hospital developed very close links with medical services at Hill End Hospital in St Albans.[17] Once the site of an asylum and then re-designated a mental hospital in 1913, Hill End was requisitioned by the Ministry of Health during the Blitz to evacuate as many civilian casualties as was feasible out of central London. Hill End staff and those of St Bartholomew's thus worked closely together. Medical personnel networked likewise with nearby Harperbury Hospital. In the 1950s, NHS staff continued to co-ordinate as they had done in wartime when the healthcare system was struggling to cope in the capital, as it was during the severe winter fog. Even so, a third logistical problem was a severe ambulance shortage in 1952.[18] There was little point ordering a transfer into central London. Its inevitable delay meant TAB might never reach on time the critical medical help he needed at either Great Ormond Street in Bloomsbury or St Bartholomew's Hospital in the City.[19] He headed therefore for St Albans in the ambulance.

A fourth logistical factor was the fact that TAB's family doctor faced a technical problem. His young patient had a bad attack of pneumonia, but there was a medical supply problem. The Chief Medical Officer (hereafter CMO) for England and Wales highlighted the key issue in the *BMJ* at the end of 1951:

There is a serious world shortage of x-ray films, due to increasing usage in all countries. In this country, usage during the first six months of 1951 was 16% greater than in the corresponding period of 1950 and was at a rate about 60% greater than in 1947. Production has been expanded and manufacturers have greatly improved their productivity. Nevertheless, it has not been possible recently to satisfy all hospital demands. New plant is shortly to be installed by manufacturers and should afford some measure of relief. Meanwhile, the present difficulties can be eased if all hospitals will exercise strict economy in the use of films and eliminate waste, particularly in processing.[20]

The CMO stressed that: 'Economy in film production should not take precedence over the efficient examination of the patient'; nevertheless, it was necessary to ration X-ray films. An NHS directive stated that 'only experienced clinicians' were to be permitted to order X-rays in general hospitals. Nobody beneath the rank of a registrar could apportion precious film. In an emergency, the patient would be triaged and sent to hospital premises that had enough X-ray film to manage the critical condition. TAB thus had to journey out of central London to Harperbury Hospital at St Albans.

Once sent farther afield, another NHS stipulation complicated the accident and emergency protocols on 5 November 1952. On the night TAB died, the radiologist on duty was not authorised to X-ray a common condition like bronchial pneumonia just because they suspected its presence in the lungs of a young patient. A consultant on call was the only person who could make TAB's case a clinical resource priority. The hospital management committee's attitude was that there was little point in filming a fatal condition which medical intervention could do nothing to heal in a pre-antibiotic era. The *BMJ* had been critical of radiologists using what it called an 'omnibus technique': that is, doing radiology on all suspected cases as a matter of course regardless of the clinical prognosis. NHS resources were scarce and the subject of intense funding debates, straining central-local relations in 1952.[21] In the case of TAB, there was an ambulance available to take him to St Albans where a supply of film was available. On arrival, there would be a specialist waiting for him with the authority to order a priority X-ray at Harperbury Hospital. Judged against these logistical criteria, moving TAB out of the Hendon area seemed to offer his best chance of survival. Even so, it is evident that the GP of the AB family had to work with a complex set of resource-allocation shortages on 5 November 1952. They explain why TAB's body became available for dissection and medical research outside inner London.

On closer inspection of the case files, what cannot be determined from the surviving medical notes is whether (or not) TAB had an underlying medical condition from birth. This may have made him more vulnerable to pneumonia and might provide a further explanation as to why he was sent specifically to Harperbury Hospital rather than Hill End in St Albans with whom St Bartholomew's had very close working relationships. Harperbury had a long history of treating those defined as suffering from mental incapacity in childhood according to the Mental Deficiency Act (3 & 4 Geo. 5 c. 28: 1913). The categories were:

a) *Idiots* – Those so deeply defective as to be unable to guard themselves against common physical dangers.
b) *Imbeciles* – Whose defectiveness does not amount to idiocy, but is so pronounced that they are incapable of managing themselves or their affairs, or, in the case of children, of being taught to do so.
c) *Feeble-minded persons* – Whose weakness does not amount to imbecility, yet who require care, supervision, or control, for their protection or for the protection of others, or, in the case of children, are incapable of receiving benefit from the instruction in ordinary schools.
d) *Moral imbeciles* – Displaying mental weakness coupled with strong vicious or criminal propensities, and on whom punishment has little or no deterrent effect.[22]

The hospital's typical patient profile also included disabled children born with genetic conditions such Down's syndrome or cystic fibrosis, impacting on their health profiles, learning needs and schooling proficiency. As one of the hospital's first medical attendants, Dr H. E. Beasley, explained in *Kelly's Directory* of 1937, Harperbury Hospital first opened as the Hangers Certified Institute in 1925. It was located on the site of an old WWI aircraft hangar, and the land was recycled to create a 'colony for mental defectives' in the 1930s:

The *Middlesex Colony*, begun in 1929, was opened on 20th May, 1936, by the Rt. Hon. Sir Kingsley Wood, M.P. Minister of Health. The *Colony* is intended for mental defectives who are socially inadaptable in the community, or who are neglected or without visible means of support. Male defectives who are capable of being employed are provided with suitable agricultural occupations on the land, or at various industrial occupations in the Colony's workshops. Female defectives are suitably employed in the laundry, general kitchen or workrooms. Children who are capable of it are given various simple occupations. The patients live in separate 'homes' of the villa or pavilion type. The Administrative Centre, consisting of the main administrative offices, dental and surgical clinics, dispensary, central kitchen, reception hall, workshops, laundries, &c. has been built on an axial line running north and south, the *Colony* buildings for male and female being placed east and west around and overlooking playing fields. An isolated site on the south side is allocated for the children's section.[23]

Nursing staff and a medical superintendent lived permanently on site. They supervised the medical cases using a wide variety of diagnostic and therapeutic interventions including art, drama, sport and daily farming activities for residents. The aim was to promote the benefits of occupational therapy for mental well-being. Under the NHS in 1948, the Middlesex Colony was renamed Harperbury Hospital in 1949.[24] There was, however, more continuity than discontinuity in its healthcare provision. It often took in mental-health patients referred from the North London area during the 1950s. TAB thus entered a well-known facility for treating physical and mental disabilities in childhood on 5 November 1952, and one in St Alban's with close wartime associations with St Bartholomew's Hospital: again circumstances that materially influenced what happened next.

When TAB died on 5 November 1952, official jurisdiction over his material body started to change medico-legal hands. This was a child, the death was unexpected and his body passed from the emergency team to the pathology department but overseen by a hospital coroner. As there would need to be a hospital post-mortem, the cadaver was preserved in formaldehyde from 5 November to 11 November. In these six days, TAB had no official legal status in the public domain. No death certificate was issued. The body did not technically belong to his parents. In property law, it was '*Res Nullius* – Nobody's Thing', as we saw in Chapter 2. The coroner with the co-operation of the pathologist now had to establish the cause of death. Ideally, they would do so with the parent's co-operation to reassure them that the hospital was not guilty of medical neglect. Even so, this was not strictly speaking a legal requirement, and such ambiguities could be misleading for the family involved. Indeed, on closer inspection it is apparent that standard procedures involving this seemingly routine post-mortem were not straightforward in 1952. As Figure 4.2 suggests, step by step TAB's body and body-parts moved into the jurisdiction of medical science, creating an elongated and hidden afterlife of the body which was not ended until TAB was buried some fourteen months later.[25] In his hidden history of the body, there are three noteworthy time gaps from detailed record linkage work. These provide important clues about the research threshold points of medical science's work on TAB.

Extra Time of the Dead

In the early 1950s, GPs made a number of complaints to the British Medical Association that the NHS seldom informed them officially about the death of one their registered patients on a hospital ward. As a result, there was a lot of concern and considerable confusion about who should issue a death certificate to bereaved families and when exactly a family doctor should do it. In the interim, a bureaucratic space opened up for the medical research community to obtain jurisdiction over the dead for longer than it appeared. The General Medical Committee Conference thus informed the *BMJ* on 17 April 1954 that to resolve the confusion, from now on: 'it has been agreed that a letter will be sent ... drawing attention to the importance of ensuring that general practitioners are promptly notified of the death or discharge of hospital patients'.[26] TAB's dead body entered this extra time of the dead in its paperwork too, as Figure 4.2 illustrates.

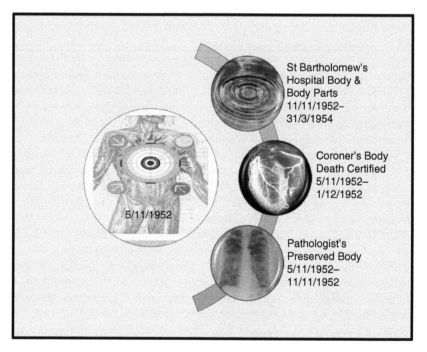

Figure 4.2 Time frame and time travels of TAB's body: death, burial and certification
Source: Reconstructed from St Bartholomew's Hospital Dissection register MS81/5–81/6 and associated detailed record linkage work in the archives. Ethical note: case details de-identified and anonymised.

Harperbury Hospital did not issue a death certificate for twenty-six days until their coroner eventually registered it officially on 1 December 1952. This happened at St Albans Registry Office, even though the child had resided prior to death with its parents in Hendon. In the meantime, TAB's body became a site of negotiation and tension over the professional remit and standing of different groups of actors in the post-death process. We see such tensions clearly played out in early November 1952, just before TAB's death. A concerned correspondent to the *BMJ* noted:

Pathologists' Fees for Coroners' Necropsies

SIR,-The salaries of the coroners in the County of London have again been increased. Everybody will approve, although the approval of the pathologists who serve them will be mixed with envy. Since the Coroners (Amendment) Act of 1926, the fees payable to pathologists for coroners' necropsies have not been increased. Are not these pathologists the only group of the community who have had no increase of pay for more than a quarter of a century?

The Committee on Coroners, under the chairmanship of Mr. Justice Jones, has reported to the Home Secretary, but, as a matter of equity, the fees payable by coroners to pathologists should be increased without waiting for the report as a whole to be carried into effect. Cannot the B.M.A. exert some pressure on behalf of the admittedly small number of its members who carry out necropsies for H.M. coroners?[27]

A matter of days before TAB's body entered Harperbury Hospital professional disputes were holding up supply-lines of bodies for potential dissection. Disagreements about fees and salaries created the context for generating implicit disputes. Liminal spaces opened up because of the delay in the official process of moving the dead whilst pathologists and coroners argued about the economic basis of their status. In TAB's case, we can explicitly observe the timeline and time-travels. Slowed down, these created a twenty-six-day gap between death and official registration. This did not mean that the body did not physically move along the chain of command or supply; it did. The crucial point to appreciate is that it had no official status in law and hence did not technically exist for its relatives. If the parents had wanted to object to what was happening to TAB's remains in the twenty-six-day gap, they would have had no official knowledge to react to. There was no record-keeping for this missing period of almost four weeks. This was commonplace and it created the potential for a series of discrete research thresholds without the full knowledge of the bereaved. Remapping what happened next brings these threshold circumstances into sharper focus.

On 11 November 1952, 'further examination' of TAB's body began once chemical preservation was completed. The hospital coroner deliberately used this legal phrasing because it was permitted by AA1832 and the Coroners Amendment Act (16 & 17 Geo. 5 c. 59: 1926), even though critics like Pearl Craigie had objected to it (unsuccessfully) in 1906 (as we saw in Chapter 3).

The same legal framework remained in force and therefore covered the removal of TAB's body on the morning of 12 November 1952 to the dissection room of St Bartholomew's Hospital in central London. Listing hospital transfers like this as a 'B' (bequest) in the dissection register (generally marked in pencil), was, however, misleading. There is no surviving evidence to suggest that this young body was the result of a written bequest. Paperwork detailing informed parental consent prior to dissection is missing, or it was never created in the first place; alternatively, the anatomist on duty may have been lazy about form-filling and did it verbally, or he was in a rush on the morning of TAB's arrival and did not do his filing properly at the end of the day. This ambiguity in the bureaucracy is nonetheless informative since it reflects the common way that many bodies were supplied at the time through an implied consent process (as we shall see later in this chapter).

Whatever the paperwork discrepancies in TAB's case, it is noteworthy that St Bartholomew's Hospital had been keen to improve its 'mechanisms of body donation' after WWII. Records show conclusively that a new scheme of bequests did not get officially under way until 1954 (Figure 4.4). This made it very unlikely that TAB's body supply involved a full bequest from Harperbury Hospital involving the parents. TAB thus appears to have been transported into central London to be dissected under an older system of supply that did not require explicit immediate family involvement, similar to what happened under the New Poor Law. There was, as we saw above, a close working partnership already established between medical staff working in the St Albans area. This made it feasible and normal for an existing network of suppliers to play a pivotal role in the presentation of TAB's body to St Bartholomew's anatomists, following long-established protocols stretching back to AA1832. A commercial transaction in TAB's case can, however, be ruled out; supply-fees were not permitted by the 1950s. On 1 July 1947, James Cave, Professor of Anatomy at St Bartholomew's Hospital, ordered that: 'Payments for injecting subjects was to be stopped.' Henceforth all such 'petty cash [was] to be handed to Miss [Dorothy] Woolaway', Cave's depart-mental administrator.[28] The old system of paying petty cash fees to Poor Law officials for dead bodies, supplied from infirmaries and workhouses, was phased out.[29] At the same time, the wartime practice of compensating hospital staff in St Albans doing chemical preservation work was revised (although actual supply-lines from the same premises renamed under the NHS did continue to the close of the 1990s: a theme we return to below). In the transition, TAB's body was not a crude commodity as it would have been under the Victorian system of supply. Rather, it was now symbolic of the changeover from the dead-end of the old business of anatomy to modern-day 'mechanisms of body donation' organised by hospital staff. The rest of this chapter examines this process in more detail.

Research Recycling

The fate of TAB's body in terms of medical teaching and study highlights three key threshold points for the ethics of the body. The first is that TAB's human remains were retained for 14 months in total before burial. That extended time frame effectively meant that the small corpse of a 7-year-old boy was dissected and dismembered extensively. In reality, there would not have been much material remains to bury at the end: less than one third at best. Seldom did doctors, coroners or pathologists explain this explicitly to grieving parents. Few could face such news on the night of a child's death in hospital. Even if the family had been amenable to a body donation (and again, there is no evidence to confirm this in the record-keeping for TAB), in their initial bereavement their primary concern would have been for the dignity of their young offspring. This would have been a life-changing moment even for the most philosophical of family members. The very fact therefore of doing so much teaching and research on TAB's human material created the potential for an implicit dispute to be generated. The process of consent was implied, not fully documented; even if it was done in some respect, it was at best ambiguous about all the research and teaching steps about to happen next. The extant evidence therefore points to the material fact that TAB's parents were not given an opportunity to make informed decisions about their child's potential to become bio-commons at this threshold point. Today, this is no longer permissible in the dissection rooms of medical schools, not simply because HTA2004 outlaws it but also because teaching facilities have now adopted a voluntary code-of-practice, which states that 'no more than one third of a "human gift" to the medical sciences will be dissected' for reasons of human dignity.[30] While we must avoid judging past practice by standards which were not in force at the time, these new standard practices help to identify the liminal spaces and research threshold points that were routinely scheduled in case histories like TAB's over the course of the second half of the twentieth century.

A second threshold for body ethics in the TAB case is the utility of the extensive dissection conducted as it became the focus of further work once teaching sessions on it had concluded. Figure 4.3 traces, through detailed record linkage work, the uses of body parts and tissue. The results are tangible. A 1961 study authored by clinicians working in the wards, pathology department and dissection room of St Bartholomew's Hospital, and based upon research over the period 1949 to 1958, provided a new analysis of pneumonia. The research team reviewed the cases of '1,330 patients, 861 were males and 469 females; 303 were children under the age of 15' who had all contracted persistent pneumonia. They concluded that typically: 'some 634 (63 per cent) of the adults and 90 (30 per cent) of the children had a pre-existing disease. Respiratory disorders, particularly chronic bronchitis and emphysema, and

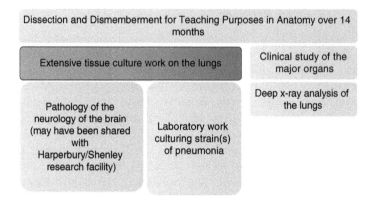

Figure 4.3 The potential(s) of TAB's threshold point(s) for the medical
sciences
Source: Reconstructed from St Bartholomew's Hospital Dissection register
MS81/5–81/6 and associated detailed record linkage work in the archives.
Ethical note: case details de-identified and anonymised.

cardiovascular diseases were by far the commonest concomitants.'[31] Further
clinical research led the research team to observe that: 'In children, associated
diseases and pulmonary complications were less common than in adults, but
the mortality was high in infancy.' Using deep X-ray equipment for which St
Bartholomew's was renowned at the time, medical evidence was found that:
'The bacteriology of the sputum and the radiological appearances were similar
to those seen in adults who did not have chronic respiratory diseases.'[32] In other
words, TAB was one of a number of cases whose lungs had been weakened by
pneumonia straining his heart, making him ideal for further medical research
study. He had thus been chosen by the hospital pathologist for 'further Special
Examination' and in so doing he became a small but no less significant part of
a medical mosaic that would eventually result in the drive for better precision
medicine in the treatment of pneumonia. Yet against this benefit we must set the
fact that the threshold points in Figure 4.3 were never mapped by medical
science for his parents. Rather, they were kept behind the closed doors of
private research facilities. This culture of secrecy was at the very least something that prevented the AB family from understanding the importance of their
son for medical research, helping them to make some medical sense of their
young son's death.

A final threshold for body ethics is also highlighted by Figure 4.3. TAB's
brain was a valuable teaching and research tool even before it left Harperbury
Hospital to travel to St Bartholomew's on 12 November 1952. As we have seen,

the Harperbury Hospital was at the forefront of occupational therapies to combat childhood learning disabilities and mental ill-health in the early 1950s. The hospital's medical records are not sufficiently detailed to reconstruct whether parts of TAB's brain may have been sliced and retained for research in-house, but nor can that possibility be ruled out either since it is noteworthy that clinical studies of brain matter happened regularly on site. It is conceivable in TAB's case that his brain became a 'control', that is, retained but not sliced extensively. Equally, it is well documented in the extant records that childhood epilepsy was a feature of extensive brain research at Harperbury, with a particular focus on 'hemispherectomy'. This method involved the removal of part of the brain, sometimes up to half in cases of severe epilepsy, on the basis that neurons in the young retain a neuro-plasticity to repair successfully after major invasive brain surgery.[33] Known as 'anatomical hemispherectomy', it was carried out on both the living and the dead on site at Harperbury's twin-research facility for brain studies called Shenley.[34] It would be uncharacteristic of the research culture on site at that time if TAB had not been brought to the attention of the in-house team, either as a 'control' or a potential discrete brain-retention. Whatever the neurological circumstances, both at Harperbury and St Bartholomew's, the actor networks existed since wartime to share in each other's research priorities. TAB was thus a potential opportunity cost for the medical sciences. His cameo role in medical history illustrates the material fate of many others that entered similar premises, and highlights the process by which implicit body disputes might develop and the complex counter-currents of medical ethics, familial knowledge, openness and closed research processes that shaped the scale and meaning of body supply for research and teaching purposes in the recent past. In turn, we can generalise the lessons to be learned from the TAB case by switching our attention to material contained in St Bartholomew's Hospital archives. This is where Richard Harrison (from Chapter 3) trained and, tellingly, what some medical students dubbed the *Ministry of Offal* in the press because it was one of the busiest teaching and research facilities in Britain. Here, we will hence bring to bear an ethnographic approach to the 'mechanisms of body donation' employed by the hospital and show how they operated both within the law and negotiated their way through it during the 1950s and 1960s. New data illustrates material afterlives, representative of the lost property of disputed bodies in modern British research.

St Bartholomew's Bodies

St Bartholomew's Hospital was a religious foundation first established at West Smithfield in 1123; thus, it is one of the oldest healthcare institutions in Britain.[35] For almost nine hundred years, it has occupied a pivotal place in the heart of the City of London. On its flank stands the City Livery Companies near the Bank of England in Threadneedle Street along Lothbury, where many of the world's leading finance houses are still located today. For centuries the hospital took in the dispossessed and sick poor, those often blighted by the hurly-burly of financial markets, sometimes bordering on the criminal that *Punch* exposed to ridicule in Victorian times. The courts of the Old Bailey were thus symbolically located just a short jaunt across the road from the hospital, which was within easy walking distance of St Paul's Cathedral. Standing opposite the hospital gate was Smithfield meat market, too. Few missed the annual fair staged nearby. Strangers, passers-by and residents all came to enjoy the entertainments at the hospital's King Henry VIII gate, erected in the Tudor period. After the dissolution of the monasteries, St Bartholomew's survived the turmoil of the Counter-Reformation to emerge by the eighteenth century as a voluntary hospital with a long-term commitment to treat the sick poor from its endowments. This entailed embracing science and promoting a culture of teaching and research. That raison d'être spearheaded the expansion of medical education in the nineteenth century, so much so that St Bartholomew's became the fourth-largest teaching facility in Britain by the close of Queen Victoria's reign in 1901. Yet, for every new medical student recruited, there needed to be a constant supply of dead bodies to dissect. London's destitute supplied the dissection table and thus helped to bring medical education at this famous hospital into the modern era.

The Medical Act (21 & 22 Vict. c. 90: 1858) stipulated that anatomical education was mandatory for every doctor. By the time those legal processes were extended in 1885, it was also a statutory requirement that each trainee should dissect a minimum of two cadavers (either whole bodies or enough body-parts to constitute two complete anatomies). This had to be done over a two-year anatomical teaching cycle at a designated teaching hospital like St Bartholomew's, in order to qualify for general practice, surgery or midwifery. There remained, however, tensions over whether bedside training on the wards or research at the laboratory bench was the best way forward for a modern medical education. This tension was not resolved until after WWI when a redesigned curriculum tried to ensure that 'medical education had a direct impact on clinical care'.[36] As Keir Waddington explains, the 'gap between science and the bedside had been bridged' as a priority by WWII; nonetheless, 'debate continued over the nature of academic medicine'. Waddington elaborates that by the early 1950s: 'If science had been accepted as an integral part of a doctor's training, old divisions between clinical and pre-clinical study were challenged as uncertainty grew about the location and content of training.'[37] In many respects, dissection was at the centre of these ongoing debates because St Bartholomew's had been extensively bombed in the war and its teaching facilities needed rebuilding to be world leading again. The NHS after 1948 tended to be slow about repairing this wartime damage, but committed staff pushed ahead to better integrate anatomical teaching with more specialised research facilities into the curriculum once more. Looking back, despite the problems of regeneration, many who worked on the premises in the 1950s recalled 'golden years, with a sense of ever-expanding horizons'.[38]

Studying the dead in detail in this period is feasible because of the remarkable longevity of the accurate record-keeping at St Bartholomew's Hospital. It has one of the best-documented archives in Britain and remains committed to sharing its past histories. Using such material, Figure 4.4 shows that 1,072 bodies were supplied for dissection from 1929, when the New Poor Law ended, until 1965. This reflected an organised network of suppliers. Four observations set in context the acquisition of these bodies and the implied system of consent that kept it functioning. The first observation is that the end of the New Poor Law had an immediate impact on the supply of the destitute for dissection from asylums, infirmaries and workhouses. As this author has documented

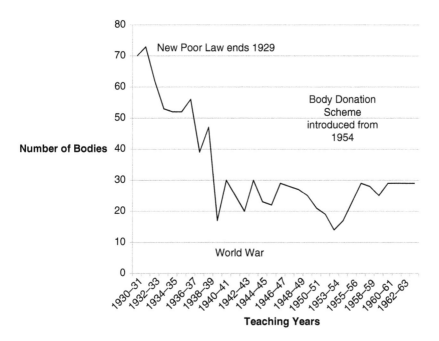

Figure 4.4 Number of bodies supplied for dissection to St Bartholomew's Hospital, c.1930–1965 (where N=1,072)
Source: Reconstructed from St Bartholomew's Hospital Dissection register MS81/5–81/6.

elsewhere, on average St Bartholomew's Hospital had been able to acquire at least 50 cadavers each teaching year from the time of the passing of the AA1832 until 1929. Indeed, in the early years of the new legislation, supply levels had peaked at 70 per year. A total of just over 6,000 bodies (from around 60,000 generated across the capital as a whole) were bought from the dead-houses of Poor Law institutions to the hospital in the period 1832 to 1929.[39] In other words, St Bartholomew's share was a minimum of 10 per cent of the entire system of body trafficking in the capital. Since these figures represent just whole bodies, another 10 per cent should be added for trades in body parts too. The latter were always more profitable because more money was made from the corpse broken up into piecemeal transactions. St Bartholomew's trading figures were thus never less than 20 per cent of the dead of London until 1930. The system functioned because generous petty cash payments persuaded people in the employ of body dealers to co-operate. It became a well-organised business of anatomy and the dead were a commodity that medical education expansion relied on.

This deep history matters, both for the interpretation in Figure 4.4 and the subsequent issues around body ethics in the twentieth-century. St Bartholomew's had a lot of go-betweens in its employ to make this trafficking in the dead operate efficiently each night. It was commonplace for a so-called 'undertaker', really a body dealer, to be employed by the dissection room. That disguise hid the fact that they were buying and selling corpses on the London streets. Once the New Poor Law ended, all of these trading arrangements had to be renegotiated, and this took time. Consequently, St Bartholomew's trading position went down from 70 bodies in 1929–30 to 52 bodies by 1934–5, a loss of nearly 20 per cent. The dissection room staff then put a lot of effort in 1936–7 to try to improve supply-lines again, but they could not prevent them dropping by another 10 per cent to around 40 per year by 1937. By the start of WWII, these figures had stabilised to about 45 bodies each teaching cycle, but it was more difficult to maintain supply-lines in the Blitz once more people evacuated out of London. Putting this trading activity into its broader perspective, the 1939–40 supply-rate was just 64 per cent of the supply levels there had been in 1929–30. This was a crucial 36 per cent reduction overall at a time when medical student numbers were expanding. When Richard Harrison (see Chapter 3) signed up for a new medical career in 1939, he was unaware of this supply problem. It never featured in the recruitment literature sent out to prospective students. As the 1930s had been a very difficult economic decade after the Wall Street Crash, everyone inside the medical profession assumed that the dead of the destitute would be available in large numbers due to startling poverty levels (as they had been in late Victorian times), but this was not the case. Subscriptions to burial clubs run by trade unions and small co-operative societies provided the means to bury the dead and hence alleviated the stress of those subsisting on the threshold of relative to absolute poverty.[40] This meant that St Bartholomew's relied on a much narrower range of former Poor Law institutions, many of which became County Council care-homes for the aged, for its regular supply needs.

A second observation is that during WWII supply levels dropped sharply. This supply pattern matched that of WWI. Those medical students, like Richard Harrison, evacuated out of London to study at Queens' College, Cambridge, together dissected no more than thirty bodies per year for the duration of 1939–45. It was thus much more common to dissect parts of bodies rather than whole cadavers over a two-year training cycle. This sets in context Harrison's recollections of daily tensions in the dissection room about when to turn a body over to make sure everyone got a chance to do an anatomical procedure. In other words, dissection was piecemeal and this reflected the fact that men recruited into the armed forces died abroad in greater numbers, rather than at home in poorer parishes where they had traditionally been sold on in death. The majority of dissections during the war were therefore on the aged. Middle-aged women did not tend to feature in the dissection registers because they had vital war work in munitions factories, took on more childcare respon-sibilities and were generally nursed at home even when seriously ill because of their value to the makeshift economies of the labouring poor. In terms then of calculative reciprocity, women until their 60s continued to be cared for by their kinship networks. Only those worn out by a life of hard work, aged, friendless and lonely would eventually come into the purview of the 'mechanisms of body donation' supply-lines of St Bartholomew's.

This situation did not improve in 1945. Until 1954 and the introduction of a new body bequest drive, supply-lines were under pressure, such that just thirteen bodies were acquired in the teaching year of 1953, and this despite the high death toll in the 'Great Fog' of 1952. At no time in the entire history of dissection had supply-lines been as difficult to sustain. Even under the Murder Act (25 Geo. 2 c. 37: 1752), supply-lines were relatively buoyant compared to this.[41] Anatomists indeed often complained that the murder rate did not keep up with demand from medical students whose numbers increased sixfold; none-theless, AA1832 resolved this situation. In the meantime, supply-lines nation-ally tended to be on average fifteen a year from 1752 to 1832. In the capital, however, by 1800 supply-lines were much worse than in provincial England: they peaked at seventeen a year in 1815 in the provinces compared to just three bodies per year in London. This meant that St Bartholomew's in 1953 found itself with a very old supply problem more akin to that of the early nineteenth century than one normally associated with modern medical research in the standard historical literature. It meant that bodies like TAB took on a symbolic importance and a lot of use was made of them, as we have seen.

Finally, it is evident from Figure 4.4 that the introduction of a body bequest scheme from 1954 had an important effect, bringing supply to about 30 per cent of its early twentieth-century peak. During the 1960s, students at the hospital would have had access to around thirty corpses each teaching cycle. Yet, this is only a partial picture because there were also important changes to the composition and character of the bodies supplied, as further detailed record linkage on individual cases reveals. They illustrate epidemiological trends. In other words, we need to compare TAB's material journey (from pneumonia death to dissection on into further research cultures) which was happening in parallel with other medical research activities at the time. It is important to examine these too because otherwise we will not gain a comprehensive enough historical picture about how a system of implied consent operated, the motivations driven by underlying disease trends, and thus nosology factors potentially shaping research priorities inside the actor network of anatomists, coroners and pathologists working together.

When each new body entered the dissection room, there was an important opportunity for the staff on duty to check the death certificate, which was often inaccurate. They stated the proximate cause of death, that is, the last ill-health episode the person died of. These were not reliable in terms of epidemiological trends in the general population because each GP would not have necessarily known the outcome of a detailed post-mortem. The poor were often signed off as 'heart problems', 'diseased' or 'dying from neglect', for instance. And, thus, expensive post-mortem costs were saved. Anatomists therefore as a matter of course always conducted their own autopsy before commencing teaching. They re-checked the pathology of death and arrived at a more accurate underlying morbidity result. This having been done, that then raised the possibility of doing further medical research on the body, its parts, organs and tissue in question. In Table 4.1 we thus see in the left-hand column the common certified causes of death before they underwent autopsy in the dissection room. In the right-hand column are listed the common ways that anatomists assessed the underlying potential for further medical research once they had arrived at more accurate morbidity results. In this way, staff on duty were able to identify a range of complications and to follow an enhanced set of research and teaching priorities. Thus, when the dead body of a male aged 70 named CD arrived on 25 March 1950, what appeared to be death due to a combination of mental and physical degeneration reflecting 'decline in old age', on closer examination proved to be caused by 'tubercular enteritis'.[42] CD had lived in abject poverty and died in the old St George's Workhouse Infirmary on Mint Street in South East London. The medical premises, even in the 1950s, were still in use. The NHS occupied them to treat some of the most vulnerable residents of Southwark, a parish traditionally linked with high levels of death in Victorian times. Today, this association with typical disease patterns of endemic poverty continues, since 'gastrointestinal and

Table 4.1 *Epidemiology of dissection cases at St Bartholomew's Hospital, 1945–1965*

Death certification date(s)	Disease classification(s)	Potential for research
1930–65	Diarrhoea, Mental & Physical Degeneration	Old Age, Dementia & Decline
1945–50	Myocardial Infarction Myocardial Degeneration Hypertension	Heart Attack Prevention
1950–55	TB (broadly defined) & Tuberculosis Enteritis Pneumonia	Lung Complaints (bacterium *Mycobacterium tuberculosis*) & Gastrointestinal Tract Treatments Deep X-Ray & Pathogenesis
1955–60	Carcinoma Colon Carcinoma Stomach	Radiology & Chemotherapy
1960–65	Cerebral Haemorrhage	Intracranial Bleed Stroke Prevention

Source: Reconstructed from St Bartholomew's Hospital Dissection register MS81/5–81/6.

peritoneal tuberculosis remain common problems in impoverished areas'.[43] Presentation of the disease TB in the abdomen has always been very difficult to diagnose. Even so, it is often present in the urban, elderly poor. Before the introduction of laparoscopy, it was hard for doctors to see the bacterium growing in the GI tract (in the ileocecal area, the ileum and the colon); in virulent cases, any area of the gut might be infected. Generally, it is still connected to poor immune levels (notably in HIV patients), but in the past tended to be a reflection of economic patterns of deep social deprivation and diseases associated with consumption.

CD was, therefore, typical of the sorts of bodies still generated for dissection at St Bartholomew's from long-established links to the basic healthcare facilities of the New Poor Law. The dissection register states CD's retention for teaching and research purposes lasted from 25 March 1950 until the start of 1951. In nine months, every opportunity was taken to culture the strain of 'tubercular enteritis' in the abdomen area, and to do further research on major organs including the heart and lungs. As with TAB, medical students cut up CD extensively. Eventually Robert Hogg (a so-called 'undertaker', really body dealer) buried what little remained. Hogg, according to the dissection accounts, also selected bodies from Guy's Hospital too and took them to the Examination Hall if he thought they would be useful specimens for students' oral tests. CD appears to have been one such case, and since the records confirm his destitution, this typical profile matches others in the sample size. It is likewise informative that the taking of his body from St George's Infirmary was part of an implied process of consent from many other similar institutions because he was friendless in death. There was nobody to dispute what was happening except the infirmary staff, and it was not in their interests to upset a network that by the 1950s was deeply embedded into a chain of body supply that stretched as far back as 1834 when the New Poor Law was established. Nobody therefore searched for CD's far relatives to check on his last wishes; although ethical standards at that time did not require this, the inaction does reveal a lot about questions of loneliness and autonomy in death, and the potential for implicit body disputes.

We often think that the current healthcare crisis in loneliness is a recent social phenomenon, but it occurred often in the early 1950s. In fact, the social anthropologist Geoffrey Gorer wrote in *Exploring the English Character* (1955 edition) about how 'most English people are shy and afraid of strangers, and consequently very lonely . . . especially in old age'.[44] Anatomists therefore deployed that social situation without fear of official censure. Indeed, the *Lancet* in one of its most forward-looking editorials in 1949 forewarned, 'The plight of old people is one of *the* [sic] biggest and most embarrassing problems facing the National Health Service.'[45] That fact of life was a boon for the medical sciences, as many similar entries to CD in the dissection books confirm. Indeed, it is feasible not only to retrace the three discrete thresholds in his case (teaching, heart-lung research, culturing tubercular enteritis) but also to reconstruct other 'undertakers' that were used to bury what little remained at the end of life because a tally of those who doubled up as body dealers was kept, as Table 4.2 shows. Many worked for New Poor Law institutions. Most stayed on the staff when premises were renamed, transferred to the NHS. The records facilitate therefore the opening of the door marked 'KEEP OUT – Private!' highlighted in Chapter 3.

The system of supply therefore afforded dignity and respect in death, and did so across religious denominations, but equally the network of body dealers disguised as 'undertakers' that facilitated a system of implied consent stretched across London, with some longevity. In the next section, we therefore explore this hidden history of the dead in further archive detail, because the historiography has tended to lose interest in the dead *at burial* – failing to appreciate that *to get to burial* could involve a complex medical research culture of pathways still to be mapped materially.

May-Die! Mayday! Mayday!

Disregarding such privacy notices personified by Table 4.2, it is notable how many healthcare institutions listed in the St Bartholomew's dissection registers had close links with the New Poor Law. Often these premises were recycled

Table 4.2 *Undertakers that buried dissections from St Bartholomew's Hospital, 1930–1965 (including those in the employ of Guy's Hospital)*

Undertaker	Trading premises	Hospital supplier
Merett & Son	**519 Hackney Road, NE London**	**St Bartholomew's**
R. Hogg	**30 St George's Road, Southwark London**	**St Bartholomew's & Guy's** **• Burials at East London Cemetery Plaistow**
J. Gaulborn	**61 Greyhound Road, Hammersmith London**	**St Bartholomew's**
J. Field	**183 Blackfriar's Road, SE1 London**	**St Bartholomew's & Guy's** **• Burials at East London Cemetery Plaistow**
J. Kenyon	**45 Edgware Road, Paddington London W2**	**St Bartholomew's** **• Burials of Roman Catholics**
Askton Brothers	**252 Clapham Road, SW9 London**	**St Bartholomew's & Guy's** **• Burials at East London Cemetery Plaistow**
E. Napier and Sons	**157 Lancaster Road, Notting Hill W11 London**	**St Bartholomew's**

Source: Reconstructed from St Bartholomew's Hospital Dissection register MS81/5–81/6.

under the NHS, continually hidden from public view. Some key examples stand in for many at the time and illustrate the sorts of network suppliers generated that made a complex system of implicit consent function over time inside the modern system of supply. The Mayday Hospital situated at Thornton Heath in Croydon did this on a regular basis.[46] For appearance's sake it was styled the Croydon Union Infirmary and then renamed the Mayday Road Hospital in 1923. This was because in an era of widening democracy, voting rights had to go hand in hand with better healthcare provision or else welfare facilities looked like an empty political promise to ordinary people. By the time that the Croydon Corporation took over the premises in 1930 and then the NHS absorbed the local healthcare infrastructure in 1948, it seemed that the Mayday Hospital had embraced the modern era of universal medical provision. Yet, many local people did not see it this way. For despite the careful rebranding of the hospital under the NHS, its popular name was the 'May-Die Hospital!' So sensitive were the local NHS health committee to this slur of medical negligence that eventually the premises were renamed the Croydon Hospital to sever all associations with social deprivation and poverty. Even so, this did not stop

St Bartholomew's lobbying for body supply there in the 1950s. Thus, when a 76-year-old female died in Mayday Hospital on 3 October 1956, her body went to St Bartholomew's at 10 a.m. on Thursday 4 October 1956. The patient had died from a 'cerebral haemorrhage' and the body was retained over 20 months for teaching and brain research until 7 July 1958. It was again buried by Hogg, the 'undertaker' and body broker go-between.[47]

This case in many respects is intriguing because of its mundane conclusion, despite a number of curious features. It resulted in a dreary death and disposal, representative of many examples in the dissection registers. The female named EF had a Jewish birth name.[48] Yet, it was a cultural taboo in the Jewish community to delay the burial or cremation of the dead for more than twenty-four hours. Ideally, the interred body would be intact. The woman lived, however, at the time of her death in a Church of England home for retired deaconesses located at Staines near Heathrow airport. The balance of the evidence suggests that this association with the Anglican faith made donation feasible. Even so, the body was not marked with a 'B' to indicate a written bequest in the dissection register. The female in question was respectable, but poor. It was common for care-homes of the elderly to offset funeral fees by agreeing to donate bodies in return for the medical school bearing the costs of burial or cremation. There seems therefore to have been an implied assumption in this case that handing over the body was conventional, given the deceased's relative poverty. Besides, if EF's orthodox faith had been strong, it is unlikely that she would have been retained for twenty months without her Jewish family's consent. Perhaps she gave such consent herself verbally and willingly, with the paperwork not processed properly. Or her 'donation' was implied from her modest personal circumstances and carried out by the care-home to save money. Whatever the motivation, Hogg buried EF at East London Cemetery in Plaistow, which was some considerable distance across the capital from her last place of residence in West London and far from the Jewish cemetery at Kensal Green. There does not therefore seem to have been any further family involvement by her Jewish kin. Here we glimpse someone connected to an Anglican community, amendable perhaps to the 'gift' of the body, but for whom the end-of-life experience was not so far removed from the friendless dead-end of others less fortunate than herself such as CD. Death was not just a common denominator; it could be a social leveller too. Determining who entered the system of implied consent often involved something as simple as slipping beneath everyone's social radar out of reach in old age, a situation that the *Sutton and Croydon Guardian* reported on even as recently as November 2013. Today, Croydon University Hospital (CUH) still faces insufficient staffing levels, substandard cleanliness and long waiting times in accident and emergency, affecting the elderly; for, according to a newspaper investigative journalist: 'CUH is not officially stated as the worst hospital in London but it is the most complained about earning the misnomer The May-Die, referring back to its former name Mayday Hospital before it was renamed University College Hospital in 2010.'[49] In hidden histories of the dead, such repeated scenarios are noteworthy. They suggest considerable longevity, little chance to dispute what was happening with regards to implied consent, and a system that was all about recovering a welfare debt in death. Others who equally were perceived as a burden to taxpayers entered the same supply chain too.

Perhaps one of the most interesting features of the body supply to St Bartholomew's in this period is that many cases came from former asylums and prisons. They thus encapsulate a central dilemma in modern medical research – namely, the exploitation of the unfortunate for scientific gain. We saw this criticism in Chapters 2 and 3 during the 1950s when articles and letters published in the medical press expressed ethical concerns about how to protect with legislation those suffering from anxiety, depression, and more serious mental-health conditions like schizophrenia. Some patients consented to drugs trials they could not comprehend fully, since informed consent was very difficult to monitor in the mentally vulnerable. The standard approach in the historical literature to this sensitive issue is to tally up all of the premises of incarceration that were involved in body-supply schemes, mapping their geo-graphical alignment to assess the business of anatomy on a regional basis. Yet in the modern era, that geo-approach could be misleading. What really mattered to modern medical research was not just the physical location of potential bodies, but the over-laying of hidden histories inside medical spaces of incar-ceration. It was possible for a patient to enter a mental health establishment for general treatment, for instance, and then get caught up in the dissection system by virtue of how research pathways had accumulated inside the premises over time. One representative case illustrates how this worked in detail.

Thus, IGH was a 68-year-old female who died on 12 September 1952.[50] She resided in a relatively affluent area of Notting Hill in London. Her home was grade-II listed and faced a garden square of some architectural merit. She was not therefore the sort of person that one would expect to end up on a dissection table unless she had agreed to a body bequest in her will, which does not seem to have been the case. So, how did she come into the medical purview of St Bartholomew's? IGH had taken a decision to enter Banstead Hospital in Sutton towards the end of her life. She had contracted cancer and needed specialist nursing care.[51] This institution, however, had a complicated healthcare history layered with meaning for the dissection system of supply. This IGH seems to have been unaware of in its entirety, but it did nevertheless have a bearing on her destination in death. Banstead Asylum first opened in 1877 with the capacity for 1,700 patients (615 males and 1,075 females).[52] It was one of three asylums in Middlesex. The premises remained open to 'mental defect-ives' (broadly defined) under the New Poor Law until WWI. However, from

1889, Banstead came under the jurisdiction of London County Council. By 1912, it was a site covering 200 acres. On its 130-acre farm, patients did occupational therapy and learned self-sufficiency. After the war, however, with so many men returning from the trenches suffering from shell shock, institutional rebranding was commonplace. The premises became Banstead Mental Hospital. In 1937, it was restyled again as just Banstead Hospital, and it transferred to the South West Metropolitan Hospital Board under the new NHS by 1948. Various NHS reorganisation schemes from 1974 until the 1980s preceded its eventual closure in 1986. Often described as a 'lost hospital of London' its hidden history in the 1950s proved to be relevant for IGH's body.

After being requisitioned during the war, by the start of 1950 the military had packed up and left Banstead Hospital.[53] It once more became a civilian facility under the NHS. The bed capacity was now '2,599', but in 1951 a decision was taken to designate the premises as a Regional TB Unit too.[54] Here men that had contracted persistent TB, and were psychiatric patients, were treated. The female wards on the Unit also contained '21 typhoid carriers who were constant excretors'. Often standard treatments had failed to stem their contagious conditions. There were likewise a small number of 'dysentery carriers'.[55] A decision was taken to designate its 15 wards (each with a maximum of 60 patients) with special areas of clinical responsibility ranging from TB, epilepsy, typhoid, dysentery, VD, senility to surgical and psychiatric care. There were also 'special rooms for disturbed patients'. An additional logistical issue was a 'chromic shortage of nursing staff' in the early 1950s. It took time to refurbish the wards to attract more specialist and general nurses, and, in the meantime, the plan was to open a new Clinical Psychology Unit from 1953. Once opened, art and social therapies were introduced. Treatments for persistent mental ill-health included: 'leucotomy, deep insulin coma and ECT'. In 1951 the TB Unit for men was expanded to house 100 patients and surgical interventions were introduced such as 'pneumo-peritoneum, pneumothorax and phrenic crush – or with chemotherapy, using a cocktail of streptomycin, PAS and INAH'. The antibiotic era had arrived at Banstead.

When IGH entered Banstead Hospital in the late summer of 1952, therefore, she came into premises deeply committed to the most modern research. Up to fifteen research pathways existed inside the hospital wards run on clinical research lines to facilitate better specialist medical work in-house. This also connected to external research facilities like those of St Bartholomew's. IGH was not thus simply a lady suffering from terminal cancer; she had a patient profile that matched research pathways of some longevity and reflecting clinical priorities. Moreover, her cancer was clearly not 'simple'. Even after extensive dissection her cause of death was described as 'secondaries [sic] of carcinoma'. Evidently, the primary tumour was not found, and this, allied to the fact that she was in late middle age, but not elderly, seems to have made her an interesting subject for further cancer study. Indeed, St Bartholomew's had an excellent reputation for cancer treatment in this period, and so she was an ideal body supply.[56] In practice, IGH's time travels were not dissimilar to TAB's when we map her hidden history, as Figure 4.5 shows. In a period of low supply, the hospital was thus taking what it could get, but equally when it did have an opportunity to self-select the bodies chosen, these matched its research focus.

One final feature of the complex network of institutions that underpinned the St Bartholomew's dissection registers is that there were increasingly very close links between this institution and the hospice movement in London. These started around 1948. One representative example involves IJ, aged 66, who died from 'carcinoma of the stomach [*sic*] on 6 December 1948 in St Joseph's Hospice in Hackney'.[57] Located on Mare Street, it still treats the terminally ill today. It was established in 1905, and the Ministry of Health recognised the dedicated work of the nuns by 1923, officially designating St Josephs 'a home for the reception of advanced cases of TB'. During wartime, the patients and nursing staff evacuated to Bath, and on their return in 1945 extensive bomb damage had to be repaired. Across Hackney, the nursing staff took in those needing end-of-life care, and they soon expanded by developing close links and clinical studies with Cicely Saunders, renowned for founding the St Christopher Hospice from 1958. The ethos of St Joseph's Hospice has always been to help the poorest and dispossessed in society regardless of their religious belief, and this very much reflected its location in Hackney, the third-most-deprived area of London.[58] Unsurprisingly perhaps it has always had close

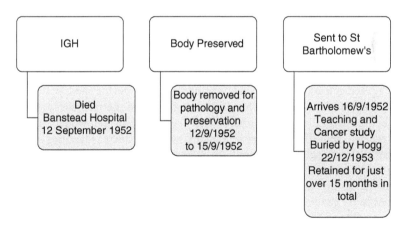

Figure 4.5 IGH material travels, 12 September 1952–22 December 1953
Source: Reconstructed from St Bartholomew's Hospital Dissection register MS81/5–81/6. Ethical note: case details de-identified and anonymised.

links to St Bartholomew's, the main hospital for the sick poor in central London serving the East End. Thus, when IJ died on 6 December 1948, her body was retained by the hospice for an initial post-mortem and then chemical preservation until 19 December 1948, a time gap of thirteen days, before being sent to St Bartholomew's for dissection. Once there, again teaching and cancer research were the features of the discrete research steps taken, with ultimate body burial some twelve months later. This was the same supply pattern occurring with KL, aged 82, who died in a hospice in Bournemouth on 14 December 1952, arriving at St Bartholomew's to be dissected and diagnosed with 'carcinoma of the colon' by the anatomist on duty, some three days later.[59] On this occasion, because KL had expressed a wish to the hospice to have a Roman Catholic burial, J. Kenyon, the 'undertaker', took charge of the internment after a total of some fifteen months of teaching and research on 7 July 1953.

Meanwhile, another major source of supply at this time was Salvation Army hostels. Thus, when MN, a male aged 56, died of 'hypertension' in a Salvation Army hostel on 20 May 1953, his last known address had a direct impact on his body going to St Bartholomew's, where he arrived on 26 May 1953.[60] It was studied until buried by Hogg in a multiple grave on 29 December 1954. The case was not dissimilar to OP, a male aged 85, 'whose last place of abode was Whitechapel Infirmary' when he died at Leavesdon Hospital on 1 December 1960.[61] This was a deprived area of London where the Salvation Army were very active in rescuing the homeless found in dire straits on the streets and placing them in whatever former Poor Law premises where available close to death. Thus, OP was moved on to St Bartholomew's within three days; his death from 'myocardia degeneration' was common but his body and body parts were still worth studying until 3 January 1962. Buried in a batch of six bodies in a common grave, there was little to inter at the end. This more extensive use of the human material reflected the much more detailed pathology from the 1960s in the dissection registers. At that time in 1963/4 when the scribe who wrote up the entries changed hands, the bodies became a surname in capital letters and just their initials. The clinical discourse of the medical sciences was being streamlined once more, and the 'gift' of the whole person disappeared into discrete research steps whose human identities were gradually downgraded to a summary in the record-keeping. The modern era of clinical research was now looking towards a more sophisticated biomedical future, and this extended the potential for an implied system of consent to be generated and re-generated, especially amongst the homeless of London. To engage with that context, it is essential now to track forward in the record-keeping to the 1990s and examine in our penultimate section the scale, scope and clinical reach of anatomical records on a national basis.

A National Picture – Remapping Donation and Dissection

The NHS public enquiries into organ retention that were the catalysts for HTA2004 established three things that are important for understanding the national scale of the implicit system of consent and its potential for body disputes by the 1990s. The first was that hospital coroners were crucial to the supply mechanisms of medical schools post-WWII. The second was that the need for high-tech pathologies on organs, body parts and tissue cultures complicated issues of consent by grieving relatives. The third was that even those amenable to donation had little material sense of what actually happened to each cadaver divided up in the name of medical science. One predominant issue was that detailed record-keeping had effectively lapsed during the 1980s because AA1984 did not reflect adequately the rapid pace of biotechnology. At the same time, the transplant era had begun and the scientific parameters of innovations, like drug-rejection therapies, were changing the course of research agendas inside the scientific community. In subsequent chapters, we will be engaging with this new biotech landscape in more detail, but before doing so, it is essential to try to understand the nature of dissection work in the recent past. The aim in this section is to examine the scale of the system of implied consent across England, and thus reflect historically on how many people could have been involved in disputing what was happening. Although some of the bereaved may have been in agreement, others might not have been; in fact, few got an opportunity to make that informed choice. Figure 4.6 thus provides an overview of rates of body donation around the country in the 1990s from figures made available by the Anatomy Office. This data is also displayed in Figure 4.7, with locations and rates of donation itemised for individual institutions in London. Then these figures are broken down again into annual rates of donation for all medical schools, and summarised in terms of regional versus metropolitan trends across Britain in Table 4.3.

Considered in the round, we can see that although London dominated the dissection scene in terms of the economies of scale that an institutional collaboration, like UMDS, could acquire (involving the United Medical & Dental Schools of Guy's & St Thomas' hospitals, London including Royal Dental Hospital of London – all merged again into King's College Hospital post-1998),[62] the capital overall generated 1,468 bodies (42.4 per cent), but provincial institutions generated more cadavers (2,505; 58.6 per cent). Training in London was no longer the guarantee of a better-supplied anatomical education that it had been in the previous 200 years. We also, however, need to engage with the demography of this supply picture because younger bodies have always been prized by anatomists over older ones. Figure 4.8 analyses the age range of all 'body donations' in the 1990s and shows that the majority were in the 50- to 100-year range. This narrows again on closer inspection. For in the

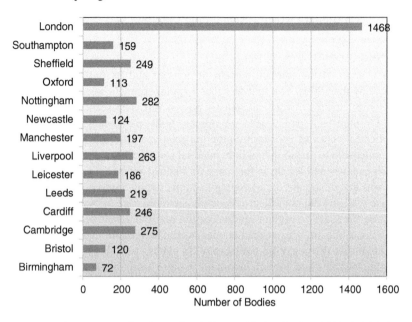

Figure 4.6 Bodies donated and dissected in England, c. 1992–1998 (where
N=3,973 [2,505 for the regions and 1,468 for London])
Source: National Archives, JA 3/1, Anatomy Office, Data-Set Returns for
England, c. 1992–98.

age range(s) 70–79, 1,067 bodies were donated; at 80–89 years-old it was 1,802
bequests; and even in the 90–99 age category there were 702 cadavers acquired.
Perhaps the most surprising outcome is that 51 bodies were aged 100 or more,
roughly equivalent to the 49 for those in the 50–59 age range and proof positive
of the crisis of ageing affecting the modern NHS. Medical students today
dissect the elderly just as much as, if not more than, their Victorian
counterparts.

Delving deeper into the demography of dissection is informative. If we
break down the figures again by gender as well as age, as in Figure 4.9, there
is evidently not a normal distribution. What becomes apparent is that 2,113
bodies (53 per cent) were generated from females dying between the ages of
50 and 84 years of age. Fewer women were dissected in the 85+ category. If,
therefore, a medical student needed to dissect someone younger in the 1990s,
that would have been a woman who had died in or near the standard
retirement age in force in this decade. This was the exact reverse of historical
trends over the previous 200 years when men, not women, dominated the
dissection table.[63] After age 84, men start to be dissected in much higher

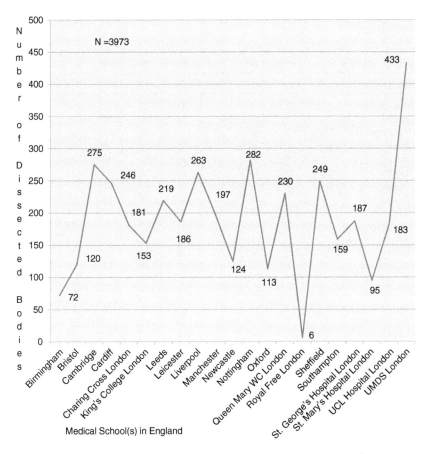

Figure 4.7 Bodies that were donated and dissected at medical schools in
England for teaching and further research purposes, c. 1992–1998
Source: National Archives, JA 3/1, Anatomy Office Data-Set Returns for
England, c. 1992–98.

numbers than women during the 1990s, when the former generated 1,860
bodies (47 per cent) in the data-set, with the majority being in the 84 to 94
age range. The interesting point about this trend is that the medical students
who recalled doing dissections from the 1940s up to the 1980s (see Chapter
3) remembered dissecting very old men, but not women. In the 1990s,
therefore, a key cultural transition occurred with females supplying dissection. There appears to have been enough bodies to devise a screening process
to select women over men, unless, that is, they were in the upper-age deciles.

Table 4.3 *Bodies donated and dissected at medical schools in England,*
1992–1998

Medical school	1992	1993	1994	1995	1996	1997	1998	Total(s)
REGIONS	100	465	435	352	343	471	339	2505
Birmingham	0	5	14	13	12	14	14	72
Bristol	3	17	22	22	17	20	19	120
Cambridge	7	65	33	50	36	45	39	275
Cardiff	11	47	55	20	29	46	38	246
Leeds	10	47	22	18	33	48	41	219
Leicester	6	35	35	25	22	42	21	186
Liverpool	20	52	44	42	45	41	19	263
Manchester	9	38	32	26	29	48	15	197
Newcastle	5	19	30	20	21	18	11	124
Nottingham	8	44	49	43	44	55	39	282
Oxford	4	24	31	18	13	21	2	113
Sheffield	8	40	47	26	26	50	52	249
Southampton	9	32	21	29	16	23	29	159
LONDON	77	212	208	225	210	311	225	1468
Charing Cross Hospital	10	19	21	16	40	46	29	181
King's College	7	25	21	18	17	29	36	153
QMWC*	12	29	33	46	30	47	33	230
Royal Free Hospital	0	6	0	0	0	0	0	6
St George's Hospital	13	37	35	33	13	33	23	187
St Mary's Hospital	9	16	19	18	16	17	0	95
UCL**	9	27	27	24	22	41	33	183
UMDS***	17	53	52	70	72	98	71	433
Totals overall	177	677	643	577	553	782	564	3973

Source: The National Archives, JA 3/1, Anatomy Office Data-Set Returns for England, c. 1992–98.
* QMWC = Queen Mary and Westfield College London
** UCL = University College London
*** UMDS = United Medical & Dental Schools of Guy's & St Thomas' hospitals London
including Royal Dental Hospital of London (all merged again into King's College post-1998)

In other words, against the backdrop of general agreement at the various
public enquiries into organ scandals in the NHS, which generated implicit
disputes because so many of the general public were misinformed or uninformed about their Coronial remains, it is evident that it was a female voice
that was lost in medical ethics during the 1990s. Medical science, which has
been a male-dominated profession, relied on women for its teaching and
research culture at that time, but then denied them full knowledge of the 'gift
relationship' they had sustained.

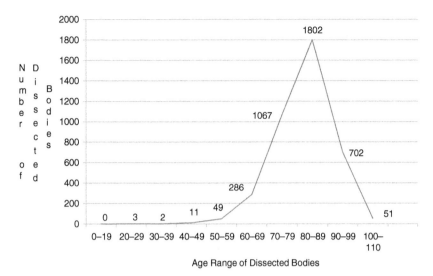

Figure 4.8 Age range of body bequests dissected in England, c. 1992–1998 (where N=3,973)
Source: National Archives, JA 3/1, Anatomy Office, Data-Set Returns for England, c. 1992–98.

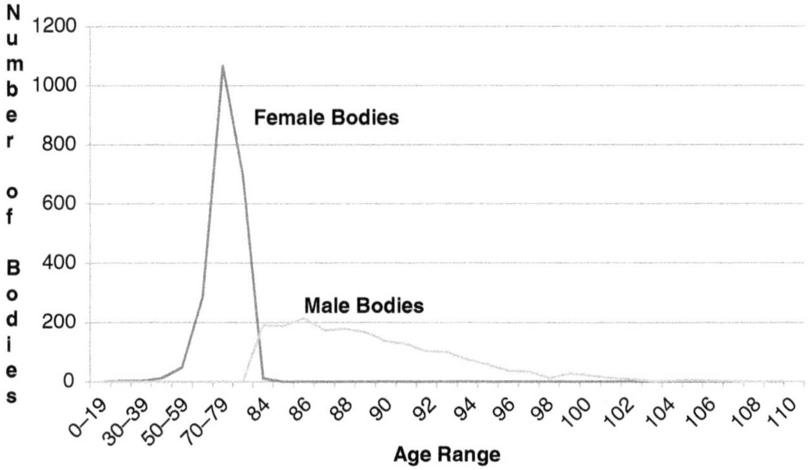

Figure 4.9 Number of dissected bodies analysed by gender and age range, c. 1992–1998 (where N=3,973)
Source: National Archives, JA 3/1, Anatomy Office, Data-Set Returns for England, c. 1992–98.

This trend has had other important consequences too, especially for organ donation. Public health campaigns to increase organ donation have tended to target the mass media in a manner akin to shooting arrows at a target, the aim being to hit anywhere on the pool of public opinion regardless of its cultural impact. Had it, however, been better understood that women, rather than men, were more inclined to bequest by the 1990s, then public money spent on speaking to a female constituency with the most take-up rate in body-donations could have been more productively spent. Indeed, the latest NHS2020 strategy to improve donation rates admits that:

The problem is with family consent (or, in Scotland, 'authorisation') rates, which have remained unchanged at about 57% for many years. This means that every year, about 4,099 organs are 'lost' because, when a person dies, their families refuse to allow their organs to be removed. The target in the 2020 strategy is to increase family consent rates to 80% by 2020.[64]

In other words, there is little point in encouraging people to join the Organ Donation Register (ODR) alone. In death, what really matters at the point of bequest is talking beforehand about the need to give in families: 'In order to achieve the 80% target it is necessary to also leverage the ODR so that new joiners go on to have conversations with their family about their wishes in the event of their death.' As the ODR2020 strategy explains:

For the first time, NHSBT will thus attempt to achieve behaviour change among donor families as well donors themselves. This will require a major cultural shift throughout the UK. NHSBT will need to tackle common myths and misunderstandings around organ donation (particularly as it relates to burial or cremation). Moreover, it necessitates that families appreciate that this is a decision that they will be asked to take, discuss it in advance and come to view donation as a natural and positive step in the grieving process.[65]

Yet, the rediscovered evidence is clear and robust. First, it is women, and not men, who have been the chief source of communication about the need to be active donors in families. Second, that important observation is based on national dissection data, which confirms that from the 1990s females have been the active givers. The ODR2020 strategy therefore currently maintains (erroneously) that to target young people and get them to effect the most change is the way forward in families. Instead, the social reality is that mothers and grandmothers are key and this social policy finding arises out of the most recent 'gift' data available in modern Britain. ODR2020 is moreover concerned that: 'Between April 2012 and March 2013, 2,918 families were asked for their consent to recover organs from their loved ones. Of these, about 43%, or 1,242 families, refused.' It goes on to comment that 'this figure is high, particularly when compared to other European countries, for example in Spain, fewer than

20% of families withheld their consent'.[66] That being the case, it is vital to get women talking to shape family decisions, not men; and to do so in terms of ethnicity because up to 68 per cent of families still refuse to donate in communities of higher net-migration.

When we therefore neglect hidden histories involving implicit disputes, it can have very real consequences for a patient on a waiting-list for an organ transplant. Dissection and its discrete research steps have remapped all our medical futures in ways that we still need to engage with and talk about openly to improve the NHS of tomorrow. Under Prime Minister David Cameron, a Behavioural Insights Team was established and staffed by economists based in the Cabinet Office. Their behavioural economics policy promoted an agenda of: 'If you want people to do something, make it easy.' Easy that is, from the policy makers' point of view. Their modus operandi was to ignore hidden histories of the body and instead create legal changes to 'tax collection, organ donation, and energy efficiency – and most notably pensions . . . where participation . . . dramatically increases when people must explicitly opt out, if they are not be automatically enrolled'.[67] This 'psychological realism', however, talks *at* people not *with* them; it lacks patience and creative imagination to find robust data to establish the appropriate historical course of action based on what we know, rather than on what we think we know. Political short-termism has failed to engage with the wider cultural meaning of death and dissection for everybody and, in particular, female voices in British society. If we do not properly model what was happening inside modern medical research cultures, then we can so easily define death in a way that is out of date – an issue that the final section turns to.

Defining Death – Out of Date?

There is one last and important aspect of these national figures that merits closer inspection, and it is disease classification. Before we begin that analysis, however, it is important to appreciate that the entire data-set for the 1990s has a number of curious features that are only discernible when tabulated. The first of these is that the medical terms used to describe the pathologies of death are rather old-fashioned and outdated. They resemble the sort of medical language used in the 1890s. Why this still occurred regularly by the 1990s is difficult to pinpoint with precision. It appears to reflect just how slow medical discourse is to change. Most anatomists and their pathologists doing dissections and post-mortem work in the 1990s trained just after WWII when an older nomenclature was in vogue in medical education. A Victorian vocabulary seems, therefore, to have survived much longer than one would expect in the record-keeping of anatomy departments. This also means that the pathologies of death were in themselves often a missed opportunity to learn more about the underlying causes of death from bequests in the 1990s, a theme we will be expanding on in Chapter 5 when we look at the work of the Coronial Office in more depth.

A second curiosity is that because these descriptions of death in the heart/ lungs/brain are rather general when one analyses them from the vantage point of those used in emergency room medicine today, the older terminology looks confusing. Often one 'mode of death' seems to overlap with another. Hence, these descriptions of death in the anatomy records do not reflect how a doctor in general practice would certify death in the NHS. The system that they use is very different (as was briefly explained above). Doctors are required to certify 'the cause of death' (its pathology, if known) but not the 'mode of death' (the part of the body that actually failed). They do so by filling in a number of official categories on the death certificate, as follows:

1 (a) what finished the patient off?
1 (b) what was (a) due to or as a consequence of?
1 (c) what was (b) due to or a consequence of?
2 what other signs of pathology may be associated with the cause of death? [68]

Thus by way of example if a patient dies of

1 (a) Acute Left Ventricular Failure – in the heart as it became strained
1 (b) It was caused by breast cancer (secondary cause)
1 (c) It was caused by bone cancer (primary cause)
2 The patient had type 2 diabetes complicating their pathology [69]

There is then a lot of potential disparity between doctors' death certificates in the NHS and those of anatomy departments dissecting inside the same system. This common situation is further complicated by the fact that in London, coroners (who liaise with GPs, the police and bequests) tend to be doubly qualified – that is, medically and legally qualified – whereas in the regions, coroners still tend to be solicitors who hold a Diploma of Medical Jurisprudence. For this reason, the requirements of the Registrar in different Coronial areas will have subtle differences. Historically, therefore, there has been a tendency for descriptions on death certificates to be more lax in the regions compared to metropolitan areas, a trend that continues in the NHS. In other words, the system of death certification and disease classification ought to be streamlined, but it is not, and this has contributed to a system of presumed consent that was implied by insiders eager to get hold of bodies to know more about their *real* death causes. There are, in other words, many gaps, and a lack of uniformity in disease causation as determined in dissection spaces. So, although a lot of research was significant, anatomists co-operating with scientific studies, it could also have been much more streamlined if the system of death certification had not been convoluted and complex. This is a core theme we will be returning to throughout this book because there were lots of lost research opportunity costs caused by a system that functioned with so much ambiguity, and deliberately so, to keep up its supply chains.

Thus, for reasons of statistical significance, the disease classifications from the 1990s data-set have been grouped around the top ten big killers (as described in the record-keeping). These are detailed in Table 4.4. Each of the major categories comprises a mixture of proxy dates – that is, deaths in which pneumonia, for instance, was the final killer or a heart attack, but causation was actually a complex combination of underlying conditions and *real* causes of death. According to that data, almost 20 per cent of people died of broncho-pneumonia, which indicates clinically people who were dying from multiple health complications. In other words, the various pathology categories if used today would have a lot of clinical overlap. In a typical heart attack patient, by way of further illustration, certified as dying of Ischemic Heart Disease (IHD), the individual would have also had three 'modes of death' that overlapped with IHD, including: Left Ventricular Failure (LVF), Congestive Heart failure (CCF) and Acute Myocardial Infection (AMI). The main underlying causes of the primary 'mode of death' and 'secondary subset' would have included little physical exercise, lack of mobility due to a sedentary lifestyle, poor nutrition, obesity, asthma and old age itself. Importantly, for the purposes of this book's focus, these are patients who will have lived longer (often in extreme frailty) with a number of underlying health problems before death, and therefore had longer to consider organ donation and a body bequest as an option.

Table 4.4 *The disease classifications of dissection bodies nationally, 1990s*

Disease classification (biggest killers)	Numbers dissected in the 1990s
Bronchopneumonia	773 cases out of 3973 in total (or **19.45%**)
Acute Myocardial Infarction	671 cases out of 3973 in total (or **16.88%**)
CVA [Cerebral Vascular Accident]	433 cases out of 3973 in total (or **10.89%**)
CCF [Congestive Cardiac Failure]	197 cases out of 3973 in total (or **4.95%**)
Dementia -Extreme Old Age – Debility	184 cases out of 3973 in total (or **4.63%**)
COAD [Chronic Obstructive Pulmonary Disease]	132 cases out of 3973 in total (or **3.32%**)
IHD [Ischemic Heart Disease, known generally as Coronary Heart Disease]	127 cases out of 3973 in total (or **3.19%**)
Pneumonia – general	93 cases out of 3973 in total (or **2.34%**)
LVF [Left Ventricular Failure]	89 cases out of 3973 in total (or **2.24%**)
Cerebral Vascular Disease/Stroke	76 cases out of 3973 in total (or **1.91%**)
Top 10 killers in total	**2775 cases out of 3 973 in total (or 69.84%)**

Source: The National Archives, JA 3/1, Anatomy Office Data-Set Returns for England, c. 1992–98.

Other major killers like cancer brought fewer into the ambit of dissection – less than one might expect given how many cases feature today in the media – 212 cases in total (or 2.26% of the total) in Table 4.5. Cancer broadly defined as *carcinomatosis* was the eleventh killer listed in the national sample as the 'primary cause of death'. Again, it is noteworthy for this book's focus that these patients had much less time to consider bequests, and therefore featured in fewer numbers in the data-set (even allowing for the fact that pneumonia could have been disguising cancer in individual cases). Overall, this would have mattered to teaching programmes and implied opportunities for further research. Whilst anatomists therefore were self-selecting women up to the age of 84, they could not control their disease classifications or background health

Table 4.5 *Disease classifications of those with cancer nationally, 1990s*

Cancer types	Area(s) of the body	Number(s) dissected
Carcinoma – general – carcinomatosis	Whole body	72
Carcinoma – specific areas of the body	Abdomen	1
	Bladder	9
	Blood	4
	Bone	2
	Brain	7
	Breast	13
	Bronchioles	17
	Colon	12
	Endometrial	2
	Kidney	8
	Large bowel	2
	Larynx	1
	Lower Hip	1
	Liver	1
	Lung(s)	65
	Oesophagus	17
	Pancreas	14
	Prostrate	23
	Rectum	2
	Skin	7
	Stomach	14
	Thyroid	1
	Tongue	1
	Uterus	5
Exhaustion following carcinoma	Whole body	3
Total cases of cancer		**212**

Source: The National Archives, JA 3/1, Anatomy Office Data-Set Returns for England, c. 1992–98.

conditions. This meant that it was difficult to predict bequests that matched research/teaching priorities. Any they did therefore acquire and shared with pathologists at the right time became exigent, a matter to which we return in Chapter 6. Thus, TAB (young body), EF, IGH and IJ (middle-aged bodies) and OP (elderly body) from St Bartholomew's represent the spectrum of cases nationally sought and harvested for extensive and valuable further work.

Another important feature of this epidemiology is that historical longevity is a vital analytical tool when examining disease trends. So, for example, the foundations of lung conditions such as COAD (Chronic Obstructive Pulmonary Diseases) and heart conditions like IHD and LVF were in reality laid in the 1950s, but came to fruition in the 1990s. This was in terms of smoking, a general decline in exercise, the rise of blue-collar jobs, city pollution and the high salt content of diets, as well as brown fat in fast foodstuffs. In other words, when we try to measure the health of the nation from dissection cases, it is always a case of being Janus-like. St Bartholomew's hence in the 1950s was really managing the remnants of New Poor Law health issues dating from the 1920s. Likewise, when looking at 1990s cases, what we are really seeing is a disease picture of the landscape of early NHS healthcare dating from the 1950s. Thus, by way of example, pollution levels, as we saw in the opening section of this chapter, were considerable in the 1950s for many people and the Clean Air Act (4 & 5 Eliz. 2 ch.: 1956) did not resolve these for some time. Consequently, lung complaints resurfaced in the 1990s. In fact, what complicates this epidemiology is the advent of car pollution that replaced coal fire smog, and has been a worse killer than, say, cigarette smoke or chimney pollution because one cannot always see car pollution to walk away from it.[70] Most demographers faced with these sorts of everyday car pollutants would therefore ask a key question of the underlying statistics, namely: Are the rates and concentrations of the causes of death random in the population?

The answer is negative for both data-sets, either at St Bartholomew's or in the national sample-set. It is a case of thinking very carefully about what the statistics are really saying, because they were the material basis of the system of implied consent and its research thresholds that we have been mapping for the first time. Examining the males in the sample base is instructive in this regard. At first glance, it looks like the anatomists were selecting by gender – this would explain why women up to the age of 84 appear so frequently in the dissection records but not their male equivalent. After 85 years of age, the number of men rises disproportionately (as we saw above). However, this was not simply about an aged-related screening programme. It reflects another social care explanation too. Men came from care-homes because they outnumbered women in social care provision during the 1990s. Historically, in fact, women have always been able to care for themselves for longer at home than have men. In poverty studies we see this continuity stretching back to the Old

Poor Law of the eighteenth century.[71] In other words, body bequests, donation rates and their gender profiling continue to rely on a basic understanding of life-cycle trends and their social care crisis points. Anatomists took what they could get, but equally they worked with what they had always known over the past 200 years. And, as they did so, what they began to do was to elongate how long they could keep hold of a body, a theme that we began to explore above and which is developed at length in Chapter 5. In this process, many questions were unasked or unanswered: Who decided what bodies and body-parts were worth keeping and what should be discarded? What got missed in this filtering process? Did access to certain research material shape medical breakthroughs and exclude other options? How did professional boundaries play out in matters of authority over the body and body-parts? And what role did financial budget setting play in remapping the 'Human Atlas'? We will be continuing to ask these thought-provoking questions throughout the rest of this book, reflecting more broadly on them in the conclusion in particular.

Conclusion

> Science and technology diminish the body's mystery, employing a discourse of instrumentality and utility to which, from a practical standpoint, it is often difficult to object. And yet there is something disturbing in this emerging consequentialist strand in discourse about the body. Non-economic values are unlikely to enjoy prominence or protection in the law's haste to take the body to market.[72]

One of the main scientific outcomes of the Enlightenment is that we have all become bodies of information in a global biotech age. This is the logic of medical proficiency and its flourishing research cultures around the world. Few would want to go back to the threats of famine, plague and war that blighted so much human endeavour for centuries.[73] Even so, the medical threat of a worldwide pandemic has become a lived experience as this book goes into press, as things that people faced in the past are becoming very real in the present. We know to follow the science, but equally we have to keep checking on its working practices and ethical credentials as they evolve. When com-modification is the primary mode of exchange in contemporary society, the law cannot always protect our physical vulnerabilities in a Genome era, whether alive or dead. There is a loophole in international law that fosters the breaking of medical boundaries, but it has seldom been discussed in relation to body disputes. In order to arrive at a consensus in, for example, the United Nations Security Council, all member states agree to comply with the principle of *qui tacet consentire videtur* [s/he who is silent, is taken to agree]. In diplomatic parlance it is known as the *silence procedure of international law* – speak up, and be heard; otherwise, it will be taken that silence means acquiescence and a tacit agreement.[74] Although scholars have concentrated on the implications of property law for body disputes in case law, in reality the equivalent and precedence of a silence procedure of international law has been, often, deployed inside the 'mechanisms of body donation'. The public never said anything about bodies being moved around and retained for up to thirty-six months, and that silence was assumed to have created a consensus in Britain. Added to which, we increasingly live in a social media world with a complex sense of community and belonging.[75] At a time, therefore, of increased loneliness in modern society, there has been little detailed knowledge of just how much the medical sciences relied on our cultural disaggregation (however benignly) to foster a flourishing research culture from behind the dissection room door. Few got the opportunity to see the editing done in the name of medical progress, how the whole became piecemeal. As Halewood elaborates:

> The conversion of the body into patentable information and the speed with which that information is processed and transferred effect a postmodern, technological transformation of the human body that undermines the stability of conventional, liberal legalist assumptions about rights and persons, and about self-ownership and the autonomy it is said to protect. Paul Rabinow . . . claims that the body is so fragmented by technology, so analysed into a 'discrete, exploitable reservoir of molecular and biochemical products', that really no conception of the person as a whole remains beneath.[76]

This is dangerous ethical territory, the equivalent of being back in the pea-soup of a London fog about to be despatched for dissection in the 1950s. For when we examine the potential for implicit body disputes in the post-WWII era in Britain, what is notable is the law of unintended consequences that follows on from the silence procedure of international law on the one hand and local research and professional practice on the other hand. The medical sciences effectively deployed their powers of acquisition to shape a clandestine culture of research thresholds that had time-gaps (between death and official registration), time delays (for post-mortem and chemical preservation to happen), and time stops (moved from one location to another), before doing morbid pathologies for up to three years before interment. It was easy to lose sight of the whole person divided up and hence bureaucracy literally left them behind, hidden inside the medical research community. TAB, CD, EF, IGH, IJ, KL, MN and OP – are now initials on the pages of this chapter, de-identified for ethical reasons, but also socially revived for medical posterity. They have been put back into research pathways that constituted their 'gift' to humanity – for, medical time was a thief that took 'who that "*me is*", or the "*you understand*" it to be, as the poet Marianne Boruch reminds us in her poem 'Human Atlas' that opened Part II of this book.[77]

Scientists hold that individual contributions and their hidden histories do not change the overall picture of medical progress. But how can we know this for certain about bio-commons, if we have never had the human information to look at properly in the first place? And what happens to us as human beings when we lose sight of each part of a whole story? Thus, Edward Thompson reminded us how the value of social history to science is a renewed sense of our 'collective conscience'. It ensures we do not lose historical sight of life stories 'of as many people as possible and as many ways of being in the world' that represent 'the complexity and content of human experiences in the past to the readership of the present', so that medical ethics are the 'engine of our collective maturity' (refer, also Chapter 7).[78] This again echoes Kwame Anthony Appiah's recent lecture as part of the Reith Lecture series for the BBC in 2016: 'Although our ancestors are powerful in shaping our attitudes to the past' and we need to always be mindful of this, we equally 'should always be in active dialogue with the past' to stay engaged with what we have done and why.[79] It is still very difficult to be engaged in, for instance, systems biology or the cultural impact of precision medicine in a meaningful way if its research processes are a disaggregated series of discrete research steps never mapped to maintain a sense of human connectedness.[80] For when deadlines shift – as they do often with biotechnology – the 'gift' recedes, farther and farther from public view. Many insist bio-commons is the price we all pay for medical progress – but it has become one with negative aspects too that require regular historical scrutiny. In organ donation today, we can observe a convincing business case for not acting as we once did in the recent past. Medical science is still miscommunicating with donor families because in neglecting the female demography of dissection in the 1990s, we overlooked a gender bias in the underlying data. Consequently, we have lost sight of misperceptions and misunderstandings that HTA2004 tried to redress but did not necessarily resolve. In Chapter 5, we thus move on to rediscover the pivotal role that the Coronial Office has played in disputing deadlines.

Notes

1. *Punch* often featured satirical cartoons about the financial ruin of a London fog. In, by way of example, 'Various & lemon feature, Mark [Editor] facts for foreigners', *Punch, or the London Charivari*, XXXVIII (18 February 1860), p. 71, it mocked stockbrokers in the city of London that would trade even the thin air of a winter fog if they thought they could profit by it. *Punch* too condemned 'foggy fortune-tellers' that misled those who could afford it least. The queues at soup kitchens and the number of pauper graves in the capital were, editorials pointed out, 'a sad testament to lives ruined by the stress and strife of swindlers'.
2. Charles Dickens highlighted the impact of London fog on graveyards. In *Little Dorrit* (London: Bradbury and Evans Publisher, 1857), he spoke of foggy weather hazards and in *Household Words* he criticised undertakers who exploited the poor unable to afford their wares, forced to sell loved ones for dissection under the cover

of a London fog at night to avoid the public shame of lacking money for a pauper burial.

3. Letters, *Daily Telegraph*, Tuesday, 9 December 1952; see also 'The fog-catcher', BBC News, 2 December 2016, https://www.bbc.co.uk/news/av/magazine-3817520 2/the-fog-catcher-who-brings-water-to-the-poor – featured an intriguing magazine item about an engineer in Peru who is using large fog-nets designed to trap water vapour found in the humidity of fog to turn it into a freshwater supply for the poorest in Lima. Modern science could yet learn from skilled engineers how to handle fog!

4. B. Luckin, 'Demographic, social and cultural parameters of environmental crisis: the great London smoke fogs in the late 19th and early 20th centuries', in C. Bernhardt and G. Massard-Guilbaud (eds.), *The Modern Demon: Pollution in Urban and Industrial European Societies* (Clermont-Ferrand: Blaise-Pascal University Press, 2002), pp. 219–238.

5. G. K. Chesterton first highlighted how the British character reflected the seasonal weather patterns in *Alarms and Discursions* (London: Good Reads Ltd, 2016), chapter 18.

6. Theodore Edward Hook, *Maxwell: A Novel* (London: R. Betley & Co, 1834), p. 10, coined the popular term a *pea-souper* for the medical hazards of a London fog.

7. See, by contrast, E. T. Hurren, *Dissecting the Criminal Corpse: Staging Post-Execution Punishment in Early Modern England* (Basingstoke: Palgrave Macmillan, 2016) covering the 1752 to 1832 period, and Hurren, *Dying for Victorian Medicine: English Anatomy and Its Trade in the Dead Poor, c. 1834–1929* (Basingstoke: Palgrave Macmillan, 2012). This Cambridge University Press book completes a trilogy by focussing on the 1930–2000 period of body supply.

8. 'Death of Dr. R. W. Moore, Headmaster Harrow Public School', *Times*, Obituary notice, Monday, 12 January 1953, issue 52517, p. 8.

9. 'Death rate in London fog', *Times*, 31 January 1953, issue 52534, p. 3.

10. Ibid.

11. B. Luckin, 'Pollution in the City', in M. Daunton (ed.), *The Cambridge Urban History of Britain*, volume III, *1840–1950* (Cambridge: Cambridge University Press, 2000), pp. 207–228.

12. *Daily Telegraph*, 9 November 2016, covered these events in 1952 as part of its celebration of the Netflix series *The Crown* detailing the year that Queen Elizabeth II was became monarch. One part in the series is devoted to the 'Great Fog' of 1952.

13. Richard Stone, 'Counting the cost of London's killer smog', *Science*, 298 (13 December 2002), 5601: 2106–2107.

14. All names are anonymised for ethical reasons, even though the parents died in 1984 and 1997, respectively. Extensive record linkage work reconstructs their family history at: St Bartholomew's Hospital Dissection register MS81/5–81/6 (1952) cross-matched to health and coroner's records of the Harperbury Hospital held at the London Metropolitan Archives, Civil Registration Death Index, 1 December 1952 for St Albans Hertfordshire, Electoral Registers for Harrow North West Ward 1945–1965, and The National Archives Census for 1911. Further cross-checking was done on local government archives of the London Borough of Harrow, Greater London Council and Mayor's Office.

15. The father was active for a time in local government and served his North London community (name withheld) in a variety of roles (anonymised here).

16. Refer, also, P. Brimblecombe, 'The Clean Air Act after 50 years', *Weather*, 61 (2006), 11: 311–314; Michelle L. Bell, Davis L. Devra and Tony Fletcher, 'A retrospective assessment of mortality from the London smog episode of 1952: the role of influenza and pollution', *Environmental Health Perspectives*, 112 (January 2004) 1: 6.
17. For an excellent appraisal of wartime arrangements see, K. Waddington, *Medical Education at St. Bartholomew's Hospital 1123–1995* (Woodbridge, Suffolk: Boydell Press, 2003), pp. 316–318.
18. This 'Rising cost of the ambulance service' and the severe ongoing shortages from 1952 to 1954 was reported extensively in the *BMJ*, 17 April 1954, p. 175. It explained that: 'The Ministry of Health has sent a circular (No. 7/54) to all local health authorities in England and Wales notifying them of advisory surveys to be made into all aspects of the ambulance service, because of the rising cost. A limited series of local surveys, covering both the authorities' organization of the ambulance service and the demands made on it by the hospitals, will be carried out by one of the Minister's ambulance advisers and one of his medical officers. Any conclusions reached, together with any recommendations, will be passed on to both the authorities and the hospitals concerned. The rules on the use of local ambulance services are reprinted in an appendix to the circular.'
19. Great Ormond Street specialised in paediatrics, whereas St Bartholomew's had the clinical expertise to treat pneumonia with deep X-ray facilities: a theme we return to below.
20. 'Economy in the use of X-ray film', *British Medical Journal* (8 December 1951): 255, column 1.
21. See, notably, on this trend, T. Cutler, 'Dangerous yardstick? Early cost estimates and the politics of financial management in the first decade of the National Health Service', *Medical History*, 47 (2003) II: 217–238.
22. Refer, W. H. Gattie and T. H. Holt-Hughes, 'Note on the Mental Deficiency Act, 1913', *The Law Quarterly Review*, 30 (1914): 202–209, quote at p. 202. The new legislation repealed the Idiots Act (49 Vict. c. 25: 1886).
23. *Kelly's Directory for Hertfordshire and St. Albans* (1937), entry on the 'Middlesex Colony'; also referred to in, Kevin Brown, *Harperbury Hospital from Colony to Closure, 1928–2001* (Hertfordshire: Harper House Publications, 2001).
24. See, http://www.hertfordshire-genealogy.co.uk/data/topics/t070-long-stay-hospitals.htm, accessed 15/11/2016. Within the NHS there was a county reorganisation in 1948 for budgets reasons, and those hospitals situated on the borders of Middlesex were transferred to Hertfordshire Health Authority.
25. In TAB's case, it has not been possible to trace either a death notice in the local papers for a funeral or the advertisement of a protracted cremation ceremony, staged fourteen months later. Usually, St Bartholomew's offered to pay the costs of burial for those in destitution, but the AB family were not in poverty. Robert Hogg, the undertaker in the employ of St Bartholomew's and Guy's hospitals, did the interment once the dissection, teaching and further research were finished. By the 1950s, grieving relatives often preferred a cremation, and this might explain the lack of church or humanist funeral. It would also explain how two parents managed their grief in their local community when they did not have the physical shell to bury but

could plan for a cremation and scattering of the ashes privately. Regrettably, no family papers, or correspondence, survive to substantiate the material facts of a funeral.

26. *Supplement to the British Medical Journal*, 17 April 1954, covered all the recommendations of the Annual Conference in detail, see p. 163 for quote, death certifications recommendations that numbered pp. 153–156 inclusive. The General Medical Committee Conference was the annual event for the Representatives of the Annual Conference of Local Medical Committees.

27. *Supplement to the British Medical Journal*, 1 November 1952, Letter to the Editor page, 'A. Piney, London WI on 'Pathologists' fees for coroners' necropsies', p. 179.

28. St Bartholomew's dissection registers, MS81/5–81/6, annotated for 1 July 1947.

29. See, Hurren, *Dying for Victorian Medicine*, on the payment system under the New Poor Law 1832–1929.

30. See, for example, Leicester Medical School, Body Donation Programme, Public Information Sources at https://cms.le.ac.uk//medicine/about/body-donation-programme

31. C. Neville, G. Oswald Simon and R. A. Shooter, 'Pneumonia in hospital practice', *British Journal of Diseases of the Chest*, 55 (3 July 1961), 3: 109–118, all working on a research study from clinical cases at or connected to St Bartholomew's Hospital.

32. Ibid.

33. For a modern surgical assessment of its effectiveness as a treatment today, see, Shearwood McClelland and Robert R. Maxwell, 'Hemispherectomy for intractable epilepsy in adults: the first reported series', *Annals of Neurology*, 61 (2007), 4: 372–376.

34. See, for instance, H. H. Fleischhacker, 'Hemispherectomy', *The British Journal of Psychiatry*, 418 (January 1954), 100: 66–84. Later Shenley in the 1960s would become a leading centre for epigenetics.

35. On the early history of the site see, Euan C. Roger, 'Blakberd's treasure: a study in 15th century administration at St. Bartholomew's Hospital London', in Linda Clark (ed.), *The Fifteen Century XIII: Exploring the Evidence: Commemoration, Administration and Economy* (Woodbridge, Suffolk: Boydell Press), pp. 81–109.

36. For a comprehensive history of trends, see, Waddington, *Medical Education*, p. 7.

37. Ibid.

38. Waddington, *St. Bartholomew's Hospital*.

39. See, Hurren, *Dying for Victorian Medicine*, chapter 4.

40. See, for example, Julie-Marie Strange, *Death, Grief and Poverty in Britain, 1870–1914* (Cambridge: Cambridge University Press, 2006).

41. See, E. T. Hurren, *Dissecting the Criminal Corpse: Staging Post-Execution Punishment in Early Modern England* (Basingstoke: Palgrave Macmillan, 2016), supply rates and their geography are detailed in chapter 5.

42. Name anonymised, St Bartholomew's Hospital Dissection register MS81/5–81/6.

43. See for example, J. B. Marshall, 'Tuberculosis of the gastrointestinal tract and peritoneum', *American Journal of Gastroenterol*, 88 (1993) 7: 989.

44. Geoffrey Gorer, *Exploring English Character* (New York: Criterion Books, 1955), p. 17.

45. Editorial, *The Lancet* (1949): 740–741.
46. Refer, John N. Mason, *Mayday Hospital Croydon, 1885–1985: A History of a Century of Service* (London: Croydon Health Authority, 1986).
47. Name anonymised, St. Bartholomew's Hospital Dissection register MS81/5–81/6.
48. Ibid.
49. Diane Jarvis, 'Is Croydon University Hospital's nickname "MayDie" a fair reality', *Sutton and Croydon Guardian*, News section, 7 November 2013, p. 1.
50. Name anonymised, St Bartholomew's Hospital Dissection register MS81/5–81/6.
51. See, 'Closure of Banstead Hospital', *Lancet*, 328 (15 November 1986), 8516: 1160–1161. HMP High Down prison opened for Category A prisoners in 1992. In 1989, a separate prison known as HMP Downview opened on the site of the old nurses' home for Category C prisoners. In 1999 it then became a closed prison for women before being refurbished again as a young offenders' juvenile unit for those jailed aged 15 to 18 years old, from 2004. See, http://ezitis.myzen.co.uk/banstead.html, accessed 6/12/2016.
52. Name anonymised, St Bartholomew's Hospital Dissection register MS81/5–81/6.
53. Niall McCrae and Peter Nolan, *The Story of Nursing in British Mental Hospitals: Echoes from the Corridors* (London: Routledge 2016) provides useful comparative histories that show Banstead was representative of trends elsewhere.
54. See, 'The lost hospitals of London', accessed 6/12/2016 at: http://ezitis.myzen.co.uk/banstead.html,
55. For a history of these clinical trends, see, Richard D. Tonkin, *Lecture Notes on Gastroenterology – Compiled Whilst Consultant Physician at the Mayday Hospital Croydon* (Oxford & Edinburgh: Blackwell Scientific Publications, 1968) and refer, again, for quotations, 'The lost hospitals of London', accessed 6/12/2016 at: http://ezitis.myzen.co.uk/banstead.html
56. A point made convincingly by Waddington, *Medical Education*, chapter 1, and Victoria Bates, 'Yesterday's doctors: the human aspects of medical education in Britain. 1957–1993', *Medical History*, 61 (2017) 1: 48–65.
57. Refer, *St. Joseph's Hospice: Our History*, accessed 26/6/2016 at: https://www.stjh.org.uk/about-us/our-history
58. Name anonymised, St. Bartholomew's Hospital Dissection register MS81/5–81/6.
59. Name anonymised, St. Bartholomew's Hospital Dissection register MS81/5–81/6.
60. Name anonymised, St. Bartholomew's Hospital Dissection register MS81/5–81/6.
61. Name anonymised, St. Bartholomew's Hospital Dissection register MS81/5–81/6.
62. United Medical and Dental Schools of Guy's and St Thomas' hospitals London including Royal Dental Hospital of London that all merged again into King's College Hospital post-1998.
63. For instance, there was a ratio of 3 men to 1 woman under the New Poor Law from 1834 to 1929 sent for dissection in London; see, Hurren, *Dying for Victorian Medicine*, chapter 4 and conclusion.
64. 'A strategy for delivering a revolution in public behaviour in relation to organ donation', prepared by 23red for NHS Blood & Transplant, pp. 1–63, accessed 6/12/2016 at: https://nhsbtdbe.blob.core.windows.net/umbraco-assets-corp/4254/nhsbt_organ_donation_public_behaviour_change_strategy-2.pdf
65. Ibid., p. 9.
66. Refer footnote 64, above, p. 18.

67. See, for example, 'Lunch with the FT, Professor Richard Thaler, Nobel Laureate talks to Tom Harford – If you want people to do something, make it easy', *Financial Times Weekend*, Life and Arts section, 3 August/ 4 August 2019, p. 3.

68. Name anonymised, St. Bartholomew's Hospital Dissection register MS81/5–81/6.

69. Ibid.; I am very grateful to Dr Paul Lazarus for assisting me with these details at the Medical Centre, University of Leicester.

70. BBC News, for instance, on 15 February 2017 led with the report 'Air pollution "final warning" from the European Commission to the UK', based on findings that 'more than 400,000 people were dying prematurely each year across major cities in the UK and Europe from car pollution and its respiratory conditions', accessed 20/02/2017 at: http://www.bbc.co.uk/news/uk-politics-38980510

71. See, for example, A. Tomkins and S. A. King, *The Poor in England, 1700–1850: An Economy of Makeshifts* (Manchester: Manchester University Press, 2003).

72. Peter Halewood, 'On commodification and self-ownership', *Yale Journal of Law & the Humanities*, 20 (2008), 2: 131–162, quote at p. 132.

73. Argued convincingly in, Yuval Noah Harari, *Homo Deus: A Brief History of Tomorrow* (London: Harvill Secker Press, 2016), pp. 1–2.

74. See, for example, Elizabeth Schweiger, 'The risks of remaining silent: international law formation and the EU silence on drone killings', *Global Affairs*, 1 (2015) 3: 269–275.

75. Refer, notably, K. D. M. Snell, 'The rise of living alone and loneliness in history', *Social History*, 42 (2017) 1: 2–28.

76. Halewood, 'On commodification and self-ownership', p. 140.

77. Marianne Boruch, 'Human Atlas', in *Cadaver, Speak* (Port Townsend, Wash.: Copper Canyon Press, 2014), p. 43.

78. E. P. Thompson, *The Making of the English Working Class* (London: Penguin Books, 2002), introduction; also cited in more recently and of relevance to this book, McCrae and Nolan, *The Story of Nursing in British Mental Hospitals*, preface, p. 2.

79. Professor Kwame Anthony Appiah, Chair of Philosophy and Law at New York University, Lecture 1, 'Creed', *Mistaken Identities*, BBC Reith Lectures (2016), at: www.bbc.co.uk/programmes/articles/2sM4D6LTTVlFZhbMpmfYmx6/kwame-anthony-appiah; review by Gillian Reynolds, 'How this year's Reith lecturer broke new ground', *Daily Telegraph*, 19 October 2016, p. 32, column 1.

80. A point made forcibly by Denis Noble, *The Music of Life: Biology beyond the Genome* (Oxford: Oxford University Press, 2006).

5   Explicit Disputes
'The Balance of Probability' in Coronial Cases

On 6 December 1962, a *Daily Mail* headline announced: '12 People get notes from a Dead Man'. The newspaper article explained how a suicide victim had sent a letter outlining his decision to take his life 'to his solicitors, his accountant, his bank manager, his next door neighbour, relatives and friends, a coroner and even the police'. Mr Herbert Jones, aged 77, resided in Southcliffe Road in Christchurch, Hampshire. He worked as a Borough engineer for his local council. Shortly after retirement, he was diagnosed with a terminal illness and his note explained that:

> *The necessity for hospital treatment is obviously becoming more and more imminent. I feel, however, unable to face the liability of causing so much inconvenience to a number of people, especially at this time of year, and so having the firm belief that my life is entirely my own responsibility, I have decided to end it by asphyxia. I am sorry to inflict this on you. . . . I wish to leave my body to Bristol University for research* [sic].[1]

His neighbour Mr Reginald Wells explained to a *Daily Mail* reporter that the eloquence of the suicide note was typical of the deceased: 'He was that sort of man, orderly, quiet and unselfish. He hated being a trouble to people.' Further police enquiries established that Mr Jones had bought his family home, in which he committed suicide, for his only son. Sadly, the son had died a few months earlier, though the circumstances were not elaborated in the press. Jones had, according to neighbours, been bereft because he faced a double bereavement. His wife had died the year before in April 1961. Like Francis Partridge in Chapter 3, Herbert Jones was unable to cope with the pain of being both a widower and bereaved parent. Diagnosed as suffering from an incurable medical condition, he saw no reason to go on. Grief and memories did not outweigh his rationale that the quality of his life had been fundamentally diminished. An Inquest concluded that suicide was a measured decision. Jones wanted to cause the least disruption to medical staff at Christmas.[2] Yet, ironically, the last request in his suicide note was to cause a lot of official consternation. As a *Daily Mail* reporter explained: 'Mr. Jones's last wish – to give his body to science – cannot be granted. The coroner has ordered a post-mortem.' This simple statement published as a byline to the headline story

150

exposed an explicit body dispute – on twelve prior occasions Jones had expressed in writing his explicit wishes to donate his body to medical research, which the coroner had the powers to countermand. As we shall see, this situation was in fact common because of the longevity of the powers, and ingrained procedural flaws, of the Coronial Office in the modern era: the central focus of this chapter.

Essentially, therefore, this fifth chapter is about these sorts of explicit disputes concerning the power and control over the dead body, body ethics and the boundaries and limits of professional practice, involving the official figure of the coroner. The chapter is thus split into two halves. In the first half we will encounter a brief history of the Coronial Office in England, before then engaging with a series of stories about explicit body disputes involving specific coroners. We will be focussing on the symbolic story of a dead girl called Carol Morris because the circumstances of her harvested human material proved to be very controversial. Her case exemplifies why tracking the material journeys of post-mortem bodies and their body parts matters in hidden histories of the dead. The details are lengthier than others presented so far in this book but that is because it was to be legally a very significant case. Thus, in the second half of the chapter, we explore why one human story is a historical prism for lots of others, and how micro-history can inform macro-trends of considerable longevity. In fact, as we shall see, the Carol Morris case made a significant contribution to establishing the legal precedent of anonymity for all donors in national and international law. Today, this remains in place, and we will be reflecting on the status quo of that standard of medical ethics, since the story behind its legal precedent is not known in the literature.

In other words, we will be asking: Does knowing the human circumstances of such cases change the way we view the ownership of the body once we know more about explicit body disputes, and what exactly were the long-term medico-legal ramifications of these stories that we have seldom thought about in the modern era of scientific achievement because they were neglected in the archives? In order not to dissect the storylines in the way that bodies were dissected and disassembled routinely inside the medical research community, with their human stories subsumed into a bio-commons, we will be looking in a little more detail this time at all the human factors and facets involved in the chosen representative cases. This means that the reader might wish to pause after the chapter's first half, before discovering in the second half of this lengthier chapter the universal lessons that can be drawn from the newly discovered source material and the reasons for their historical longevity.

Our central analytical focus therefore is the palette and power exercised by coroners once a dead body was in their jurisdiction, despite explicit body disputes that were being generated between medico-legal officials and grieving relatives wanting to fulfil their loved ones' dying wishes. It is also the case that in a transplant era the technical ability to harvest organs brought the Coronial Office into open conflict with the medical sciences. Historians of medicine have only very recently begun to examine these professional stand-offs through detailed case study, with most accounts still overly reliant on broad brush central government papers.[3] Meanwhile, the lack of efficiency of the Coronial Office meant that important evidence about causes of death on coroners' death certificates got lost inside the systems of forensic medicine and pathology, which should have been a 'treasure trove of information'. Instead 'real causes of death' remained 'hidden because of indifferent post-mortem examinations' conducted hastily and which were often 'obscured by deficient recording of data'.[4] That common situation did not come to full public attention until the publication of the *National Confidential Enquiry into Patient Outcome and Death* in 2006 (hereafter NCEPOD). The National Patient Safety Agency commissioned the NCEPOD report into the professional conduct of the Coronial service because there were serious misgivings about its extensive powers of retention. It concluded that the system of certified autopsies had structural flaws throughout the twentieth century. Paradoxically, the history of explicit body disputes co-ordinated by the Coronial Office was one of many missed research opportunities for biomedicine too. We begin therefore with a short overview of the history of the Coronial Office in England.

Part I

The Coronial Office in Context

The history of the Coronial Office in England is one of slow expansion from the twelfth to early nineteenth centuries, during which the majority of coroners were legally, rather than medically, qualified.[5] On average in England, they consistently dealt with about 5 per cent of all reported deaths from the early modern to modern period. Their main official responsibility was to investigate 'unnatural deaths' in the community. They did so by sifting gossip, and retrieving any relevant physical evidence at the scene of a death until foul play could be ruled out, or not. Coroners were under legal instruction, however, to wait until a suspicious death was reported to them. They had no official powers to investigate an unusual death. Legislation did not permit them to act just because they suspected that an unnatural or violent act of some description had occurred in their area of authority. Once, however, a suspicious death was reported officially to them and they had retrieved a dead body in their jurisdiction, they had a great deal of discretionary power. They could, for instance, decide how much to cut open the deceased or to leave the body intact. Each coroner could also waive the need for an Inquest if a cause of death in their opinion was obvious at a suicide or the scene of an accident at work or in the home. In this way, Coronial justice was often 'remade from the margins' because it involved a lot of discretionary powers of decision-making delegated to individual coroners.[6]

In suspicious circumstances, coroners have always been required to co-ordinate a 'view of the body'.[7] Normally from the thirteenth to the early twentieth century, this occurred within twelve hours of death. It involved calling a jury to service, composed of up to twelve local ratepayers respected for their social standing. The jury would congregate at a public house or another convenient place such as a gaol room or town hall. Here, a coroner's assistant laid out the dead and jury members undertook a visual inspection of the deceased, looking for flesh wounds and suspicious bruising. This autopsy meant literally looking at the external appearances during the 'view of the body'. At it, the coroner gave a verbal report that summarised for those assembled the physical evidence-gathering and general gossip garnered in the community. The jury under the coroner's direction would then assess the circumstances surrounding the unexplained death and arrive at a verdict before releasing the body for burial. Disinterring bodies after Inquest was rare, even with new subsequent evidence. In the early Victorian era, formaldehyde replaced mummification and alcohol preservation of the body and tissues, respectively. Even so, it was hazardous to hold on to a corpse for long; contamination by contagious diseases, like cholera or diphtheria, was common. The smell of formaldehyde was also difficult to stomach and thus at the 'view of the body' chemicals tended to distort lingering synaesthesia impressions. The aim was thus to look quickly and get the body buried as soon as possible. By the 1880s, French morgues were introducing refrigeration techniques, and soon this was copied everywhere across Europe by the early twentieth century.[8] Before then, it was vital for English coroners to conduct efficient enquiries in the thirty-six hours after death before the human material started to decompose. Putrefaction devalued human material from a forensic standpoint.

English coroners were under instructions to conduct themselves according to the legal principle of 'the balance of probability'.[9] In other words, provided the available evidence seemed to indicate that a death 'probably' looked 'natural', then the coroner had the discretion to pass a verdict without the need for an expensive Inquest. In the case of a drowning, this would be a suicide verdict, by way of example. Coroners were not required in law to prove that someone was guilty of causing that death. Nor did they need to abide by the legal stipulation that the accused was innocent until proven guilty in a court of law. Their role was to establish that neither manslaughter nor homicide was suspected, and, if it was, to refer on that serious matter to the local forces of law and order to investigate further and arrest the culprit. In which case, if it looked like a capital charge might go to the Quarter Sessions court, the coroner was duty-bound to ask a surgeon to perform a post-mortem on the dead body and report back to an Inquest jury.

From the 1830s, and following a concerted campaign in the *Lancet*, coroners slowly started to be medically qualified.[10] They also tended to adopt standard post-mortem methods. Generally, this involved making a crucial incision from the neck to the naval, and across the chest cavity.[11] An appointed surgeon would handle the heart and major organs, as well as closely examine the brain, for any suspected violent injuries. Coroners might also call additional medical witnesses who had the requisite expertise in, say, the forensics of poisoning to establish a death by misadventure.[12] Likewise, an 'unnatural' cause of death could have been caused by a stabbing or a drunken brawl that got out of control. In which case, they could call on a medical man with a lot of experience in doing post-mortem examinations for high-profile cases tried at the Old Bailey in London. If subsequently at an Inquest a verdict of 'murder' was based on reliable medical evidence, the coroner would refer the matter to the appropriate legal authorities, and the dead person would be buried without further delay.[13]

The role of the coroner has always involved a very visual method of working. Looking at the surface of the body was important before medical science had X-ray technology, CT and MRI scans. There is therefore a long art history of the Coronial Office because such visual methods interested artists trained in life drawing who liked to sketch and paint dead bodies, and thus record coroners' working-lives. For this reason, it is feasible to trace their broad development from the early nineteenth to early twentieth centuries through the medium of iconography. In Illustration 5.1, for instance, we see a typical satirical cartoon mocking the bumptious nature of the Coronial Office from the 1820s when arguments started to be made about the need to have medically, rather than just legally qualified coroners. The image thus lampoons an inept and legally qualified coroner who has little expertise in the metabolic mysteries of medical death. In this case, we can observe a blazing fire that may have warmed up a body, seemingly dead, but capable of resuscitation. To the disquiet of the surgeon on duty, it appears that the post-mortem he has been called in to perform in his clean pale apron might involve human vivisection. He wants to halt proceedings at the 'view of the body' because the so-called victim has in fact started to wake up. If the surgeon continues to cut the body in front of the assembled jury, he would be breaking the Hippocratic Oath 'to do no harm'. Even so, the Coroner insists he carry on:

Surgeon [dressed in a yellow frock coat and apron] informs the Coroner: *'The man's alive. Sir, for he has opened one eye'.*

Coroner [dressed in wig & dark coat and depicted as fat from his office fees] replies by deploying his discretionary justice: *'Sir, the doctor declar'd him Dead two hours since & so he must remain Dead Sir'*

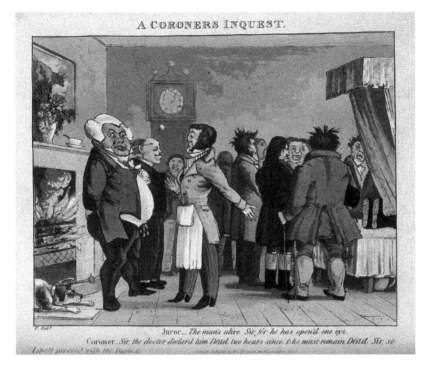

A CORONERS INQUEST.

Juror__ *The man's alive Sir for he has open'd one eye.*
Coroner__*Sir the doctor declar'd him Dead two hours since & he must remain Dead Sir, so*
I shall proceed with the Inquest.

Illustration 5.1 ©Wellcome Images, Reference Number V0010903, *A Juror Protesting that the subject of the Coroner's Inquest is alive; showing the dangers of blind faith in doctors when declaring medical death* – Coloured aquatint by Thomas McLean, 26 The Haymarket, London, c. 1826, copyright cleared under creative commons Attribution Non-Commercial Share Alike 4.0 International, reproduced here under (CC BY-NC-SA, 4.0), authorised for open access, and non-profit making for academic purposes only.

By the late nineteenth century, the Coronial Inquest was held in private, away from prying eyes in a specially designed morgue. Seldom were the jury present by this time. Reporting the facts of forensic science at an Inquest court became accepted practice. Cutting the corpse involved hence a close working partnership behind closed doors between coroners, pathologists and anatomists working in tandem. We see this typical situation in Illustration 5.2. A coroner handed over a man to the St Bartholomew's Hospital dissection room who died a 'natural death'. The coroner had the discretion to rule that the death was obvious as the man died in the care of the Poor Law authorities and thus there was no need for an expensive Inquest. On 7 July 1894, when the corpse

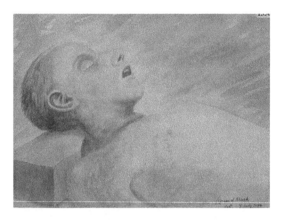

Illustration 5.2 ©Wellcome Images, Reference Number L0062513,
Watercolour drawing done by Leonard Portal Mark on 7 July 1894, depicting
the face and chest of a man (unnamed) to show the appearance caused by rapid
post-mortem decomposition. It was made about twelve hours after death,
during the hot weather of July 1894 at St Bartholomew's Hospital dissection
room, copyright cleared under creative commons Attribution Non-
Commercial Share Alike 4.0 International, reproduced here under (CC BY-
NC-SA, 4.0), authorised for open access, and non-profit making for academic
purposes only.

arrived, an artist skilled in pathology sketched the face and chest of the
friendless man in order to study the nature of decomposition, represented
here with the grey-scale area of shading, spreading down the right side of his
torso, in reality a blue hue. The weather was hot at mid-summer and this
accelerated putrefaction, despite the corpse being injected via the carotid artery
with formaldehyde to replace bodily fluids over a forty-eight-hour period.

Further record linkage work from data previously collected by this author
confirms that the corpse was that of William Smith, aged 64, who died in
Islington Infirmary at Highgate Hill, North London.[14] Supplied by a Poor
Law dead house, he was dissected, then buried. Initially the coroner concluded from a visual examination of the body that William Smith the pauper
had died from a common disease of poverty, namely 'phthisis' [tuberculosis].
This made his body ideal for study because it came into the dissection room
without extensive post-mortem cuts. We can thus observe in Illustration 5.2
how the head supported by a brick has no lancet marks on the chest, where
normally a crucial incision happened at autopsy. In other words, this is
exactly the sort of supply mechanism that coroners were co-ordinating with
medical schools on a regular basis and it placed the Coronial Office at the

forefront of the expansion of medical education in the growing Victorian information state.[15] In total, anatomists dissected William Smith for '250 days' until 11 March 1895. His remaining body parts were interred into a shared pauper grave, next to six other bodies. This status quo was to remain largely intact for the poorest people in society at the behest of coroners even after WWII.

In a third image, Illustration 5.3, we glimpse the modern situation during the late twentieth century. Instead of the coroner conducting a post-mortem in-tandem, the forensic examination has now been delegated entirely to a hospital pathologist. We can observe the cross-like pencil lines of the crucial incision down and across the torso. The equipment is sterile and resembles the design of an operating theatre, rather than an old

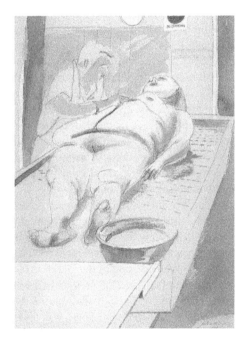

Illustration 5.3 ©Wellcome Images, Reference Number L0029414, 'Royal Liverpool University Hospital: a pathologist cutting open a body in the mortuary', original drawing on site by Julia Midgley, Liverpool, 1998, artwork dimensions 42 x 29.7cm, copyright cleared under creative commons Attribution Non-Commercial Share Alike 4.0 International, reproduced here under (CC BY-NC-SA, 4.0), authorised for open access, and non-profit making for academic purposes only.

late-Victorian morgue. There is a basin at the foot of the steel table to collect the major organs and any tissue samples retained for further pathological study or transplant surgery. Notice, too, the ridges on the steel table to scrub down the equipment after each post-mortem. The pathologist likewise wears surgical gloves and a disposable apron. To the rear are the large refrigeration units that keep the body fresh. Here there is little physical indication of putrefaction of the sort seen in Illustration 5.2. The coroner's role is cleaned up, with the aid of biotechnology. The facial identities of both the pathologist and the body on the dissection table are indistinct: anonymity is an ethical choice here, but it also distances medical science from human stories and their hidden histories.

Further record linkage work confirms that at the Royal Liverpool University Hospital in the 1990s this unnamed body in Illustration 5.3 was one of nineteen bequests (see Chapter 4, Table 4.3) that passed into the official ownership of the medical sciences. Its donation point was coordinated and delegated to a pathologist on duty via the Liverpool Coronial Office. This third image is hence the logical expression of a century of scientific co-operation – by coroners, the forensic sciences, pathologists and dissection rooms – in order to cement professional status. It represents what happened to Mr Herbert Jones in our opening story too. The coroner for south Hampshire examined his body; a hospital duty pathologist confirmed the cause of death; but there was no further dissection at Bristol medical school. The coroner had the discretionary justice to decide otherwise in an explicit dispute about the deadline and its dead-end of life: one of many cases we will be encountering in this chapter.

One of the main reasons the coroner did not send Mr Herbert Jones automatically for dissection was that at the time of his death old legislation outlawing suicide had recently been changed. To allow for suicide (no longer illegal) but prevent euthanasia (still illegal), the coroner was now legally obliged to make sure that nobody else was involved in the decision of the victim to take his life, even those patients facing an imminent fatal medical prognosis: a context from 1962 that still occupies policy-makers today. The Suicide Act (9 & 10 Eliz. 2 c. 60: 1961) had only recently legalised 'self-murder'. There was thus extensive debate in the press and medical journals at the time whether 'doctors should prolong dying or not'.[16] Debates about what constituted medical euthanasia appeared often in the media. Against that liberalisation of suicide backdrop, it remained, however, still illegal to assist an individual dying from a fatal prognosis in making the decision to end their life, termed 'complicity in suicide'. According to Section 2 of the Act, which still remains in force in Britain: 'A person who aids, abets, counsels or procures the suicide of another, or attempt by another to commit suicide shall be liable on conviction on indictment to imprisonment for a term not exceeding fourteen years.' Legally this can result in a charge of 'conspiracy' in 'assisted dying'. The twelve letters that Mr Herbert Jones penned to his bank, legal representative, coroner, police and neighbours seem, therefore, to have been some sort of legal safeguard to make sure that this eventuality was ruled out at Inquest. The paper trail implied that he alone made the decision to commit suicide and donate his body to medical research. He was a careful and meticulous man, and thus his actions were in character. Even so, the coroner was sensitive to what amounted to his first case of this sort of suicide situation under the new legal guidelines. He acted conservatively, investigating the full circumstances of death and the 'gift relationship' attached to it. Using his discretionary powers, he ordered a post-mortem to clarify Coronial Office guidance, as to:

- Whether the action which caused the death was done deliberately
- Whether the intended consequence of the action was their death
- If the individual did not intend to take the action, their death may have resulted from an 'accident' to be recorded by the coroner's verdict
- If the individual action was deliberate but the consequence was not intended to be fatal, then the coroner should record 'a verdict of misadventure'
- If the individual's intention was unclear, the short-form conclusion by the coroner would be an 'open' verdict[17]

In other words, legally coroners could recommend verdicts according to the 'balance of probability'; in practice, suicide and its assistance (or not) made it imperative for the coroner to dispute Herbert Jones's explicit wishes.

Complicating this situation was the fact that the coroner was also working with another important context, and one of material significance to the eventual destination of the cadaver in this sad case. Herbert Jones self-evidently wanted to bequest his body to medical research. But whether it was suitable for donation or not could be disputed by those the coroner might decide to hand the corpse over to. If the cancer about to kill Herbert Jones riddled his dying body, then in death this made it of less material use for anatomical teaching. In which case, the body would be sent for cremation without delay once the coroner passed his verdict. If, however, the specific cancer was of research interest to medical science, then parts of the body and human tissue could still be used in part for further patho-logical study. Another alternative is that if the body did not have significant secondary tumours, but a key organ had deteriorated to such an extent that it threatened a patient's life, then 'parts of' that dead body were still a very useful teaching and medical research resource. In other words, in hidden histories of the dead, the coroner had a very important role indeed to play in starting off the post-mortem after-life of human material that came into the Coronial Office jurisdic-tion: a factor seldom traced in the archives, and one which we will be elaborating on later when we encounter the detailed case of Carol Morris. In the meantime, the critical point to appreciate at this point in this chapter's developing argument is that the type of Inquest ordered, given the diseased condition of the dead body, mattered a lot to its eventual destination for harvesting. Coroners typically faced two competing tensions in this situation – how much the pathologist *should* cut to complete death certification procedures and how a coroner *could* prioritise anatomists' need for a clean corpse to dissect.

There is one final operational issue that many coroners had to work with. Most experienced moral pressure from grieving families to alter upsetting suicide rulings. Coroners thus typically recorded 'accident', 'misadventure' and 'open' verdicts on death certificates. In other words, disputed bodies were contested sites of multiple research agendas and reflected family sensitivities. That said, in Mr Jones's case his wife and son had pre-deceased him. He died without family involvement. This case's explicit body dispute was thus exclusively between the coroner and a dead person: the former over-ruled the latter because the dead, as we saw in Chapter 2, are *Res Nullius – Nobody's Thing*. Herbert Jones's post-mortem was thus akin to those of Keith Simpson, a leading pathologist who told the *Listener* magazine in 1977 that for all pathologists: 'My patients never complain to me. If their illness is perplexing, I can put them in the refrigerator and come back later on.'[18] Silent conversations in cold storage facilitated the medical sciences co-creating with the Coronial Office; yet these actor networks and their working arrangements remain opaque in the historical literature. Explicit body disputes involving those such as Herbert Jones sent for cremation rather than further study remain too often undisclosed in the paper trail of a bureaucracy that made these 'mechanisms of body donation' both function and malfunction. It is to this paper trail that we now turn. We begin by examining first some of the common systemic flaws in the system that processed and recycled the dead.

Auditing a System with Systemic Flaws

At the various public enquiries into the NHS organ retention scandals that led to HTA2004, a considerable weight of evidence was presented that the paper trail relating to dead bodies and co-ordinated by coroners, pathologists, anatomists or medical researchers was inadequate. At the time, the Chief Medical Officer Sir Liam Donaldson concluded that it was essential to carry out a full audit of all human material held in medical schools and Coronial facilities, as well as museums, to ascertain the extent of both historical and recent retentions. In a previous chapter we briefly discussed how the final report revealed that there were '105,000 organs, body parts and fetuses that had been retained in 210 English NHS trusts and medical schools'.[19] Of these 210, 'around 25 leading institutions accounted for nearly 90% of the body parts retained'. Michael Redfern QC, who conducted a separate public enquiry into organ retention involving the nuclear industry, likewise concluded there was: 'a weak and poorly understood legal framework that had allowed bad practice to flourish'.[20] It was difficult not to reach the conclusion that medical scientists of all descriptions had intentionally kept patients and their families in the dark. In response, the Royal College of Pathologists issued a statement defending their position and proposing to conduct an extensive internal investigation into working practices. Even so, a concerted press campaign reported on how some pathologists with the co-operation of coroners had conducted 'their business by stealth'. This use of emotive language to describe medical research as a 'business' drew widespread criticism from inside the medical profession. Many were stung by the quoting of an old English proverb: 'A thief is a thief, whether he steals a diamond, a purse, or a small part of you.' There was soon a cultural stand-off. Yet it was established by a series of timely new historical studies that the term 'business' was an accurate depiction of dissection and its hidden histories, which were closely associated with the Coronial Office and its pathology partners.

The 'business of anatomy' flourished because AA1832 permitted it to do so until HTA2004 became law (see Chapters 1 and 2).[21] However, because the medical sciences had very little historical sense of their own inner workings, the paper trail that was created to make this system of supply function was never retained by those in charge. As a result, when scandals about the retention of human material reached the press, there was a tendency to apportion blame to HTA1961 or HTA1984 without appreciating that AA1832 had stated transparently the need to keep records. The original legislation did have a tracking system for its mechanisms of body supply. Until at least the 1930s this monitored human material much better than any modern legislation, with up to twelve certificates issued each time a body or part moved from source to dissection table. The flaw in the system was that, once audited, usually every three months, destroying paperwork became the norm to avoid unwelcome publicity. Civil servants misunderstood therefore what happened inside the system by the 1950s. They assumed there had never been a system of accountability in the past because they could not find evidence of it when drafting new parliamentary bills. Their modus operandi was thus to tinker with statutes, instead of overhauling them. As a result, histories of anatomy often assume, incorrectly, that AA1832 had no paper trail and audit procedures. The opposite was the case. There was a complex system with detailed paperwork: a classic case of the medical sciences needing to look forward to the past.

The anatomy 'business' was also enterprising and inventive. Staff sought practical solutions to overcome any operational issues in the most pragmatic way; and, it was logical to do so. That status quo reflected the fact that, as Joanna Innes points out, parliamentary statutes for centuries were written with 'a sufficient level of generality to cope with diverse local circumstances'.[22]

From the Georgian era onwards, successive governments drafted legislation in a cursory manner because what was proposed 'often did not commend' itself 'to eighteenth-century Britons'. This meant that when it came to medical reforms, discretionary powers shaped procedures. There was a high degree of discretionary justice deliberately written into 'orders' and 'guidelines' accompanying any new legislation. Coroners soon used those powers to develop close working relationships with anatomists and pathologists. So much so, Coronial officials often made up procedures as they got on with the task in hand. Over time, this created a sense that medical paternalism mattered more than death's customary rituals in Britain. A lack of public accountability had a ripple effect in other parts of the global community too, notably in Canada, Australia, New Zealand and other Commonwealth countries, where the British legislative framework continued to shape medico-legal standards until the 1990s.[23] The odd thing about this backdrop is that AA1832 never intended this outcome.

When the NHS was created in 1948, new legislation gave the impression that teaching hospitals were now meticulous about the retention and disposal of human remains, but this was not always so. One example is illustrative of what could go wrong when procedures in morgues became disorganised. On Friday 14 December 2001, the *Evening Standard* reported on a case where procedures in a teaching hospital went awry. Paperwork was not properly attached to a dead fetus:

A baby has been found dead among hospital laundry in London. Scotland Yard were called just after 5am yesterday after reports of a 'human foetus' at the Laundry in Acre Lane, Brixton. Police are checking which hospitals provide the unit with laundry. One report said the body was that of a foetus of about seven month gestation. They are trying to establish whether the baby was born naturally or as a result of a miscarriage or abortion. A post-mortem will be carried out today.[24]

The *Times* some weeks later, on 13 January 2002, explained the events in more detail:

The body was that of a baby boy, J. K., who had died one hour after being born at Queen Mary's Hospital, Sidcup. He had been born at 23 weeks gestation, some 17 weeks prematurely, his weight at birth having been 1lb 1oz. After death the child had been wrapped in a sheet and taken to the mortuary and placed in a refrigerated drawer. Next to the drawer was a bag for laundry from the mortuary and the wrapped body had accidentally been transferred to the laundry-bag. From there it had been taken to the Sunlight laundry, Brixton and had been put through a boil wash. The father, aged 36, and mother, aged 25, were both named, the latter being a Spanish national who had since returned to Spain to recover.[25]

In reviewing this case, and the circumstances that led to it, Robert Bruce-Chwatt MBBS, MFTM RCPS (Glasg.), Senior FME, Metropolitan Police, concluded that there had been 'an error of omission' in the paperwork process when the fetus was placed in the fridge next to the laundry basket. He did not find 'an error of commission' involving organ and tissue harvesting of the sort practiced at Liverpool Children's Hospital at Alder Hey by Professor Dick van Velzen.[26] The fetus had self-evidently come under the jurisdiction of HTA1984. When it was moved after being stillborn it should have thus been sent to the hospital morgue with the standard paperwork attached to it. But this had been 'mislaid' in 'either theatre, the labour ward, or mortuary, with the soiled laundry'. It is thus a historical prism of the sorts of material anomalies that happened inside the system as soon as the dead were moved from one jurisdiction (hospital ward) to another (morgue, Coronial facility, pathologists' lab). Along the way, parts of the person might be consigned as 'clinical waste' due to carelessness. For in the case under discussion, nobody could explain how exactly the stillbirth was taken out of the refrigerated drawer in the morgue and dropped into the laundry basket by mistake. Something had gone wrong, but who was involved remained undisclosed.

The fetus was found to be '5–6 months old' when examined for forensic purposes, and it now had to be disposed of according to current regulations. But these were not necessarily what the general public would have expected either. There were three legal options. If the stillborn fetus was still intact (it was in fact in a poor state having been through a boil wash in the washing machine), then it came under the Burial Laws Amendment Act (43 & 44 Vict. c. 42: 1880). Where it was instead to be cremated (after its post-mortem), then this would be carried out in accordance with the Cremations Act (15 & 16 Geo. 6 & 1 Eliz. 2 c. 31: 1952).[27] Even so, if the pathologists found the fetus to be incomplete in terms of its identity, and thus its body was, strictly speaking, in parts (again, having been through a double-spin cycle), it was then in law defined as 'clinical waste'. In which case, it could only be disposed of according to the Control of Pollution Act (Eliz. 2 c. 40: 1974), or the Environment Protection Act (Eliz. 2 c. 43: 1990). In other words, there should have been a careful paperwork trail, but it was omitted. All those involved expected the Coronial Office to use its extensive discretionary powers to put things right after a dereliction of duty.

These overlapping agencies and statutes are illustrative of the sorts of misunderstandings that could occur about the bureaucracy attached to the movement of the dead and their disposal in England. It exemplifies how the paperwork attached to the deceased was often delegated by default to the coroner, especially when things went wrong in NHS hospitals. Indeed, as Chapters 1 and 2 pointed out, the central flaw in HTA1961 was that everyone assumed that each hospital owned human material that died on its premises. They thus had the authority to dispose of their mistakes with the help of any coroners and pathologists on duty. Even after HTA1984 tried to correct this, the situation was further complicated by clause 42 of the Coroners Rules (SI 1984

No. 552), which 'expressly provided that no verdict' should be framed in such a way as 'to appear to determine any question of criminal liability on the part of the named person or civil liability'.[28] In other words, even when things went wrong and hospital negligence was self-evident, Coronial rules meant that at a public Inquest there was no legal leeway to name either a negligent medical professional or an NHS facility as substandard. The facility staff might look morally culpable of contributing to a death, but it was not up to the Coronial Office to determine whether this constituted a criminal offence. The *Times* newspaper thus explained that if, for example, a man having a very bad asthma attack died as a result of a severe delay in the arrival of an ambulance, even when there was evidence of medical negligence and an 'unnatural' death, the coroner could not apportion blame.[29] The pathologist doing the post-mortem was correct to state that the deceased had died from '*status asthmaticus*' [a prolonged asthma attack], but whether the circumstances surrounding the death decreased the patient's survival chances or not, and to what extent these constituted 'a lack of care', was open to legal interpretation. Technically in dispute was not 'the cause of death' in such a case, even if the circumstances surrounding the outcome were in doubt. This common situation recurred often during the 1990s in landmark cases like that of *Regina* v. *the Coroner for North Humberside and Scunthorpe* involving a prisoner put on a suicide-watch because he threatened to take his life.[30] Due to a staff shortage, the man went unobserved for periods in his prison cell, and so died of asphyxia. Whether this was, strictly speaking, 'self-neglect' or due to 'a lack of care' was 'blurred'. The question of how long the body should be retained and which parts of it should be taken for a criminal case (or not) remained contentious.

Coroners thus continued to act conservatively and often asked their designated pathologist to remove what 'might possibly' be required to determine 'the balance of probability': a judgement call based on their individual career experiences, as we saw in this chapter's opening story of Mr Herbert Jones. To understand how this complicated medico-legal situation worked in practice, however, it is necessary to examine a broader selection of representative cases than the ones we have encountered so far in this chapter. In each, we can observe a coroner in conflict with those that claimed agency over the dead. The Coronial Office would nonetheless prove to have extensive powers of discretionary justice in the transplant era of the 1970s. The explicit disputes that occurred often exemplified the frustration that bereaved families felt to determine the material fate and resting place of their loved ones. Since this backdrop shaped a political consensus to pass HTA2004 and those new standards were adopted in many parts of the world, a detailed analysis of the role that coroners played in the circumstances that led to a system of informed consent to correct explicit disputes are of some relevance to this book's central focus.

Coroner's Explicit Disputes and Organ Donation
Cards – The Alcock Case

In 1983, the Department of Health and Social Security (hereafter DHSS) had taken a strategic decision to re-launch a national organ donation campaign: outlined briefly in Chapter 2 and now elaborated with human stories here. The Conservative government of Margaret Thatcher was concerned that just 15 per cent of the population were carrying organ donation cards in Britain. As a result, the British Medical Association reported that transplant waiting lists were getting longer. The DHSS commissioned a number of social surveys to measure public opinion. These indicated that NHS patients were broadly in favour of donation, but this cultural trend did not translate into positive action. The DHSS therefore allocated a budget to raise the media profile of carrying organ donation cards, taking out expensive one-page advertisements in the national press. On the eve of the campaign, the actions of a coroner from North Staffordshire brought instead unwelcome publicity about explicit body disputes. The case was to highlight the extensive powers of coroners to requisition and hold on to human material without government or familial interference.

Thus, in December 1983, *The Times* reported on 'a dispute over a Staffordshire coroner's decision to stop the heart of a maintenance fitter being used in a heart transplant operation'. He had been 'killed accidentally' at work.[31] The facts of the story were that:

Mr Graham Alcock, aged 28, a fitter at an excavator factory in Rocester [*sic*], had carried a donor card with him. Before he died last Tuesday, he told his relatives that he wanted his heart and kidneys to be used for transplants.

As a result of the request doctors at the Royal Infirmary in North Staffordshire kept him alive until suitable recipients could be found for the heart and kidneys. Tests were carried out on his organs to match those of patients waiting for a transplant.[32]

Several hours later a 'suitable patient was found at Harefield Hospital in Uxbridge, West London' and an air ambulance was ordered. A helicopter flight was the quickest way to get the donated heart from Staffordshire to London. At the last minute, however, the deputy coroner for Stoke-on-Trent, Mr John Wain, informed the head of the transplant team that he had 'unexpectedly called a halt to the removal of Mr Alcock's heart'. The Coronial Office issued an official statement that 'the pre-existing condition of the deceased's heart might be relevant to the Jury Inquest in due course' and this necessitated halting the transplantation. If the man had an underlying heart complaint, then his employers might be guilty of a breach in health and safety standards at work where he had died from an accident. There could therefore be legal implications from the case and his human material needed to determine liability or not.

The widow of Graham Alcock was upset by this turn of events. She disputed the moral right of the coroner to prevent what her husband had explicitly requested in writing on his organ donation card. Interviewed by David Cross of *The Times* newspaper, she complained 'that the dying wish of her husband had not been honoured'.[33] As she stressed: 'It seems he died in vain.' The rest of her family were also critical of the decision. They thought it was counter-product-ive for the medical sciences. Mrs Dorothy Alcock (mother of the deceased) told the press: 'Many people with organ donor cards could be dismayed that their wishes were not carried out. This has lost them hundreds of donor cards.' Likewise, Mr Ray Alcock, father of the dead man, disputed the coroner's actions, and in calling for a public enquiry declared: 'It seems pointless to carry a donor card if the parents cannot carry out the wishes of their dead son.' The transplant team supported their moral position. However, as a hospital spokesman explained, they had no choice. They had to 'pay attention to what a coroner decided – We cannot argue about it.'[34] The Coronial Office was all-powerful at the dead-end of life: a procedural fact that would be debated extensively in the 1980s, as we shall see later in this chapter when we examine similar representative cases.

The coroner in this case, Mr John Wain, did in fact have a very good reputation for representing people in his local community over his thirty-year career. On his death aged 77 in 2014, after 'a long battle with cancer', the *Stoke Sentinel* described him as 'a much loved character' whose 'life touched many in Staffordshire'.[35] He was regarded as fair-minded, and an advocate for the underdog, according to his colleagues. It was reported that he: 'sprang from humble roots in the city's *neck-end* [*sic*] and took his first fumbling steps into the legal profession as an articled clerk without even a law degree (back then)'. He obtained two A-levels, worked as journalist for a short time and eventually rose in the legal profession to run one of the busiest Coronial Offices in the country. In Stoke-on-Trent he was renowned for his human empathy, as a local obituary writer elaborated:

Because he came from the same humble origins, he had a deep affinity with ordinary families as he helped them to seek answers to how their loved ones died. As their champion he would fearlessly take on at times protected interests of the establishment to get to the truth. That could be anything from top surgeons messing up operations, and social workers ignoring alarm signs from the vulnerable, to deaths in police custody. At times he stretched coroner's legal flexibility to its limit to announce verdicts which brought maximum benefit to those left behind.[36]

John Wain was also a keen advocate of opening up Coronial records if they could help further medical research into, for instance, the underlying causes of suicide in his district. In January 1999 he thus co-operated with a large-scale study covering North Staffordshire in which Wain had been the presiding coroner. Data was collected on 'all cases of suicide' and 'undetermined injury' between '1991 and 1995' in which '212 cases and controls' were identified.[37]

The study team concluded that 'the risk of death due to suicide and undetermined death was associated with: recent separation, relationship difficulties, experience of financial difficulties, history of past criminal charges or contact with the police, a past history of deliberate self-harm, being on psychotropic medication at the time of death and a diagnosis of bipolar affective disorder'. In a similar refrain, Wain had assisted with an NHS study into whether 'pre-hospital deaths from accidental injury were preventable'.[38] Again he released Coronial records covering the period '1 January 1987 to 31 December 1990' in which there were '152 pre-hospital deaths from accidental injury (110 males and 42 females)'. The important conclusion of this study was that: 'Death was potentially preventable in at least 39% of those who died from accidental injury before they reached hospital. Training in first aid should be available more widely, and particularly to motorists as many pre-hospital deaths that could be prevented are due to road accidents.' Wain was thus not the sort of coroner who would routinely hold up a heart transplant unless he believed it was necessary.

Nevertheless, the Alcock family thought he was guilty of having 'stretched coroner's legal flexibility' (to use his obituary writer's precise phrasing). Even so, whether the bereaved family had legal grounds to challenge what happened or not, what really mattered in the end to them was that Wain had the discretionary justice to act as he did and he brought about a dispute at a key discrete research threshold point in a donation process. Generating explicit disputes in a transplant era was, seemingly, often part and parcel of a coroner's normal working-life. Since cases like this raise the issue of representativeness, it is important to explore general trends regarding the retention of human remains involving the Coronial Office covering elsewhere in England. As we shall see, other coroners also took a similar view of their extensive powers to be advocates for the bereaved but also to query organ donations and hold them up if necessary. An important case of Carol Morris outlined next is illustrative of general trends in the Midlands. It is, moreover, a significant story because it was to make medico-legal history by changing the law on the anonymity of organ donation in Britain and around the world (as we shall see in Part II of this chapter, where we discuss the case's ingrained lessons and their historical longevity involving coroners).

The Carol Morris Case

On 6 August 1977, the *BMJ* carried a detailed report on the modus operandi of the coroner for Leicester City and South Leicestershire.[39] Since what he wrote was to have far-reaching consequences just three years later in another explicit body dispute, it is important to pause and consider the coroner's detailed letter to the *BMJ* to set the scene in what became known as the Carol Morris Case. Mr Michael Charman explained in 1977 that he was legally qualified. On average, he oversaw about '1400 unexplained deaths' every year in a busy area of the Midlands. He paid careful attention to the bereaved and tried where possible to relieve their stressful situation, as he explained:

Of necessity the reports issued to me by my pathologists are all couched in medical terms and when I first became a coroner I had to unravel this terminology to discover the cause of death. I also determined that to be efficient I would need to obtain explanations from my pathologists. I therefore not only view the body but also, in cases in which there is some difficulty or peculiarity, will view the body while the necropsy is taking place and my pathologists are kind enough to demonstrate to me the actual cause of death. In cases of death from a cause other than a natural one, I find this very helpful indeed when taking the inquest. Since usually the only medically qualified person at an inquest is my pathologist he is also careful to give an explanation in non-medical terms of the cause of death so that those present, including the jury, understand precisely what has happened.[40]

Charman told the *BMJ* that he worked with one of four pathologists, and he carried on the tradition at Leicester of allowing the duty-pathologist to pass on a copy of his report to the bereaved family's general practitioner once an Inquest had been finished. He was not legally obliged to do this, but he felt that it did alleviate grief. Often the GP was in a better position to reassure a family that the deceased had not suffered or been in a painful condition. In terms of the grey areas of these legalities, he elaborated that:

It must be remembered that in England the post-mortem report on any sudden death is prepared by a pathologist appointed by the coroner and that the report is the coroner's and belongs to no one else; furthermore it is not a public document until after the inquest or the issue of the coroner's certificate that the death was by natural causes. It therefore follows that it would be very difficult indeed for the pathologist conducting the examination to give any explanation to a relative except in the vaguest of terms until the legal formalities have been completed. Once this has happened I personally, as coroner, would be very happy indeed to permit any of my pathologists to alleviate distress by giving simple explanations, but at the same time I know they are very busy people. . . .[41]

It would be precisely this medico-legal situation – a coroner having extensive powers to withhold information if he judged it to be in the public interest – and with the co-operation of his pathologist often pushed for time – which was to cause an explicit dispute that made national headlines. Events at Leicester by 1980 would prove contentious and ultimately change the terms of reference of working coroners everywhere in England. We begin with a tragic accident in the Carol Morris case files.

On 25 January 1980, Carol Morris, a young woman aged 16, was driving a moped in the early rush hour at Houghton-on-the-Hill village about 6 miles from Leicester city-centre.[42] It was a cold and icy winter's day. Near a crossroads in the centre of the village close to a garage, Carol Morris tried to join the oncoming traffic down the lane from her home. The location was notorious for car accidents where the B3129 crossed the A47. Tragically, in the inclement conditions a 40-foot lorry collided with the moped as it exited from a side road into the main arterial route into the city. Carol lay on the ground seriously injured. She was soon taken unconscious by ambulance to Leicester Royal Infirmary, where three days after the accident she died from her injuries. Carol Morris was carrying a donor card. Dr David Riley, a surgical registrar on duty, thus began the formal medico-legal process of checking on whether the accident victim was a suitable transplant donor. He needed to liaise with a transplant team at Papworth Hospital in Cambridgeshire to carry out a tissue match with patients on the organ donation waiting list covering East Anglia and the Midlands NHS regions. Because Carol Morris was aged 16, there were two lifestyle factors to assess. An evaluation of her general health condition prior to the accident was undertaken. The doctor found in her case-notes that it had been generally very good before the fatality. She was a fit and healthy young woman. There was every chance therefore that her kidneys (specifically ticked by Carol Morris on her organ donation card) would be healthy and ideal for transplant. The medical team also needed to assess the wishes of her bereaved parents and their familial relationship with Carol. She was aged 16 and so over the legal age of adult consent, but she was not yet 18 years old; therefore, her parents had guardianship of their daughter as next of kin. They wanted to respect Carol's wishes to donate, and so the transplant team prepared the body without further delay. What happened next nevertheless was to cause considerable controversy – so much so that it generated a national debate in Parliament about the need for a change in the law to enshrine the principle of anonymity into organ donation programmes across Britain. The catalyst was the actions of the coroner for Leicester City, Mr Michael Charman, and the involvement of some journalists working for a number of popular daily newspapers who acted unscrupulously to get a news scoop.

Carol Morris remained on a ventilator until 'her heart, kidneys and eyes were all removed for transplant'.[43] The heart was despatched by plane and car to Papworth Hospital in Cambridgeshire on the night of 28 January. The transplant team were waiting on it. The pathologist on duty did a careful tissue crossmatch. Then the leading surgical consultant, Mr David English, and his colleagues completed a successful operation on 'Mr Nigel Olney a 35 year old man' from Bedfordshire, a patient desperately in need of a new heart. He was in due course to be the fourth heart transplant patient at Papworth after the relaunch of its surgical programme in 1979. Olney lived for almost nine years before he needed a second (unsuccessful) heart transplant in December 1988.[44] He was thus one of the longest survivors at that time.[45] Meanwhile, the Papworth team had recalibrated their working practices with some success from 1973, as recent histories of the hospital explain:

During 1973, 162 open heart operations were undertaken with a mortality rate of 5%. However, surgical activity increased rapidly and, after visiting Stanford [University], Terence [English] decided Britain needed a heart transplant programme. A major problem was lack of support from the cardiologists. However, after research at Huntingdon Research Centre where techniques for preserving the donor heart prior to its implantation in the recipient were developed, the first heart transplant was performed in January 1979. This was not successful, but four of the next five cases lived between three and eight years. Funding was also a problem in the early years, but help from the National Heart Research Fund and the Robinson Charitable Trust helped until Papworth Hospital was designated a national centre for transplantation.[46]

In addition, in 1980, around the time of Carol Morris's death, a British Heart Foundation Research Group established itself at Papworth. This initiative funded the additional staff needed to expand innovative heart transplant work. Indeed, from 1981, they were able to undertake heart-lung transplants on site for the first time. In no small measure then the heart of Carol Morris was to contribute to Papworth's becoming the preeminent heart and lung transplant unit in the UK. Even so, although the staff that led the unit feature as 'Papworth's heroes' today on the hospital's public engagement website, and the fund-raising efforts of Mr Nigel Olney after his first heart transplant are detailed (with Christopher Hubbard), no mention is made of Carol Morris. She never became an official Papworth heroine. Evidently, once removed, a body part became a discrete research step – 'Nobody's Thing'. That remapped the whole person into a series of hidden histories of the body, the equivalent of a consignment in the cul-de-sac of history, omitted from the success story of biomedicine.

Once Carol Morris's heart was transplanted, the rest of her body was still technically under the official jurisdiction of the Leicester City coroner. He was required to commission a post-mortem from his duty-pathologist since the road accident might later result in the police charging the lorry driver with death by dangerous driving. There would need to be material evidence of sudden death, made available at any subsequent prosecution. An Inquest was thus scheduled. Before it convened, however, the coroner noticed that there was a discrepancy in his pathologist's paperwork. Dr David Riley, the surgical registrar on duty at Leicester Royal Infirmary the night that Carol Morris died, asked the coroner to authorise the removal of her kidneys. Carol stated this option explicitly on her organ donation card and so her parents decided to comply with their dead daughter's wishes, as we have seen. However, the deceased did not tick any other organs for donation. There were separate cards for each organ at the time. The bereaved parents searched their dead daughter's belongings in her bed-room but found nothing. Carol's intention seems to have been to donate her kidneys, probably because (her parents thought) there had been a number of media campaigns to improve their donation in the national press over the previous three years or so under the auspices of the DHSS (as described above). The coroner, Mr Michael Charman, was very mindful of being sensitive to the parents' shocking bereavement. Indeed, he had a long history of sharing pathologists' reports with grieving families shocked by the sudden death of their relatives in tragic circumstances, as he had previously explained to the *BMJ*. He felt he was now in a very difficult medico-legal and ethical situation. He had been officially asked for the kidneys of Carol Morris but not her heart and eyes which, it seemed to him, had been harvested as 'extras' for organ transplant and grafting purposes, respectively. The parents told the hospital staff in Leicester that they were 'keen' for '*all* the organs to be donated'; they interpreted the fact of their dead daughter's having a donor card as confirmation that she was a supporter of transplant surgery per se. The coroner nevertheless believed that in case of the need for a subsequent prosecution involving the lorry driver and the question of his legal culpability on the morning of the fatal collision, the dead body had to remain solely in a Coronial officer's medico-legal jurisdiction. He felt the transplant team at Papworth Hospital was deliberately ignoring this legal consideration, with the support of their surgical liaison at Leicester Royal Infirmary. Together they had harvested more than he had authorised. There would soon prove to be a very difficult professional stand-off between all the interested parties at the Inquest.

The Inquest opened on the Thursday after the death of Carol Morris. Charman was mindful of the stressful situation for the bereaved family, but there were a number of pathology discrepancies that in his opinion required action. He stated that he felt very uneasy about what had happened and how much was harvested from the body of Carol Morris, having ordered that: 'no organs could be removed in his area without his written consent, countersigned by the surgeon carrying out the removal'. This claim by Charman that the 'body of anyone who had died suddenly was his to decide upon' was, however, 'contested at the Inquest'. Carol Morris's father stated categorically that as far as his family was concerned his daughter wanted to be an organ donor, stated so explicitly on a donor card, and they needed to comply with her wishes under the tragic circumstances. To do otherwise would mean she had died in vain (echoing the sentiments of the Alcock case outlined earlier in this chapter). Even so, Michael Charman replied:

His contention is that coroners should have the ultimate power of decision over how the bodies of potential organ donors are to be handled. The law, which is based on the Human Tissue Act of 1961, is at best open to interpretations, and at worst confused, say medico-legal experts.[47]

As the atmosphere at the Inquest was adversarial, Charman took the unusual step of calling a press conference afterwards. This upset the bereaved family, and with good reason, for since the death of Carol Morris they had been the focus of considerable unwelcome media attention. Before examining in more detail what the coroner said to the media, we first need to factor in what had been happening to the Morris family since the night of the fatality.

The Morris family had been under a media siege at Houghton-on-the-Hill since the death of their daughter on the night of 28 January 1980. So intense was the media intrusion that George Morris made an official complaint to the Press Council (hereafter PC) in London.[48] He told them that: 'on the 1 o'clock news on 29 January it was reported that a heart transplant operation had taken place at Papworth hospital and that the family of the donor particularly wished to remain anonymous'.[49] He elaborated that 'a [news] leak occurred and within three or four hours' from someone working at Leicester Infirmary, Papworth Hospital or a PC news agency. The *Evening News* was the first media outlet to telephone the family for further information about the heart transplant that had taken place. Then the phone started to ring and ring. George Morris described how the phone 'rang continuously' from 1 p.m. to 5 p.m. when the family finally decided to 'take it off the hook'. Events were, however, to get worse, as he explained:

However, that did not alleviate the position. The newspapers that had been told by telephone that the family were not prepared to comment sent reporters to the door. To add insult to injury, most reporters attempted to obtain additional information and a photograph of the dead girl from the villagers, despite the family's request for anonymity.[50]

The family felt that 'particular newspapers, such as the *Daily Mail* ... behaved especially badly'. They even contacted their 'next-door neighbour, Mr. Stephen Turnbull, giving the impression that they were friends of the family requesting information'. George Morris explained that the way that the reporters worked was to inquire 'about the donor card' and only later admit that they were journalists seeking a news scoop. In the family's opinion at such a sensitive time, they all felt understandably: 'That is a despicable way of obtaining information.' Yet, worse was to come.

George Morris alleged that one determined reporter for the *Daily Mail* (Sally Brompton) waited outside the Morris family home 'from 10 am on 30 January until 6 pm'.[51] She then 'canvassed the village from door to door in an attempt to buy a photograph of Mr. Morris' daughter Carol'. George Morris subsequently relayed to his member of Parliament how 'Miss Brompton even attempted to persuade a 14-year-old girl to go into her elder sister's bedroom to remove a photograph of Carol'. She finally toned down her actions when 'at about 6 pm Miss Brompton left a card with Mr Morris requesting an interview at a later date'. The family had taken enough. They requested and were granted police protection by the Leicestershire constabulary. A police officer, posted outside the family home at Weir Lane in Houghton-on-the-Hill, also arranged for

British Telecom to make the home telephone number ex-directory until further notice. Mr Morris did acknowledge to the PC that although the *Guardian* newspaper and the *Leicester Mercury* had obtained photographs of his dead daughter, they decided not to print them once it came to light that they had been obtained by unscrupulous means. Their editors had acted, in his opinion, with common decency, unlike all the other newspaper tabloids which had 'not acted in a professional manner' at such a tragic time. The family now found themselves in the middle of a media storm not of their making and one which the coroner for Leicester city centre was about to exacerbate by calling a press conference after the Inquest about an explicit body dispute.

Michael Charman explained to the media that he felt obliged to call a press conference about the circumstances surrounding the death and harvesting of the organs (heart, kidneys and eyes) from Carol Morris because he believed procedures were unethical and technically illegal. He clashed with Mr Bernard Hargrove, head of a legal team who appeared for the three transplant surgeons involved: one at Leicester and two at Papworth Hospital. The Medical Defence Union funded Hargrove. He insisted that since 1977 the Home Secretary had taken the view that 'no coroner could refuse for the removal of an organ unless it was needed for criminal proceedings or had been faulty'.[52] In the case of a fatal road accident arising from careless driving causing brainstem death, the retention of the brain in question would suffice as material evidence of medical death at a criminal prosecution. Hargrove also insisted that in the opinion of most doctors it was their medico-scientific duty to facilitate '*all* organ donation'. Yet, as a newspaper reporter for the *Guardian* who was present at the Inquest press conference explained, it really came down to one key question in this controversial case: 'Who has the ultimate right to decide' on organ donation in a Coronial case – 'the coroner or the family?' Moreover, this raised an important procedural point too – 'Could a coroner refuse permission for the removal of organs, even if the deceased carried a donor card?' Charman defended that he was very concerned that the surgeons who removed the heart had effectively 'disregarded the law of the land which says that my consent must be obtained'. He clarified that he was not accusing the transplant team of deliberately flouting the law – 'What they did was make assumptions which didn't exist and thought that they had got consent when it wasn't there at all.' Soon, the storm created encouraged other medical bodies to get involved in the widening debate about this and other explicit body disputes involving the Coronial Office in England.

The British Medical Association (hereafter BMA) was quick to respond, issuing a press statement that they were worried that the adverse publicity could dissuade other organ donors from coming forward in the future. If all coroners requested a written rather than a verbal consent (the latter was standard practice in some transplant units), then that might also delay the removal of a heart and render it unsuitable to transplant in time. But Charman pointed out that this was nonsense, since written permission from the coroner delayed matters for no more than 'an hour at the most'.[53] Besides, he pointed out, in practical terms most donor patients were kept 'on a heart-lung machine and time is not so vital, except at the moment of removal'. The Coroners' Society for England and Wales (hereafter CSE&W) nevertheless joined in with the BMA's concerns since both professional bodies were pro-transplantation. Dr Burton, a spokesman for the CSE&W, told the press that he had been a member of the Transplant Panel which had been convened to monitor the progress of transplantation, and in his experience: 'For years we have been slowly moving towards the general public's general acceptance of transplants as a routine matter of course. Every time this sort of thing happens', where there is a stand-off between a coroner and the bereaved involving an explicit body dispute, 'it sets the progress back years'. The assembled reporters thus asked Charman how he felt about contravening the family's wishes. Did he consider whether he was going against the wishes of the bereaved and making things much more difficult for them? In reply, Charman defended: 'No, I don't. They must of course consent before my consent is asked for. I don't think that in any way asking them for written permission affects it' (that is, the decision to donate or not by the bereaved). He told the packed Inquest that the police had found that 'there was not sufficient evidence to prosecute anyone for contravening the Human Tissue Act 1961'. Moreover, after hearing all the evidence collected from the roadside scene, there was no evidence that the lorry driver was guilty of dangerous driving. It was a tragic case; in the end, the coroner recorded a verdict of 'accidental death'.

At the close of the public controversy, the BMA issued a further statement. They did so to clarify that each Coronial official should have sole jurisdiction of bodies in unexplained circumstances. And yet, they went on to state that HTA1961 gave 'the next of kin ownership of their loved one' when they were a whole person, whereas 'the removal of parts of it must be up to a coroner'.[54] This meant that as far as all the medico-legal officials involved were concerned Carol Morris had been a person with a family history that gave her a sense of community and belonging – until, that is, in death, she had become a cause célèbre because she wanted to 'gift' part of her body as a bequest. Consequently, her lack of agency in death and dwindling material integrity because of becoming a transplant target meant that she became recycled for public consumption: an outcome that her family found painful to come to terms with. They now had a very difficult decision to make about whether they should retreat into private grief or seek public redress from the press for being hounded. Given how much their privacy was breached, few onlookers would have blamed them for closing ranks and never speaking again about the dreadful circumstances of Carol Morris's donation. Yet, with emotional fortitude, they decided to contact their local member of Parliament and asked him on their behalf to highlight the dreadful experience they had been through as an organ donation family. For, they did not want others to be in the same position of exposure to such intense public censure. And thus, we see how an explicit dispute came to national attention.

Donor Anonymity – A National Issue

On 5 March 1980, the Right Hon. Mr John Farr, MP for Market Harborough in Leicestershire, tabled an early day motion in the House of Commons. He did so on behalf of his constituents the Morris family:

I beg to move, that leave be given to bring in a Bill to provide for protection of the identity of donors of human organs. My reason for rising to present this Bill to the House is to respond to a request from one of my constituents whose daughter was recently tragically killed. After her death my constituent and his family underwent what can only be described as persecution by the media in a most improper way during their time of sorrow.[55]

Farr explained that he had 'cross-party support' for an amendment to the new Health Services Bill about to come before Parliament. The proposal was to attach to it a revised Code of Practice introduced in 1979, with the support of the BMA, to better regulate the transplant surgery of hearts by making all donations anonymous. There were thus two ways forward, as Farr explained: 'First, again in order to assist anonymity, could not all the cards of those who wish to remain anonymous have the word "anonymous" printed diagonally in large type across the top? Secondly, in these days when organs of all types are so pressingly needed, could not we have a single donor card for all organs, which would greatly simplify the system?' Farr had consulted the Secretary of State for Health, who was supportive. There was general agreement that the new procedures would protect families like the Morris's from such public exposure for an altruistic act at a time of tragedy.

During the early day motion debate, Farr explained to his fellow MPs that the pace of transplant surgery in terms of its new techniques was moving faster than the law in Britain.[56] So, whilst a Code of Practice for the Organ Donation (s) of kidneys was well known and had been operating efficiently for some time, the surgical ability to do spare-part surgery with hearts had exposed explicit body disputes that would become more contentious. The heart seemed to rouse public sensibilities because of its important cultural symbolism in Western society. It meant that any lack of clarity in the Code of Practice left heart transplant surgeons exposed to media harassment. Families that donated faced a maelstrom of press intrusion too. Yet, the Code's language was loose when transplant techniques were influx. The press were thus quick to quote any lack of clarity in the wording. It was now important, in Farr's opinion, to alter the discourse to reflect the changing realities of biotechnology by 1980. This would then ensure that compliance was transparent. He gave an example of how 'paragraph 37 of the Code' states that: 'The staff of hospitals and organ exchange organisations *should* always try to maintain the anonymity of the donor and of the recipient.' He reiterated: 'I do not believe that that goes far enough today. I *should* like to see a fresh code drawn up.' If the Code was redrafted in 'plainer language' – replacing *should* with *must* – this would guarantee anonymity for all involved on both sides of the donation exchange. The time had come to no longer fudge the pressing 'question of anonymity'. It ought not to be dealt with 'in a cavalier manner' of the sort that the Morris family had experienced. In a final gesture that acknowledged the stressful situation his constituents found themselves in, Farr closed his speech by clarifying the current law according to HTA1961: 'That Act clearly lays down that coroners have the right to require consultation before organs are secured. However, I understand that most organs are obtained after telephone consultation with the coroner, which I believe is a proper and correct procedure, which does not take up very much time.' This reiterated that although the Leicester coroner was correct in medico-legal terms, others were working their way around the law in practical ways to facilitate transplant surgery. Reforms to working practices would thus ensure the Coronial Office avoided generating explicit body and body parts disputes.

In due course, as *Hansard* confirms, 'Mr. John Farr accordingly presented a Bill to provide for protection of the identity of donors of human organs: And the same was read the First time; and ordered to be read a Second time upon Friday 14 March and to be printed. [Bill 160].'[57] He did so successfully because he had widespread support in the Commons, including amongst the ranks of an influential lobby of leading exponents of transplant surgery:

Mr. Greville Janner Labour MP for Leicester West (1974–1997), Mr. Tony Marlow Conservative MP for Northampton North (1979–1997), Mr. Jack Ashley Labour MP for Stoke-on-Trent (1966–1992), Mr. R. A. McCrindle Conservative MP for Brentwood and Ongar (1974–1992), Mr. Tam Dalyell Scottish Labour Party MP for West Lothian (1962–82) and then Linlithgow (1983–2005), and Mr. Michael Hamilton Conservative MP for Wellingborough (1959–64) and then Salisbury (1965–1993).[58]

Of these, Tam Dayell had been one of the most high-profile spokespersons in Britain. He wrote a regular column for the *New Scientist* in which he often featured the need for more transplants and the lobbying on this issue that he was undertaking in Parliament.[59] Likewise, Jack Ashley was a lifelong exponent of disability health issues and he promoted the re-enablement of those who could benefit from new medical treatments. All the others had strong local political connections to the East Anglian and Midlands regional areas of the NHS where many of the explicit Coronial disputes were being generated during the 1970s and early 1980s.[60] Together they thus constituted a powerful faction that could substantiate the unpalatable position of donor families from across the social and political spectrum. As John Farr emphasised, the issue of anonymity was an emotive one because it had real consequences:

Mr. Morris alleges that the behaviour of the media caused more pain and anguish to my wife and daughter. The newspaper reporters even had the nerve to challenge Mr. Morris when he wished to leave his house, as if he were a criminal on the run. Mr. Morris said if transplants are to continue donor organs are essential. Families will not consent to the use of deceased relatives' organs if the media continue to act in such a disgraceful and unsympathetic way. If families are to be badgered in this disgraceful and unsympathetic way by the media even when requests for anonymity have been made, the source of organs for transplant will dry up. I agree with Mr. Morris, and though I am in the van of those who believe in the need for a free press, I believe that the conduct that I have described is evil. We must therefore make it as difficult as possible for such ghouls to gain any clue as to the identity of sorrowing families.[61]

'Evil' was a strong term to use – too strong for some newspapers editors – and so soon events would prove that anonymity was not necessarily as straightforward as was implied in Parliament; for, there was another side to the Carol Morris controversy that came to light too.

The Controversial Nigel Olney Case

The PC and its media outlets were somewhat stung by the criticism being levelled at them in the Carol Morris case. Indeed, it was clear that the disputed actions of some journalists could lead to a change in the law. This would give donors, and their recipients, anonymity in transplant surgery on a permanent legal basis. If the press were to make a case for more public accountability, then they needed to take a new tack. They soon found a news angle. Reporters were despatched to investigate the personal circumstances of Mr Nigel Olney who had received the 'gift' of Carol Morris's heart. The *Guardian* newspaper was one of a number of the broad sheets and popular dailies that opened with a report that was positive in its tone. It informed readers that Nigel Olney had been sitting up in his hospital bed at Papworth, and he was recovering well from the heart transplant operation, which took 'five hours and seven minutes and was led by the South African-born surgeon Mr Terence English'. Then lead articles turned into an exposé:

Mr Olney, a Leighton Buzzard, Bedfordshire, chiropodist, had separated from his wife and two young children and lives with his parents. His severe heart complaint was amongst the factors that had saved him from being sent to prison last year after he was found guilty of obtaining £5, 553 from two local health authorities by deception. At Bedford Crown Court he admitted claiming money for patients who had died or moved.

Suspending an 18-month sentence for two years Judge David Lowe said: *You are a man of no previous convictions and we take into account your medical condition* [*sic*].[62]

The unwitting testimony implied in this editorial line was that this was a man with questionable morals by virtue of his pending divorce (allegations of adultery and child custody rights for men were still a sensitive social issue in the 1980s). He was also a convicted fraudster that had benefitted from being in an NHS facility paid for by the same taxpayers he had defrauded in his chiropody work in the community. The *Guardian* newspaper was nevertheless careful to balance its editorial slant. Interviews were obtained from Mr Olney's soon-to-be ex-wife, his near-relations, and a Papworth Hospital spokesman about the costs of his operation and aftercare. All stressed that he was a suitable donor recipient. A neighbour of the Olney family in Leighton Buzzard, Mary Campbell, described Nigel: 'He is a hell of a nice guy. Nobody deserves to live more than he does. He's been so weak recently he's had to be carried when he goes out.' In mitigation, she alleged: 'I think his illness and his marriage problems would account for some of his other troubles.' Likewise, Nigel Olney's separated spouse who had moved to a Hertfordshire village with 'her two children Jason and Nicole' told a reporter on her doorstep: 'I am extremely concerned and hope Nigel makes a steady recovery.' It was a dignified response from his separated wife in the face of full public exposure. Nigel Olney's parents similarly ignored the accusations of his unworthiness and stressed instead in a statement to the press: 'We are most grateful to the hospital for accepting our son and taking such good care of him.' A Papworth Hospital spokesperson meanwhile explained that recently the transplant team received a charitable grant of £50,000 from the National Heart Research Fund and this money, not NHS resources, was funding the transplant and aftercare required. When pressed, the transplant team estimated that 'the operation and a year's aftercare would cost about £15,000' in each case. In other words, the Carol Morris explicit dispute with a coroner was now being recycled into a much wider set of other body part disputes about the future medical ethics of transplant surgery in a modern world.

It was well known at that time that the NHS had refused to fund such risky surgical procedures as heart transplant. On the one hand, then, the newspaper coverage was being duplicitous in connecting Mr Olney's fraudulent behaviour to his alleged exploitation of public healthcare funds. On the other hand, the NHS had built Papworth Hospital in the first place from central taxation and so Nigel Olney was technically receiving a benefit in kind by being cared for in that facility. Evidently, the assessment of the case on financial, medical and moral grounds rested entirely with the transplant team and the charity in question. Indeed, the medical team stressed that they examined the best surgical chance for a tissue match and, provided the pathologist on the transplant team found that the immunology looked favourable, it was judged prudent to go ahead. There would have been a sound medical case for the transplant to proceed. It was not, moreover, for transplant surgeons to investigate the moral grounds for proceeding in individual cases. However, this question of the morality of transplant work did not abate, either at the time of the Olney case or subsequently once liver transplants became feasible. Often the media would ask: Should an alcoholic (for instance) receive a liver transplant? It was an ethical question that featured in many high-profile cases such as the ex-footballer George Best, famous for his hedonistic lifestyle and family history of alcoholism.[63] Yet, Nigel Olney's brother in response to the considerable media storm, and the very personal criticisms being levied, reiterated to the *Guardian*: 'the family are very distressed that Nigel's past has been *"raked up"* when he was still in intensive care'.[64] In many respects then Nigel Olney was a test case for what would prove to be ongoing 'moral' debates surrounding transplants and the anonymity for recipients in Britain and Europe. What Carol Morris's bereaved family felt when they discovered the personal circumstances and criminal record of Mr Nigel Olney was not recorded publicly at the time in the newspapers; yet, it cannot have been palatable to be part of an ongoing press exposé, even by association, during the first stages of grief.

The balance of the evidence in this symbolic case makes it clear that heart transplant surgery was an emotive issue in the British media – journalists tapped into a long history of the heart being a central and enduring symbol of humanity in histories of the body for many cultures.[65] Yet, it was also a litmus test for many of the procedures put in place when the Victorian Information State established working arrangements, aspects often neglected in standard historical studies.[66] Coroners had extensive powers of discretionary justice, and they had worked hard to promote their image as protectors of law and order in the community. As they moved from being legally to medically qualified, and worked alongside pathologists more regularly, it enhanced their professional status. Their individual sense of personal agency increased too. So much so, that by the modern era they had become the fulcrum of advances in forensic medicine and pathology. In an era when medico-legal jurisdiction over the body was to become contentious as researchers inside the medical sciences competed for better access to cadavers and 'live' donors (in kidney transplants, for instance), coroners began to clash with those they had co-operated with in the first place to raise their professional status. The Carol Morris case exemplified that trend and soon led to international scrutiny too. In this way, explicit disputes had a global impact.

International Impact

There had been an initial 'transplant fever' across the world from 1968. As the *Observer* reflected there were 'more than 100 heart transplants by 64 teams in

22 countries. But most of the patients died, succumbed to infection or rejection, the biochemistry of which was not clearly understood, and the fever never faded'.[67] In the mid-1970s, many thought that the transplant era 'was over' because the new technology had 'left in its wake considerable distaste for the eagerness with which some surgeons had joined the transplant rush'.[68] An added logistical issue was that governments saw such risky operations as an electoral liability. Few wanted to divert their healthcare budgets to fund the research and development of transplant units, even though survival rates and immunosuppressive drugs had improved by the end of the 1970s. Papworth had raised the profile of heart transplants in Britain, but whether they could sustain their success depended on more funding by medical charities and better management of the attendant media publicity. This is what made the Carol Morris case noteworthy. For, it exemplified that public relations were an intrinsic aspect of the transplantation era whether the medical community liked it or not.

It was in many respects ironic then that those involved in the Carol Morris/ Nigel Olney heart swap expressed surprise about the negative coverage after the coroner's explicit dispute exposed the details of the case to media scrutiny. For, in an interview with Christian Bernard (who carried out the first heart transplant in the world) for *Tomorrow's World* televised on the BBC in 1968, the audience of medical experts and church leaders assembled from across Britain kept making repeated criticisms of his team's 'mishandling of the media publicity'.[69] He was asked 'why he had made available pictures of the donor and his relatives', and 'why had he made the personal details of the donor made known to the recipient' when this was unnecessary? It could be interpreted as a breach of the Hippocratic Oath's commitment, to maintain patient confidentiality at all times. Bernard defended:

'If you could do that you're a better man than I am. ... It was just impossible'. He elaborated on how: 'We tried to stop all publicity to start with but you will well remember that when you heard the first reports of this no names were mentioned. But after this it was completely impossible, it just snow-balled, we had no control over the matter. It's just something that you can't control'.[70]

Bernard then threw down a challenge to whoever did become the first heart transplant surgeon in Britain. If they and their team succeeded in controlling, limiting or stopping the publicity of the inevitable media frenzy, then he would, he said, 'Take my hat off to them!' The transplant team at Papworth Hospital soon found themselves in an equivalent situation in the early 1980s. Yet, they could have designed a better and more confidential transfer handover process. Precedents in kidney transplants were established, and the controversial South African heart transplant situation meant professional lessons had been publicised. Equally, the Coronial Office could, and sometimes did, countermand new procedures that were put in place because they had the individual discretionary justice to do so in England. Explicit disputes were thus literally 'the heart of the matter' in many localities outside of London.

The change in the law that the Carol Morris case created to protect the anonymity of donor families, and by extension their recipients, was to have far-reaching sociocultural consequences, but not necessarily ones that were anticipated at the time. There did appear to be strong ethical grounds for checking media intrusion, especially in Britain where the tabloid press were persistent in pursuit of a newsworthy medical breakthrough. There was also a reasoned medical case put forward that some recipients who knew their donor's identity did experience psychological pressures, which included feeling guilty about being the beneficiary of someone's death. Recipients likewise expressed concern about not having the physical energy for any emotional involvement in another family's trauma. Yet, it is equally apparent that around the world as countries adopted British standards, the sociocultural distance between donor 'gift' and recipient got wider and wider as transplant techniques improved. So much so that eventually 'Red Markets' have been created in countries like India, as Scott Cairney points out (see Chapter 1), which have facilitated organ 'vendors'.[71] It is a disturbing irony that anonymity, which was introduced to protect the Morris family and many others like them, also shields unscrupulous body brokers operating as spare-parts traders via the Internet in many of the poorest parts of the world today. This socio-medico reality has recently been the subject of renewed debates in transplant surgery circles about whether to rescind or keep anonymity. Briefly, we consider this outcome of the human stories we have been examining in this first half of the chapter, and which reflects the importance of their wider historical lessons.

In Belgium, politicians debated in 2009 whether better communication should be facilitated between 'live' donors (and/or grieving families in cases of sudden death) and their living recipients.[72] They commissioned studies to test public sentiments. In one leading example, a representative sample was identified of 249 transplant patients, and, of these, 176 people took part in an opinion survey. Some 70 per cent of those participants (n=123) wanted to maintain the status quo for the psychological reasons stated above, namely, the recipient would find it very difficult to cope with any emotional engagement with the donor family. Around 19 per cent (n=11) were keen, however, 'to obtain some information about their donor' and would at some point wish to 'express their gratitude'. Meanwhile about 42 per cent (n=72) of the sample 'would worry about the donor having a different background to them', and what differences would mean (there was no suggestion of racism but rather concerns about socio-economic status, class and educational differences) in terms of relating to each other. Nonetheless, 36 per cent (n=55), having considered the survey carefully, thought there probably should be a change in the law to connect people in the 'gift' relationship and make it more ethically transparent. Eventually, it was concluded that: 'Prudence to change the law is warranted, as only a minority of patients are in favour of rescinding the anonymity.' The matter was tested again in the Netherlands in 2015, and a survey of about the same size and scope (again involving liver donations) came to the conclusion that: 'There is no need to change the current legislation on anonymity of organ donation.' However, it also found 'that most liver transplant recipients would like to receive *some general* [author's emphasis] information about their donor'. Therefore, 'clear guidelines on the sharing of donor data with recipients needs to be established'.[73] Moreover, in countries like Israel and the USA, studies have recently been delivering similar messages. Provided transplant co-ordinators take the initiative and facilitate appropriate contact between donor families and recipients in all types of surgical interventions (heart, lungs, kidneys, eyes and liver), then there is a public appetite for promoting more personal interactions, paced properly and sensitively handled.[74] The Carol Morris case continues hence to be the focus of global ethical debates, even by those who are unaware of how the powers of an explicit body parts dispute by her Leicester City coroner were to change the terms of reference in transplant history for everybody in Europe and beyond. Having therefore engaged with these human stories we now need in Part II of this chapter to evaluate their ingrained historical lessons to reconsider how and with what outcomes the power and palette of the Coronial Office endured for so long. To do this, we need to look in more detail at the systemic flaws in the Coronial system of handling the dead – picking up on themes we have encountered in Chapters 2 and 4 and now expanding on them – namely, the extra time coroners spent with human material, how it was harvested, and in what ways the flawed system of death certification potentially undermined the precious information that could be generated from 'causes of death' pathologies to further medical research in the modern era. In other words, the next section is concerned with how micro-stories, reassembled from their dissected remains, have macro-lessons of significant longevity in hidden histories of the dead.

Part II

More Extra Time of the Dead

Adverse publicity generated by the Coronial Office was placing anatomists too in a very uncomfortable professional position by the 1980s. In the media, they had been busy promoting body bequests as the ethical way forward since 1954. Few relished being tarnished by the sorts of explicit body disputes happening routinely in organ donation. Practically speaking, however, anatomists had to find a way to continue to work with coroners involved in sensitive explicit disputes to keep up their supply-lines. As a result, most anatomists became evasive and publicity shy when asked about the specifics of their workload, fearful that being honest could undermine their campaign for more body bequests. This atmosphere of public engagement on the one hand and public retreat on the other hand, sometimes created the misimpression that all cadaver work was suspect, when, in fact, anatomists were just being cautious to protect essential supply-lines for better medical education. An added operational difficulty was that in the Thatcher era, all NHS facilities were under intense financial pressures to cut budgets. Staff were being made redundant or leaving voluntarily to train in another career. Hence, the medical research sector started to contract. Often administrators were hit by the first rounds of budget squeezes. As a result, the bureaucratic time it took to process dead body bequests inside the medical school system was elongated. By 1993, it could take up to an extra thirty-one months in some training facilities to get human material signed off officially by the Anatomy Inspectorate at the DHSS. These bureaucratic inefficiencies not only created the potential for discrepancies to occur from time to time but also started to alert the public to paperwork slippages. Those covered in the media created a climate of mistrust by the end of the 1990s when the tide of public opinion turned against the medical research community. To appreciate that context, and how it was to shape debates surrounding HTA2004, it is important to engage with how much extra time with the dead was first created inside the system (as we did in Chapter 4) and then extended (as we will do here).

The way that the system of supply worked was that when a death occurred on the wards of a teaching hospital, it was reported to a coroner. S/he then asked a pathologist to do a post-mortem to rule out medical negligence, as we saw above. If the cause of death was obvious, then the body could be passed on as a bequest, or a body part such as the heart could be retained for future research. This was entirely in the 'gift' of the coroner, provided the donor family had been consulted beforehand. That then opened up the possibility for dissection. Provided there was no reason not to go ahead, a medical school would receive a bequest body in the usual way. For up to two years, medical students would train on the corpse. Once this had finished, the human remains went for 'disposal', generally by cremation authorised by the anatomist on duty (see Chapter 2). All of the paperwork so far inside this system of supply looked straightforward, until, that is, one examines the official returns to the Anatomy Inspectorate for the 1990s. These reveal minor but important paperwork discrepancies.

In a significant number of cases, the signing-off certificate that should have been issued at the time of cremation was delayed – sometimes for up to another three years post-cremation. Grieving families generally assumed that at cremation, 'disposal' was certified and then the case closed as signed off by the dissection team, but this was not always the case. The coroner, for example, could delay issuing a final sign-off certificate if body parts, human tissue or cell-lines had been retained for 'further consideration'. Hence, these were not cremated with the residual corpse after dissection, a situation exposed during the NHS organ retention scandals in 1999. The absence of a final signing-off notification was in fact ample proof that parts and pieces of the corpse might be used to push past a deadline. The anatomy auditors either did not notice this discrepancy on the part of pathologists (who kept the retentions), or by convention chose to ignore what was not their business. Either way, the system of supply did not operate in such a way that officials could easily take an overview of all the discrete research steps involved, reiterating the autonomy and discretionary power that has often featured in this book. The power and palette of the coroner was pivotal to this system of retention and recycling.

A further complication is that even though most anatomists worked within the law according to HTA1984 (keeping detailed records and ensuring that bodies were signed off locally before cremation to complete paper trails), the DHSS centrally was not necessarily following suit. Serious underfunding of the Anatomy Inspectorate during the Thatcher era meant that if for any reason paperwork related to a dead body that then went for cremation got held up inside the reporting system (the local sending in returns to central control that got delayed), it could remain in an overworked official's in-tray (now that staffing had shrunk) and not signed off centrally, sometimes for as long as three years. Under normal circumstances, this would not have mattered. After all, it was an internal procedure. The body in question had finished being dissected and was cremated properly with an appropriate ceremony. Yet, it also left open the opportunity for future criticism of anatomists that they were not in full control of their internal audit mechanisms: facets of their working-life that would be closely scrutinised in the run-up to the HTA2004. Anatomists also kept little track of Coronial material designated for 'further consideration' that might involve more research study for an extended time period. Several cases are illustrative of this sort of routine gap in the record-keeping.

An elderly man aged 85 died of a stroke on 22 March 1993. His body went to King's College medical school. This was done with the co-operation of the Coronial Office on 25 March 1993.[75] The original cadaver was then sent for 'disposal by cremation on 23 May 1994 to the South London Crematorium'. Thus, it underwent dissection study for 14 months in total. The final signing-off certificate was not, however, issued by the Anatomy Inspectorate, centrally (having been originally counter-signed locally by King's College anatomy department) until 12 December 1996, another 2 years and 5 months post-cremation. Whether this involved the 'further consideration' of any human material taken from the Coronial supply-chain was not disclosed or recorded. Similarly, when a female aged 75 died of 'MI [myocardial infraction, a heart attack due to lack of blood flow] on 3 January 1993', with the co-operation of a hospital coroner, she was passed over to St George's Hospital medical school for dissection on 7 January 1993. That is, once the pathology had been done on her defective heart over 5 days, the original body shell was then dissected until 6 October 1993 before being 'disposed of by cremation', again at South London Crematorium. Once more, however, the signing-off certificate was delayed, not issued in this case until 12 November 1996, another 3 years and 1 month post-cremation. In terms of the complete paperwork trail, this body looked like it had been retained for a total of 3 years and 11 months, whole and in part(s). Again, whether this covered human bio-commons taken for 'extra consideration' is not clear.

The anatomical sciences, without anticipating how public perceptions might view this bureaucratic slippage, were leaving themselves wide open to future criticism that they had lost sight of a series of all their discrete research steps, when in fact it was the central authority that was letting them down. It was unfortunate that systemic flaws in the bureaucratic system for signing off the dead (the result of understaffing problems) made it look like what was happening was that hidden histories of the body were designed to deliberately flout HTA1984. Generally, they were not, but the gap between the public rhetoric denying systemic problems (everything is fine and functioning well – the official DHSS line) and the reality of financial constraints (constant financial cuts, and corners cut in paperwork by exhausted personnel) was never properly explained to the general public to protect the supply-lines of anatomists from coroners. As a result, when we look at the official figures from this time period, they look odd. It appears that anatomists were spending more extra time with the dead than may always in fact have been the case. Figure 5.1 illustrates this common situation by using the example of UMDS medical school (one of the biggest in London, combining anatomical, medical teaching and dentistry training) which first featured in Chapter 4. A sample year of 1993 has been chosen to illustrate trends in the time lag of signing-off procedures. However, although these figures show that the creation of this extra time of the dead was not the fault of those working in individual medical schools, it does raise the question: Did these time lapses created by the central authority become something that later those that wanted to keep hold of more human material for 'extra consideration' took advantage of? In other words, did the systemic flaws in the system of processing the dead, after Coronial, pathological and anatomical work, create the canvas on which explicit body disputes were to be played out? To answer this question, we need to delve deeper into the archive material.

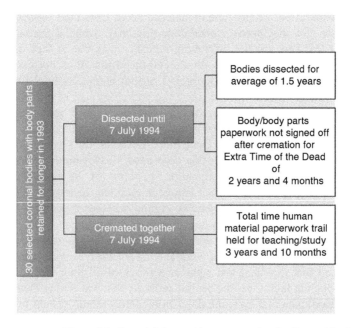

Figure 5.1 Coronial donated human remains (bodies and body parts, human tissue and organs) supplied to, but not officially signed off on behalf of, UMDS medical school, 1993
Source: National Archives, JA 3/1, Anatomy Office, Data-Set Returns for England, c. 1992–98.

Returning to the large anatomy data-set of national trends that under-pinned Chapter 4 (data displayed in Figures 4.6 and 4.7, and Table 4.3), it would appear that from 1993 onwards it became normal to delay the sign-off of human material post-dissection.[76] This happened as a matter of course not just at leading London medical schools, like King's College, St. George's and UMDS, but also at Bristol, Manchester and Liverpool medical schools too. Consequently, in the record-keeping one can observe the broad contours of what would become the prime locations of NHS organ, heart and human tissue scandals, some seven years before they came to public attention. Thus (by way of example), there were 55 bodies in the 1993 teaching cycle in which 'extra time' was created after initial crema-tion. Again Figure 5.1 focusses on 30 of those 55 bodies donated to UMDS, since it illustrates the typical time frames of retentions that may have involved more recycling of material. Altogether the human material was not officially signed off for 3 years and 10 months, even though the corpses supplied from Coronial officers were cremated after 1.5 years. In other words, in cases that were potentially already explicit disputes inside the system of processing for teaching and research purposes, there is an extra time of the dead of 2 years and 4 months which is unaccounted for. It might be a bureaucratic slippage as a result of financial factors constraining less staff to sign off the paperwork centrally, or we could be viewing a process of 'extra consideration'. We will probably never know which because the archival record is so patchy, but nonetheless we are glimpsing a hidden history of the dead arising out of explicit disputes, and one of some longevity. Today this is no longer legal, as Figure 5.2 explains.

Any attempt (intended or by default) to elongate the authorised paper-work trail that processes the donated dead is no longer permissible under HTA2004. As Figure 5.2 shows, the maximum retention period is three years for the body, though generally most are cremated after two. Significantly, no more than one third of the donation bequest is used for 'teaching and/or further examination'. This code of practice is to guarantee human dignity in the dissection room. Provided, however, that the donor and their relatives have agreed to it, body parts can be subject to a bequest for 'an undetermined' period. This must nonetheless have been the result of fully informed consent. In other words, there is still an 'extra time of the dead' inside the system, but it is now a transparent process rather than a covert one. Altogether the old system of 'extra consideration' that we saw in Figure 5.1 has now been outlawed by the new system of 'an undetermined period' with fully informed consent in Figure 5.2. This means that the explicit disputes of the past have now been redressed, but before we leave behind that context we need to pause and appreciate what all this extra time with the dead (intended and unintended) meant. Thomas Laqueur writes: 'Death in culture takes time because it takes time for the rent in the social fabric to be rewoven and for the dead to do their work in creating, recreating, representing, or disrupting the social order of which they had been a part.'[77] We can only know this, however, in terms of how medical research recycles the dead by first finding and mapping material fates found in the death certification processes of dissection, its pathologies and the performance of actor networks. If we are to follow explicit disputes from human story to advancement in medical science, then we need to also ask two related research questions in the final stages of this fifth chapter. If Coronial remains were pivotal for anatomical teaching and practice, the expansion of pathology and forensic medicine, as well as more wider research cultures, what role did their death certification process play in improving public health in Britain after WWII? In this way, were body disputes the bedrock of better medicine for everybody, and did this justify their bio-commons?

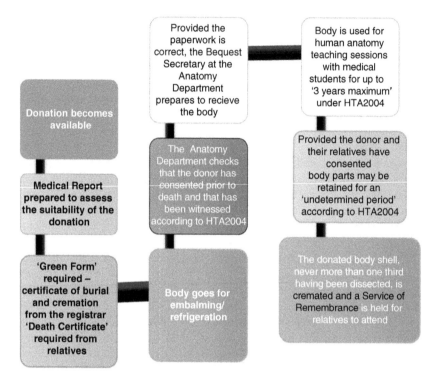

Figure 5.2 The official procedures for donation to a medical school anatomy department under the Human Tissue Act 2004
Source: National Archives, JA 3/1, Anatomy Office, Data-Set Returns for England, c. 1992–98.

Coronial Necropsies – Missed Opportunities and Their Public Health Costs

In the early 1980s, the National Patient Safety Agency (hereafter NPSA) commissioned a series of annual reports paid for by medical charity funding under the auspices of the National Confidential Enquiry into Patient Outcome and Death (referred to from now on as the NCEPOD), which we touched on in the introduction to this chapter.[78] The aim of the initiative was threefold: first, to better understand why patients died in large medical facilities, such as NHS teaching hospitals. Second, to ascertain what Coronial reports indicated about 'real' causes of death on a national, regional and local basis in order to improve healthcare standards. Third, to identify whether pathologists could help improve autopsy reports and assist with auditing perioperative deaths. Professional bodies like the Association of Anaesthetists and Surgeons and the Royal College of Pathologists and the Coroners' Society agreed to co-operate with the NCEPOD to try to improve best practice. It was, however, the NCEPOD report for 1990 that would cause the most controversy by identifying that with respect to autopsy reports, 'communications between pathologists' (whether working in hospitals or with coroners) 'and clinicians is so poor that useful lessons cannot often be learnt'. As a result, a Joint Working Party of the Royal Colleges convened in 1991. It recommended that there should be a more 'systematic monitoring of the discrepancy rates between ante-mortem [patients' health profiles] and post-mortem diagnoses', with this vital clinical information being made 'more widely available to consultants'.[79] In other words, there was a recognition that explicit body disputes existed, they were generated by Coronial cases, and yet, not enough was being done to learn from them. Cases that attracted a lot of adverse publicity had therefore no balancing mechanism of a public gain for the medical scientific community. Bio-commons was not necessarily beneficial for everybody.

Further complicating this common situation was that central government defended its position about a lack of public health gains by pointing to better clinical audit procedures that were enshrined into the National Health Service and Community Care Act (Eliz. 2 c. 19: 1990). That new legislation had created self-governing NHS trusts, as well as GP fund-holding practices. They were now responsible for managing healthcare and welfare services in the community, including their financing.[80] This was creating serious resource issues for the Coronial Office, with central government finance re-diverted to NHS front-line need. With less in local budgets for coroners and pathologists to spend, fewer healthcare lessons were passed on. The situation was a missed opportunity cost. It was becoming unaffordable for the dead to improve medical outcomes for the living. There thus remained uncertainty inside the reorganised NHS system as to whether autopsy results were in reality informing clinical practice or not, with many practitioners sceptical that they did so.[81] Against this backdrop, the fact that autopsy rates declined significantly between the 1990s and the passing of HTA2004 appeared to be a worrying trend. Consequently, the NCEPOD in 2006 undertook a new investigation styled: 'The Coroner's Autopsy: Do we deserve better?' Its ramifications were to be far-reaching.

The NCEPOD 2006 audit highlighted that the *Broderick Report* (1971)[82] and the *Lucre Report* (2003)[83] had both indicated that there were persistent problems with autopsy reporting procedures across the United Kingdom. It remained the case that as late as 2006 there was 'no single body or department that oversees death certification and coroners'. Exacerbating this situation was the fact that 'the service is part local and part national'. Although most pathologists worked for the NHS, 'coroners are appointed by the Lord Chief

Justice and come under the Department of Constitutional Affairs'. So even when a coroner and pathologist worked side by side, each had a different reporting mechanism, as well as different systems of audit and accountability. In addition, the Registrars of Death responsible for monitoring the accuracy of death certificates remained the responsibility of 'the Office for National Statistics ... under the aegis of Her Majesty's Treasury'. The NCEPOD thus concluded: 'There is no centralisation or unification of responsibility and accountability' involving the Coronial Office. As a result, potentially many sorts of body disputes were being generated by a lack of communication, sporadic co-ordination, and ad hoc customary practices in Coronial autopsies, even post-HTA2004. They hence asked a pressing question: 'What level of quality in the Coronial autopsy service does the public want?' Answering this conundrum proved to be provocative because there was a mismatch between public perceptions and actual Coronial working practices of some longevity.

NCEPOD 2006 set out that there was a historical problem with the basic cost of autopsies to the taxpayer – a controversy stretching back to the 1830s – which had never been resolved.[84] It had continually undermined the official reach of the Coronial Office in England and Wales. The public expected a high standard of service and coroners to be accountable, but such aspirations did not match adequate funding allocations. As NCEPOD pointed out, 'when considering the variable quality of the current autopsy process, several pathologists and coroners commented: *What do you expect for £87.70* [the current fee for a standard autopsy without further investigations]?' Low fees meant spending no more than thirty minutes on an autopsy. Coroners paid pathologists to do their pathology work but had to factor in the opportunity costs associated with budget shortfalls. This had given rise to what this book calls a system of presumptions. That is, over time the public made assumptions about coroner/pathologist working relationships that did not match realities. For instance, most coroners on cost grounds continued to tolerate a certain level of amateurish procedures due to underfunding. Many autopsies had the official appearance of a forensic examination, but they are nothing of the sort, as the standard modus operandi of a detailed 'post-mortem' remained undefined in law. Consequently, the NCEPOD found that there were significant levels of misinformation inside the autopsy system, exacerbating a lack of clinical clarity. Very basic and routine mistakes happened a lot because of poor or illegible handwriting on rushed reports written hastily by coroners and pathologists. It was impossible to engage with autopsy outcomes because they were often indecipherable. In a digital age, this was unquestionably outdated and represented an opportunity cost for researchers to better engage with both the demographic and geographical subtleties of mortality rates in community medicine. Against this backdrop, the NCEPOD report in 2006 became the focus of a national debate about the future of the Coronial Office.

In 2005–6, the NCEPOD audited 114,600 autopsies (some 22 per cent of a total of 513,000 deaths that year) in which the Coronial Office was involved in England and Wales. In terms of those demographics, one headline announcement that was to shape media reaction was that 'the advisors had concerns over the quality of autopsy examinations in the very elderly'. They concluded that 'these were done less carefully than those on younger patients'. In an ageing population, this was a noteworthy trend, especially since anatomy teaching and research were reliant on the gerontology of necropsy bequests. There was little joined-up thinking between coroners/pathologists/anatomists of the sort that had characterised the Victorian era. A summary of the audit study also observed how:

- One in four autopsy reports was judged as poor or unacceptable
- In one third of mortuaries, the pathologist failed to inspect the body before the anatomical pathology technologist commenced opening it and removed the organs
- In one in seven cases, the brain was not examined
- In one in sixteen cases, it was deemed that histology should have been taken in order to determine the cause of death
- In nearly one in five cases, the cause of death as stated was questionable
- The extent of the examination of the heart, in those with abnormalities that might be due to cardiomyopathy (some of which are inherited), was poor
- The extent of the examination of patients with known epilepsy who died unexpectedly was poor
- There was poor recording of the presence of external injuries
- The examination of decomposed bodies was of poor quality
- There was poor communication between coroners and pathologists
- There were significant gaps in the information provided to the pathologists by the coroner[85]

Since WWII, it ought to have been the case that Coronial necropsies were a potential 'treasure trove of information' (as this chapter argued earlier). Instead, 'real causes of death' remained 'hidden because of indifferent post-mortem examinations'. Done hastily, they were often 'obscured by deficient recording of data'. Such basic flaws had not been resolved for over fifty years.[86] It was thus self-evident to many inside the profession why disputed bodies came about from the 1960s to the 1990s. As one coroner described it: 'The system is confused chaos [run] more by default than by design.' Hidden histories of the dead thus mattered and still matter for the living. For every explicit dispute, there needed to be a much better public health gain. Central government's solution was to launch an inquiry into the power and palette of the Coronial Office, but this soon proved to be controversial too.

Around 2006, after the NCEPOD report was published, the media turned their attention to a central government proposal to create a new Chief Coroner for

England and Wales. Extensive newspaper coverage debated whether this was justified on costs grounds or not. Central government proposed that the person appointed to the new role must get rid of a lot of wasteful bureaucracy and instigate a reformed system. Only this approach, it was argued, would begin to counteract explicit body disputes and the lack of public health gains: the latter was occurring on a regular basis. Everyone agreed with the NCEPOD main findings. Public health schemes should be better informed by Coronial statistics in a biomedical era. Yet, how this was to be counterbalanced with the desire to strengthen the impact of the Inquest process was unclear. What complicated the contemporary debates was that a global recession occurred in 2007. It would require a large budget to set up a new Chief Coroner's Office at a time of severe government cutbacks. Exacerbating this budget issue was that after the Coroners and Justice Act (Eliz. 2 c. 25: 2009), there was an expectation that the new legislation would overhaul a Coronial system with three inherent structural problems. First, there needed to be unambiguous leadership at the top of the Coronial service to direct future policy making. This strategic focus should be in line with central government thinking and reflect the range of stakeholders that coroners had to work with on a regular basis, including the public, pathologists and the police. Second, there had to be a better system of public accountability that would involve streamlining diverse local working practices so that these were co-ordinated around strategic priorities to improve the Coronial service overall. Third, the devolution of funding and its historical discrepancies had to be rectified. What then complicated this tripartite juggling act was a political commitment in the new Bill. It promised to uphold a new *Charter for the Bereaved*, which 'set out a range of service standards and consumer rights'.[87] The general public wanted more medical information, better consultation and improved communication channels, with the option to appeal against a coroner's verdict when, for example, 'viewing a body' or attending an Inquest.

In considering this insider/outsider set of stakeholders and their different perspectives, Alexander Pitman was one of a number of expert commentators who highlighted the inherent flaw with central government's public engagement aspirations. He told the press, 'The possibility remained that the *Charter* might raise expectations beyond the capabilities of the service, offering bereaved people *a list of laudable but unenforceable empty promises* [sic].' The latter was discussed at length during the second reading of the Bill.[88] In other words, the question of how to bridge rhetoric (legislation) versus reality (working styles) was a significant Coronial hurdle. As a result, a three-year consultation process began against the backdrop of the global financial crisis.[89] The Coalition government (2010–15) threatened to cancel the new office of Chief Coroner to help meet the budget deficit, but then did another volte-face when confronted with concerted opposition by Parliaments' Public Administration Select Committee, influential pressure groups such as INQUEST and the House of Lords. After much political wrangling, the new Chief Coroner, appointed from the judicial circuit, was told to prioritise cost analysis right from the start of taking up office in July 2013. Reviewing the subsequent annual returns of the reformed Coronial Office is instructive about how exactly the new changes would redress explicit body disputes, improve public health gains from Inquest information and streamline procedures that were still ad hoc in the regions. The simple answer is that this was an impossible task. Findings explain the longevity of ingrained problems with the power and palette of Coronial Office responsibilities, as we approach the conclusion to this chapter.

The Coroners' Statistics Annual Report for England and Wales is issued in May each year as a Ministry of Justice bulletin. It is the main legal instrument by which leadership, accountability and devolved budgets of the Chief Coroner are measured. These three facets of the working portfolios of all Coronial offices also feed into the Office for National Statistics mortality figures. In 2015 some

234,406 deaths were reported to coroners . . . an increase of 12,565 (6%) from 2014 . . . [with] just under half (45%) of all registered deaths [being] reported to coroners . . . [in] the last ten years, this proportion has been generally consistent within the range of 45% to 47%.[90]

In terms of post-mortems, some '89,206' were ordered by coroners, or '38% of all cases reported to them'. That said, not all post-mortems required that an Inquest come to court. Some are now 'a paper inquest' – a process that used to be known as a 'non-Jury' inquest in the past. In fact, since '1995, the proportion of post-mortem inquests has decreased by 23 percentage points, from 61% to 38%'. Examining those statistics in Figure 5.3, it is evident that there had been a decline in post-mortem work (broadly defined) after the mid-1990s, from 126,398 cases in 1995 to 119,610 by 2003. Yet after the passing of HTA2004, there was a further falling off of post-mortem work, with a downward trend of about 5,000 Coronial cases in every biennial accounting cycle. Chapter 6 will be exploring the impact of these trends on the work of pathologists, too. Meantime, the overall picture of post-mortems from 2011 to 2015 now has stabilised, with 95 per cent of all coroners' cases requiring a standard post-mortem.[91] Generally, 20 per cent required histology and 14 per cent toxicology (to ascertain class A drug or alcohol abuse, as well as poison from a drug overdose in cases of suicide). These are therefore the remaining potential explicit body disputes still in the system, though many have now been modified by the HTA2004's fully informed consent provisions. It remains, however, to be seen whether public health measures will improve because the system is still not uniform, remains underfunded and still operates by a considerable amount of discretionary justice: we conclude by reflecting on these historical observations of some longevity from Part I (human stories of explicit disputes) and Part II (their creation by the Coronial Office) of this chapter.

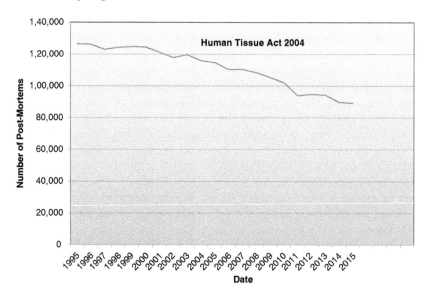

Figure 5.3 Number of post-mortems held on behalf of coroners in England
and Wales, 1995–2015
Source: https://www.gov.uk/government/statistics/coroners-statistics-2015,
accessed 31/03/2015.

Conclusion

Delays have been a very big problem, and they continue to be a big problem. If
there is one thing that comes across my desk on a regular basis, which is more
distressing than anything else, it is families writing, saying: Why has there been
three years' delay? Why has there been five years' delay? Why has there been
seven years' delay? Why has there been no date? Why don't I have a date for
anything? When is my inquest going to be? What about my family? We are all
distressed. One case came in my direction recently where the High Court had
ordered a coroner to resume an inquest. He had decided that there was no need
to resume the inquest, and was going to leave it at that. But the High Court
decided otherwise. So they ordered the coroner to resume the inquest.
Unfortunately that case got forgotten about. The papers got put on a shelf in
the back of the office for six and a half years. When it was brought back, the
family not surprisingly wanted a new coroner to conduct their inquest. I helped
them, and they got one. So delays are really poor, and they need to be reduced.[92]

In a history of explicit disputes, it was the sense of more 'extra time of the dead'
inside the Coronial system that created the context for families to become
frustrated by the amount of bureaucracy involved. Many expressed cultural

reservations about losing control of a loved one's body, especially once the transplantation era opened. And, as the above quotation by the Chief Coroner for England and Wales confirms from 2013, this historical problem of procedural delays has not necessarily been resolved in the intervening years. Hence, in 2015 the *Criminal Law and Justice Weekly* reported that: 'The most recent report of the Judicial Conduct Investigations Office showed 556 complaints were made about coroners in 2015–2016, up from 262 in 2014–2015 and 51 in 2013–2014.' By way of example, they cited the following case:

Mary Hassell, senior coroner for Camden, Islington, Hackney and Tower Hamlets, in a letter to Camden Council, extracts from which were quoted by the *Mail on Sunday* last year, alleged bullying and intimidation by the Orthodox Jewish Community in the wake of her decisions to order autopsies against the wishes of some members of devout religions. Following investigation of a complaint against her, to the Judicial Conduct Investigations Office, the Lord Chancellor and the Lord Chief Justice concluded that Ms Hassell had not misrepresented or distorted the position in her letter, as had been alleged, and dismissed this aspect of the complaint. However, they found that her decision to disclose the 'private letter' to the media demonstrated a serious lack of judgment, amounting to misconduct, and issued a reprimand.[93]

This question of tense relationships with the media and what public statements an individual coroner could make has remained one of the most challenging for the Coronial service in its long history. Indeed, at the heart of the all the representative cases cited in this chapter involving organ donation cards was the problem of how to manage the bereaved wanting agency over their dead loved one, transplant stakeholders in NHS facilities and media interest in new biotechnologies, which was often intrusive at the most tragic moment in family life. It was no easy task for coroners to be public advocates and protect the privacy of the grieving. An added difficulty has been the way that coroners were appointed, and then authorised to work on an ad hoc basis. Again, as the Chief Coroner explained in 2013:

There are also signs of a lack of a modern approach amongst some coroners' offices. I went to one coroner's office in the north, I won't say where, where there had been problems with delays, and they were using typewriters. That was a symbol, it seemed to me, of a problem of lack of organisation, and of efficiency. If you don't have efficiency, you will have delays. You will put that case at the back of the shelf and forget about it because it is a bit troublesome. So there are procedural reforms which have a rather more modern look to them. They involve opening inquests in public, recording all the hearings, setting a date for the next hearing, hopefully the final hearing, at an early stage, and giving directions to experts to provide reports and statements within a short period of time. One coroner said to me: '*I have a pathologist who's a bit slow. Usually it takes her a year to produce a report.*' I said '*That's not a report. That's a guess about what her notes mean*' [*sic*].[94]

The only way to resolve this situation is to acknowledge that coroners have, for far too long, relied on underfunded post-mortems, often scribbled down, frequently illegible, and these have represented missed opportunities for bio-medicine to learn from the dead for the living with fully informed consent. Inside the system, any legal loopholes created by inefficient bureaucracy also shaped public misperceptions in the run-up to HTA2004 that medico-legal staff acted duplicitously with taxpayers that paid their salaries in the NHS. Most did not do so deliberately, but it was nonetheless the impression fashioned in the public imagination. Anatomists suffered from this situation too when their final certificates after cremation were not signed off efficiently or officially by the Anatomy Inspectorate during the 1990s, in some cases by as much as three years at the DHSS. It looked like they were as guilty as pathologists of working their way around the law, when in fact most had been meticulous. Anywhere inside the system in fact, where too many overlapping agencies had been created, gave rise to a potential pathway for a future body dispute – a trend that medico-legal officials lost public sight of. Some medico-legal staff took advantage of this situation to conduct 'extra considerations' – a slippery medical research term – that we can only glimpse happening in an imperfect historical record filled with gaps and paperwork consigned for shredding.

The case of Carol Morris (and many others like it) is hence symbolic of heightened disputes about when to 'call death' and who could officially vie for disputed body parts from the 1960s through to the end of the 1990s. Herbert Jones (who opened this chapter), for instance, expressed in writing to numerous officials, close friends and remaining relatives in his life his wish to donate post-mortem and give the 'gift' of new ways of seeing his body. Yet, once *peri-mortem* (at or near the point of death), he was frustrated by the Coronial Office involved. This was because he was (strictly speaking) one of the first legal suicide cases in Britain once any foul play and assisted suicide was ruled out: and the ramifications of that Coronial dilemma are still unresolved in Britain today. As we shall see in Chapter 7, the ethical boundaries between suicide and assisted dying remain very controversial – even more so than in Herbert Jones's day. A painful prognosis like fatal cancer continues on many occasions to confound caring and understandably cautious medico-legal staff. Nonetheless, his explicit dispute is informative about the number of officials that had an official opinion in processes of decision-making. These actor networks could be very extensive indeed. Yet, it has always been vital for coroners to work collaboratively whatever the circumstances of their working-lives. Indeed, this is a commonplace situation that the Chief Coroner acknowledged in 2013, when he commented: 'It is no good for the coroner to sit back in his office, with the typewriters clicking away in the next room. He has got to work with that rather peculiar triangle within which he has to operate.'[95] Unquestionably, he elaborated, one of the main procedural difficulties is that:

A senior coroner is appointed by the local authority but not employed by them, so their line manager is the Chief Coroner, or possibly the Lord Chief Justice. Then you have coroners' officers, employed by the police. Their line manager is a detective sergeant, or some other officer. Then you have administrative staff, who are employed by the local authority, and line managed by someone there.

In other words, there was, and has continued to be, a: 'peculiar triangle and it only works if everybody is working together.' The solution, the Chief Coroner believes, especially when dealing with disputed bodies and complaints about coroners on the rise, is: 'talking about problems, making sure where there is a disciplinary problem in the office and getting that sorted out, keeping a review of cases on a monthly basis, discussing, collaborating'. The 'balance of probability' has always been decided by public engagement, and it thus remains one of the most important communication tools in explicit body disputes involving the Coronial Office.

In the next chapter, we thus explore in more detail why it was that pathologists got that balance wrong in their working-lives and protocols of medical research. We turn next to consider brain retention work because it is even more emblematic to families in body disputes than organs and tissues taken from those involved in tragic accidents like that of Carol Morris that were to make national and international headlines in transplantation with far-reaching consequences for medical law and bioethics. Our final substantive chapter is going to focus on missed disputes that involved research on the brain and its controversial nature in the modern era. For as professionals, pathologists looked very guilty of working their way around the law because the time constraints they operated with proved to be very different from those of everyone else in hidden histories of the body.

Notes

1. '12 people get notes from a Dead Man', *Daily Mail*, 6 December 1962, issue 20720, p. 11.
2. Detailed record linkage work on this case reveals an odd discrepancy in the record-keeping. Mr Herbert Thomas Jones was born in 1885. He married Amelia Joan who pre-deceased him in 1962. Probate records after his death confirm that his legal will still stated that he bequeathed '£7,241 14 s[hillings] to his widow' on 15 February 1963 at Winchester Probate Division – see Ancestry, National Probate Calendar (1963), Index of Wills and Administration, p. 159 entry. Yet, his widow and only son were already dead according to the Coronial records. Despite extensive checking, this author cannot explain the legal inconsistency; around £7,000 was also a large sum of money to bequest at that time.
3. See Helen MacDonald, 'Guarding the public interest: England's coroners and organ transplants, 1960–1975', *Journal of British Studies*, 54 (October 2015), 4: 926–946; MacDonald, 'Conscripting organs: "routine salvaging" or bequest? The historical debate in Britain, 1961–75', *Journal of the History of Medicine and Allied Sciences*, 70 (2014), 3: 425–461.

4. A point made convincingly by. K. Chen, 'The coroner's necropsy – an epidemiological treasure trove', *Journal of Clinical Pathology*, 49 (1996): 698–699, quote at p. 699.

5. For historical context, see, notably, E. T. Hurren, 'Whose body is it anyway?: trading the dead poor, coroner's disputes, and the business of anatomy at Oxford University, 1885–1929', *Bulletin of the History of Medicine*, 82 (Winter 2008), 4: 775–818; Hurren, 'Remaking the medico-legal scene: a social history of the late-Victorian coroner in Oxford', *Journal of the History of Medicine and Allied Sciences*, 65 (April 2010), 2: 207–252; and Hurren and S. A. King, 'Courtship at the coroner's court', *Social History*, 40 (2015), 2: 185–207.

6. Peter King, *Crime and Law in England, 1750–1840: Remaking Justice from the Margins* (Oxford: Oxford University Press, 2010), p.1.

7. Detailed in Ian Burney, *Bodies of Evidence: Medicine and the Politics of the English Inquest 1830–1926* (Baltimore: John Hopkins Press, 2000).

8. See, for example, Wellcome Collection, blog, 'Paris Morgue', 1 June 2015, accessed 18/01/2017 at: https://wellcomecollection.org/articles/paris-morgue/

9. Refer, Crown Prosecution Service, public information website, 'Coroners and their legal responsibilities', accessed 18/01/2017 at: http://www.cps.gov.uk/legal/a_to_c/coroners/

10. Refer, Elizabeth Hallam, Jenny Hockey and Glennys Howarth, *Beyond the Body: Death and Social Identity* (London: Routledge, 1999).

11. Refer, E. T. Hurren, *Dissecting the Criminal Corpse: Staging Post-Execution Punishment in Early Modern England* (Basingstoke: Palgrave Macmillan, 2016); chapters 2 and 4 detail standard methods.

12. See, notably, Katherine Watson, *Poisoned Lives: English Poisoners and Their Victims* (London: Hambledon Continuum Press, 2006).

13. Outlined with case material in Ian Burney and Neil Pemberton, *Murder and the Making of the English CSI* (Baltimore: John Hopkins Press, 2016).

14. St Bartholomew's Hospital Archives, Dissection registers, MS/81–6, Body Number 9, 7 July 1894, William Smith from Islington Infirmary. See also E. T. Hurren, *Dying for Victorian Medicine: English Anatomy and Its Trade in the Dead Poor, c. 1834–1929* (Basingstoke: Palgrave Macmillan, 2012), chapter 4.

15. Refer, Edward Higgs, *The Information State in England: The Central Collection of Information on Citizens since 1500* (Basingstoke: Palgrave Macmillan, 2003).

16. See, for example, in the same week that Mr Herbert Jones died: 'Argument in the News Feature: should doctors prolong death', *Daily Mail*, 7 December 1962, p. 1, which responded to debates in the *Lancet* with the Euthanasia Society. It gave coverage in 'A professor talks about 30,000 who want to die', *Daily Mail*, 10 December 1962, p. 6, quoting G. M. Cairstairs, Chair in Psychological Medicine at Edinburgh University, who said that 'more than 5,000 people will have committed suicide in Britain this year [1962] and at least 30,000 will have tried to'. Giving the 5th BBC Reith Lecture, Professor Cairstairs noted higher rates of depression in British society, reflecting how in his professional experience: 'Human beings need something more than physical comfort and mental tranquillity; they need a sense of values to give significance to their lives.' In a fatal prognosis, hope often diminished with a poor quality of life.

17. See notable recent ruling in the Royal Court of Justice, Queen's Bench Division, Lord Justice Leggatt and Mr Justice Nicol, [2018] EWHC 1955 (Admin), Case No: CO/367/2018, which recommended 'all cases of suicide' be decided on 'the balance of probability'.

18. Cross refer, feature article, Keith Simpson, Guy's Hospital Pathology Department, 'Their death in your hands – the life of a forensic pathologist', *The Listener*, Thursday, 22 September 1977, issue 2527, p. 371.

19. Refer, E. T. Hurren, 'Patients' rights: from Alder Hey to the Nuremberg Code', *History and Policy Papers* (6 May 2002), accessed 3/11/2016 at: http://www.hist oryandpolicy.org/policy-papers/papers/patients-rights-from-alder-hey-to-the-nur emberg-code

20. *The Redfern Inquiry* delivered to Parliament, Tuesday 16 November 2008, by Right Hon. Chris Huhne MP, Secretary of State for Energy & Climate Change, The National Archives (hereafter TNA), at: http://webarchive.nationalarchives.gov.uk/ 20101214091701/http://www.theredferninquiry.co.uk/

21. Refer, Hurren, *Dying for Victorian Medicine*.

22. J. Innes, *Inferior Politics: Social Problems and Social Policies in Eighteenth Century Britain* (Oxford: Oxford University Press, 2009), p. 105.

23. See, notably, Arthur L. Caplin, James J. McCartney and Daniel P. Reid, *Replacement Parts: The Ethics of Procuring and Replacing Organs in Humans* (Washington, D.C.: Georgetown University Press, 2015).

24. 'News section: baby found dead at laundry', *Evening Standard*, 14 December 2001. Please note: There are two ways to spell fetus (the one used in this book's text) and foetus (generally appearing in original quotes).

25. N. Hawkes, 'Hospital is sorry over baby's body', *Times*, 13 January 2002.

26. Robert Bruce, 'The laundry foetus; disposal of human remains, the Anatomy Act 1984 and the Human Tissue Act 2004', *Journal of Forensic and Legal Medicine*, 17 (2010): 229–231.

27. Revised subsequently by the Cremation (Amendment) Regulations (2006).

28. Refer, *Times*, Legal section, Regina versus Poplar Coroner, ex Parte Thomas (Dorise), 'Limit on Power to hold an Inquest', 23 December 1992, issue 64523, p. 22.

29. Ibid.

30. *Times*, Law section, Law Report, Court of Appeal Report, 'No function of Inquests to apportion blame', Thursday 28 April 1994, issue 64940, p. 40.

31. A medical fact recorded on his gravestone, see Staffordshire Local History Archives, *Memorial Inscriptions Freehay Staffordshire, St. Chad's Churchyard*, Grave 0.60, 'Graham Alcock, Accidentally Killed, 12 December 1983, Aged 28, Husband of Jean and Father of Tracey and Joanne'.

32. David Cross, 'Coroner halts heart transplant', *Times*, Saturday, 17 December 1983, issue 61715, p. 3.

33. Ibid.

34. 'Coroner halts heart transplant', *Times*, 17 December 1983, p. 3.

35. 'Tributes paid to former North Staffordshire Coroner John Wain', *Stoke Sentinel*, Obituary section, 9 December 2014.

36. Dave Blackhurst, 'John Wain's was a life that touched so many in Stoke-on-Trent and beyond', *The Sentinel*, Obituary section, 16 December 2014.

37. A. P. Boardman, A. H. Grimbaldeston, C. Handley, P. W Jones and S. Wimlott, 'The North Staffordshire Suicide Study: a case control of suicide in one health district', *Psychological Medicine*, 29 (January 1999), 1: 27–33, with an acknowledgement to Mr John Wain, North Staffordshire Coroner.
38. See, L. M. Hussain and A. D. Redmond, 'Are pre-hospital deaths from an accidental injury preventable', *British Medical Journal*, 308, (23 April 1994): 1077–1080, again with an acknowledgement to Mr John Wain, North Staffordshire Coroner.
39. Mr Michael Charman died on 15 November 2009, aged 89. He had been coroner for Leicester City and South Leicestershire for over thirty years, see *Leicester Mercury*, 20 November 2009, funeral notice section. Charman was also a keen exponent of new research into sudden infant death syndrome. He gave a conference paper at the Foundation for the Study of Infant Deaths convened in Leicester in 1987. It featured as a notice in TNA, Home Office, and Memorandum CRN/84 28/29/1, dated 19 February 1987, and annotated in pencil CC5/3/53, issued by R. B. Snow, HM Coroner, central London, as a newsletter to regional HM Coronial offices.
40. 'Physician to the bereaved' – follow-up letter to the lead article, by Mr Michael Charman, HM Coroner for Leicester City and South Leicestershire, *British Medical Journal*, Saturday, 6 August 1992, p. 384. He worked with four pathologists, a detective and two constables to resolve his 1,400 Coronial cases per annum.
41. 'Physician to the bereaved', p. 384.
42. A moped is a small motorcycle. UK citizens cannot drive a car until aged 17 or over, but can drive a moped at aged 16 or over. Typically, mopeds travel about the same speed as electric bicycles on public roadways.
43. Gareth Parry, 'Coroner's order puts doubts on transplant surgery: doctor's spokes-man calls for closer co-operation after row over remarks at an Inquest on girl in heart case', *Guardian*, 1 March 1980, p. 20.
44. See, 'Nigel Olney, transplant patient, 44', *New York Times*, 22 December 1988. Nigel Olney was a divorced father of two teenage children, aged 35 at his first transplant and aged 44 at his second failed one. See also report 'Nine year heart transplant survivor', *Los Angeles Times*, 22 December 1988, which elaborates that during his second transplant he did initially well but then deteriorated after day three and did not recover. He was an active fund-raiser for the Papworth Heart Transplant Team.
45. See, Fred Roach, 'A new beginning: memories of a volunteer worker, 1981–1996', *British Cardiac Patients Journal, The Official Magazine of the British Cardiac Patients Association*, 189 (April–May 2013), p. 10. Fred Roach knew and worked with Nigel Olney at Papworth Hospital where they raised money and worked as volunteers for the British Cardiac Patients Association. He visited him just before his second transplant and he expected to survive but did not after the third day post-operative.
46. See, *Papworth Hospital*, 'Papworth heroes', public engagement webpages, 'Terence English', accessed 21/02/2017 at: http://www.papworthhospital.nhs.uk/papworthheroes/papworth-hero.php?hero=9/
47. Parry, 'Coroner's order puts doubts on transplant surgery', p. 20.
48. See, Tom O'Malley and Olive Soley, *Regulating the Press* (London: Pluto Press, 2000), chapter 5, 'Nothing resolved: self-regulation and survival, 1972–98', pp. 71–96, which explains that the PC was under significant public pressure by the early

1980s to put its house in order or face a privacy bill entering Parliament. It never resolved its internal workings and was by the 1990s to be replaced by the Press Complaints Commission, and then from 2014 by the Independent Press Standards Organisation after the phone-hacking scandal.

49. The PC Complaint was reported in full to Parliament, see, *Hansard*, HC, vol. 123, cols. 456–91, 5 March 1980, 'Human Organs (Anonymity of Donors)', presented by the Right Hon. Mr John Farr MP, for the Market Harborough Division.

50. *Hansard*, HC, vol. 123. cols. 456–91, 5 March 1980, quotes at col. 498.

51. *Hansard*, HC, vol. 123. cols. 456–91, 5 March 1980, quotes at col. 490.

52. Parry, 'Coroner's order puts doubts on transplant surgery', p. 20.

53. Ibid., p. 20.

54. Editorial lead, 'Coroner tightens transplant rules: heart swap "shrouded in mystery" inquest on schoolgirl donor is told', *Guardian*, 29 February 1980, p. 3.

55. *Hansard*, HC, vol. 980, cols. 488–91, 5 March 1980, early day motion.

56. Ibid.

57. *Hansard*, HC, vol. 980, col. 491, 5 December 1980, 'Human Organs (Anonymity of Donors)', brought forward by Mr John Farr, Rt. Hon. Member for the Market Harborough division.

58. Ibid.

59. Refer, Tom Dayell, 'Westminster scene: to tidy up transplant procedure', *New Scientist* (27 May 1971): 525, explains that he first got involved in the spare-part surgery debate because of delays in kidney transplants and their lack of supply which resulted in the death of 'a 22 year old teacher in 1965' whom he knew personally who lived in his Scottish constituency. He introduced a 10-minute ruling bill into Parliament to highlight the problem across Britain. As a result, he worked closely with the Royal Society of Medicine, Richard Crossman, then Minister for Social Services, and prominent surgeons such as Sir Michael Woodruff, Professor Ray Calne and others. See, also, Tom Dayell, *The Importance of Being Awkward: The Autobiography of Tom Dayell with a foreword by Professor Peter Hennessy* (Edinburgh: Birlinn Publishers Ltd, 2012 edition), chapter 9, 'The 1980s', recounts his involvement in new medical enterprises of transplantation.

60. This issue has been recently investigated from a national perspective, too, in David Hamilton, *A History of Organ Transplantation: Ancient Legends to Modern Practice* (Pittsburgh: University of Pittsburgh Press, 2012), chapter 10, 'Experimental organ transplantation', pp. 195–220.

61. *Hansard*, HC, vol. 980, col. 491, 5 December 1980, 'Human Organs (Anonymity of Donors)', brought forward by Mr John Farr, Rt. Hon. Member, Market Harborough division.

62. Stephen Cook, 'Sitting up with a new heart', *Guardian*, Lead article, 30 January 1980, p. 1.

63. Refer, Ian Sample, Science Correspondent, 'Alcohol abusers should not get transplants says Best's surgeon', in which it was explained that the transplant surgeon, Nigel Heaton (Head of the Liver Transplant Team at King's College Hospital London), who performed George Best's liver transplant in 2002 expressed his view that 'those who abuse alcohol should be kicked off waiting-lists', *Guardian*, Science section, Wednesday, 5 October 2005, pp. 1–2. See, also, for instance, 'Transplant row over organs for drinkers', *Observer*, Sunday 15 February 2009,

which reported on p. 1 that: 'Heavy drinkers are receiving nearly one in four of the UK's liver transplants, it was revealed last night, igniting a furious row about the ethics of allocating organs to people with alcohol problems. Figures show that transplants for heavy drinkers have risen by more than 60% in the past decade, while waiting lists have lengthened. In December 1997, 180 people in the UK were awaiting a liver transplant, compared with 325 in the same month last year. Dr Tony Calland, chairman of the British Medical Association's medical ethics committee, said surgeons are within their rights to refuse transplants to anyone with alcohol-related liver disease if they do not demonstrate a genuine desire to stop drinking.'

64. Stephen Cook, 'Heart man stable', *Guardian*, 31 January 1980, p. 26.
65. See, for instance, Ole M. Høystad, *A History of the Heart* (London: Reaktion Books Ltd, 2007), which places the heart in a European-wide cultural context.
66. Thus extending the scholarship of Higgs, *The Information State in England*.
67. Christine Doyle, 'The return of transplant fever', *Observer*, 3 February 1980, p. 9.
68. Cook, 'Heart man stable', p. 26.
69. BBC Archive Collection, *Tomorrow's World Special*, 'Barnard faces his critics', televised 2 February 1968, accessed 22/02/2017 at: http://www.bbc.co.uk/archive/tomorrowsworld/8006.shtml. He was also criticised for a lack of clarity on how he claimed 'success' given that 'only 25 of the first 100 heart transplant patients were to survive more than a few months'. He clarified that it would be more accurate to describe it as 'some success'.
70. 'Barnard faces his critics'.
71. Scott Carney, *The Red Market: On the Trail of the World's Organ Brokers, Bone Thieves, Blood Farmers, and Child Traffickers* (New York: William Morrow, 2011).
72. See, F. Dobbels, F. Van Gelder, A. Verkinderen, et al., 'Should the law on anonymity of organ donation be changed? The perception of live liver transplants', *Clinical Transplant Journal*, 23 (June–July 2009), 3: 375–381.
73. C. Annema, S. Op den Dries, A. P. van den Berg, A. V. Rachor and R. J. Porte, 'Opinions of Dutch liver transplant recipients on anonymity of organ donation and direct contact with donors' families', *Transplantation Journal*, 99 (April 2015), 4: 879–894, the sample size was n=177/244 liver transplant patients who agreed to take part in the survey.
74. P. Azuri and N. Tabak, 'The transplant team's role with regard to establishing contact between organ recipient and the family of a cadaver organ donor', *Journal of Clinical Nursing*, 21 (March 2012), 5–6: 888–896 on the Israeli context; P. Gill and L. Lowes, 'Gift exchange and organ donation: donor and recipient of live kidney transplantation', *International Journal of Nursing Studies*, 45 (2008), 11: 1607–1617.
75. TNA, JA 3/1, HM Anatomy Inspectorate Returns on Dissections, 1992–1998.
76. TNA, JA 3/1, Anatomy Office, Data-Set Returns for England, c. 1992–98.
77. Thomas W. Laqueur, *The Work of the Dead: A Cultural History of Mortal Remains* (Princeton: Princeton University Press, 2015), p. 10.
78. Refer, Julian L. Burton and Guy N. Rutty (eds.), *The Hospital Autopsy: A Manual of Fundamental Autopsy Practice*, 3rd ed. (London: Hodder Arnold, 2001), p. 317.
79. Burton and Rutty, *Hospital Autopsy*, p. 320.

80. See, Graham Thornicroft, 'The NHS and the Community Care Act 1990: recent government policy and legislation', *Psychiatric Bulletin*, 18 (1994): 13–17.

81. See, notably, James Underwood, 'The future of the autopsy', in Burton and Rutty (eds.), *Hospital Autopsy*, chapter 2, pp. 11–16.

82. See, TNA, HO375, Committee on Death Certification and Coroners (Broderick Committee) minutes and papers, 1964–71 – 'The Committee was appointed by the Home Secretary, the Rt. Hon. Frank Soskice on 17 March 1965, under the chairmanship of Mr Norman Brodrick QC (as he then was) and its terms of reference were to review: (i) the law and practice relating to the issue of medical certificates of the cause of death and for the disposal of dead bodies and; (ii) the law and practice relating to Coroners and Coroners Courts, the reporting of deaths to the Coroners and related matters, and to recommend what changes are desirable. The impetus for setting up this Committee was provided by the publication of a report prepared for the Private Practice Committee of the British Medical Association by some of the members of its Forensic Medicine Sub-committee. The report entitled *Deaths in the Community* argued that such were the loopholes in the existing law regulating death certification and the coroners system generally, that it was possible for homicides to go undetected, a claim the Committee dismissed quite early into their investigations. The Committee published its report in November 1971, amidst considerable criticism about the amount of time it had taken over its deliberations.'

83. Refer, TNA, HMSO, CM 5831, 'Death Certification and Investigation in England, Wales and Northern Ireland: The Report of a Fundamental Review (*Lucre Report*) 2003', pp. 1–361, accessed 16/03/2017 at: http://webarchive.nationalarchives.gov .uk/20131205100653/http:/www.archive2.official-documents.co.uk/document/c m58/5831/5831.pdf. It explained that: 'In our Consultation Paper of August 2002 we offered an analysis of the systems' defects, and a set of aims for their reform. We concluded that the death certification and coroner services were not "fit for purpose" in modern society. This conclusion and the aims we suggested for their reform were widely supported in consultation responses'.

84. On this historical problem, see Ian Burney, *Bodies of Evidence.*

85. Refer, NCEPOD website (www.ncepod.ork.uk) where all reports are available online on open access – 2006 report, accessed 26/6/2016, pp. 1–176, quote at p. 113 at http://www.ncepod.org.uk/2006Report/Downloads/Coronial%20Autopsy% 20Report%202006.pdf

86. A point made convincingly by K. Chen, 'The coroner's necropsy – an epidemiological treasure trove', *Journal of Clinical Pathology*, 49 (1996): 698–699, quote at p. 699.

87. Refer, *Ministry of Justice: Draft Charter for the Bereaved Who Came into Contact with a Reformed Coroner System TSO* (London: HM Stationary Office, 2008).

88. A. Pitman, 'Reform of the coroners' service in England and Wales: policy-making and politics', *The Psychiatrist* (2012): 1–5, quote at p. 2.

89. There were sweeping changes made to government funding of a lot of quangos at the time, and there was the suggestion that the Coronial Office could be downsized too; see, for example, J. Wise, 'Government axes a further 11 health quangos', *British Medical Journal* (2010): 341.

90. These are the latest figures available (as this book goes to press) in *Coroners Statistics Annual 2015 England and Wales Ministry of Justice Statistics Bulletin* (London: HMSO, Stationary Office, 12 May 2016).
91. Ibid., table 4.
92. Statement by HHJ Peter Thornton QC, Chief Coroner for England and Wales, on 'Reforming the Inquest' to the All-Party Penal Affairs Parliamentary Group held on 5th November 2013 at the House of Commons, Minutes reported verbatim by the Prison Reform Trust website, accessed 4/4/2017 at: http://www.prisonreformtrust .org.uk/PressPolicy/Parliament/AllPartyParliamentaryPenalAffairsGroup/ Nov2013ReformingtheCoronerService
93. Veronica Cowen, 'Feature article "coroner's update"', *Criminal Law and Justice Weekly*, 80 (10 September 2016), 34: 1–2, accessed 4/4/2017 at: https://www.crim inallawandjustice.co.uk/features/Coroners%E2%80%99-Update-11
94. See, again, Statement by HHJ Peter Thornton QC, footnote 92 above.
95. Ibid.

6   Missed Disputes
Brainstorming Neuroscience

Introduction

On 15 March 2017, the BBC reported the controversial case of John Culshaw deceased. Greater Manchester Police (hereafter GMP) had retained his organs for over twenty years.[1] An investigation found that there had been no official audit of his retained human material by the Home Office, despite HTA2004. The facts were that after Mr Culshaw was stabbed to death in Wigan on 23 October in 1993, Manchester Coronial Office appointed a senior forensic pathologist from Birmingham to his case. The bereaved family were not informed of the extent of the subsequent histopathology; effectively John Culshaw's 'stomach, liver and other organs and tissues had been retained after two post-mortem examinations' – one to establish the cause of death and the other to gather evidence for a criminal prosecution of homicide. Contemporaneous and subsequent harvesting meant that around 50 per cent of his entire body mass had been taken, much more than was required to satisfy legal evidence standards in court at the time. The victim's family meanwhile thought they had buried him mostly intact. The GMP thus told the press that they had 'agonised over a number of months' whether to tell the family or not that 'a significant amount of extra human material of John Culshaw' had been stored in a police laboratory ever since his death. On balance their ethics committee concluded that they had a moral duty to do so. The retentions had been before HTA2004 came into force, and were not therefore, strictly speaking, illegal. Nevertheless, GMP wanted to be transparent about the pathology error in keeping the body parts for so long without doing anything with them.

This chapter's central focus is therefore a third type of body dispute compared to those we have encountered in Part II of this book so far. In Chapter 4 we examined disputes that arose because consent was implied but never done properly with incomplete post-mortem paperwork inside the system of bequest or donation that supplied anatomical schools and medical research facilities. In Chapter 5 we examined two further types of explicit body dispute involving the Coronial Office: cases in which loved ones wanted to donate a dead relative's organs but were stopped by the coroner who owned the dead body in law if there was an outstanding legal case to be decided as a result of an unnatural death such as a fatal road accident. And another type involving cases where someone carried a kidney donor card but then after they died their body was harvested for the heart, lungs, brain, and other associated human tissue too. Taking these extra donations resulted in explicit body disputes between grieving relatives, coroners, their pathologists and transplantation teams needing more human material to save lives. In this sixth chapter we now explore missed disputes. A typical missed dispute, as we shall see, arose because of delayed, missing or withheld information about the extent of the harvesting of human material and its long retention period that relatives of each dead person expected to be kept informed about, but were not. Instead, pathologists involved in checking on causes of death for coroners often took the opportunity to harvest brains to do further research. Although families knew that some human material had been retained for legal purposes to secure a court conviction in cases of dangerous driving, homicide and manslaughter charges, not everything about the extent of human harvesting was disclosed. The Culshaw case that opened this sixth chapter is emblematic of that commonplace situation.

Like, therefore, our longer Chapter 5, which contained human stories to illustrate common dilemmas, this chapter is likewise divided into two parts. Part I sets in context the liminal space of medical death and how biotechnology made calling the time of death much more complex in the modern era. It was not an exact science as the ability to monitor even the smallest traces of life-signs in the brain-stem became feasible, complicating the medical ethics of death's door. This discovery reflected the rise of neuroscience and its *brain banking* activities that became the new frontier of medical science in the late twentieth century. To appreciate how this new medical landscape gave rise to missed body disputes, Part II of the chapter investigates the controversial case of the Isaacs family, which created a national outcry in 2000 after it was found that Mr Isaac's brain had been retained with 23,900 other brain material deposits for ten years or more without fully informed consent (themes first introduced in Chapter 2). Families missed an opportunity to know what was happening to the brains of their loved ones because of a controversial and covert system of brain supply by pathologists. For whereas *brain banking* usually was done with the consent of families, generally what was described by pathologists as *brain accumulation* and *brain collection* was not. It was thought that after HTA2004 those missed body disputes had been resolved, but by the time GMP in 2017 got in contact with bereaved families about human material they had held in forensic pathology facilities around the UK for a decade or more, the time gap between the rhetoric and reality of informed consent was obvious for all to see. We return, therefore, briefly here to the story of John Culshaw deceased that opened this chapter and the reaction of his grieving family to a missed body dispute since it is a historical prism of many of the themes and human situations which we will be exploring together in this sixth chapter.

Jenny Culshaw, mother of John Culshaw deceased, told the BBC that she was shocked to learn that so much of her dead son, who had been murdered in 1993, was still in closed storage in 2017, supposedly supervised by a senior Home Office pathologist for almost a quarter of a century. Had she known, she would have asked questions about what was happening and why. Instead, she now found herself involved in a missed body dispute. It was evident she had not been told the full material facts relating to her son's fatality and subsequent criminal investigation in 1993. Being kept in ignorance for twenty-four years had prevented her from asking the right sort of questions and querying the ongoing situation. She knew that some human material had been taken because it was very necessary for a court case (and thus this was not an implied process of consent that she was objecting to); instead, it was the extent of human harvesting she was querying and the length of time such information was withheld from her, which she would have objected to had she known. As she put it:

He's my son. And he's been left – half of him – If he'd have died and they'd asked me if they could use his parts to help somebody, then yes. But just to be sat in a lab for 23 years doing nothing, that's just horrendous – Somebody has made a big mistake. Not just me but a lot of other families are suffering as well – I don't want anyone else going through this. It's devastating.[2]

Further inquiries by a journalist working for the *Manchester Evening News* revealed that '180 dead victims of crime in Greater Manchester had been discovered during a recent audit of organ retentions' under the official jurisdiction of GMP.[3] Again, Jenny Culshaw questioned the reason that her son's body had been harvested for so many organs that did not relate to how he had been murdered and could not therefore have informed the victims' court case in 1994:

I thought I had buried the son that I gave birth to. In fact I buried a shell. Why? He was stabbed through the heart. Why would they need to retain other parts? We don't know we've got everything back. That's what we are panicking about. Are they going to come back and say they have found some more? The officer who visited us apologised to us. But there are other people out there suffering like I am. We have been visiting him at the cemetery every two weeks. But he's not there. He's not at rest.[4]

Jenny Culshaw was not alone. An audit of all human tissue stored on behalf of police forces around the country, carried out in 2012: 'revealed 492 whole organs or *significant* body parts [like brains] were kept at police stations, labs and hospitals mortuaries on behalf of the police in murder or suspicious death cases'. These related to cases across England, Wales and Northern Ireland

(Scotland has a different legal system). When pressed by angry families about missed body disputes (and their human parts), the Home Office took the view that: 'this is an operational matter for the police'. In the case of GMP, its former Forensic Science Service came under the audit spotlight in 2014, leading to the rediscovery of John Culshaw's potential missed body dispute. The description of his human material in clinical terms ('one of 180 samples') is noteworthy given our discussion in previous chapters about the need for the human life to be put back front and centre to the body 'gift' process. In this case, GMP appointed a dedicated team of detectives familiar with the original case files. They worked methodically to identify the retained human remains of all of their 'police cases' and to contact their respective families. A spokesperson for the GMP review confirmed to the *Manchester Evening News*:

In this case we have been to visit John Culshaw's family twice and had several open and honest conversations with them. Every family we visited has reacted differently to this difficult conversation and in this case they were clearly upset by the news. As with all cases we have offered them specialist support and will continue to do so. We have now spoken to dozens of families and in many cases they have thanked us for the personal visit, but we accept that everyone reacts differently.[5]

In response, Jenny Culshaw told the press that there needed to be more human understanding of the impact that such delayed news would have on the majority of families. She refuted the accusation that her emotional response was either exceptional or excessive. Mrs Culshaw conceded that she was perhaps more outspoken than others about feeling pained, but all those she now knew in similar circumstances were equally shocked. Indeed, she and the other families resented the corporate-speak used to describe how the GMP press office was engaging with them in 'open and honest conversations'. Repeating that phrase several times made it feel like the opposite was happening and the GMP staff were out of touch. The Culshaw family's expectation was that HTA2004 had sorted out '*all*' potential missed body and body parts disputes, not just in the NHS. Now they learned that John Culshaw's human material was located at a forensic science laboratory in Birmingham:

Honestly, this has put 10 years on my life. We've kept this quiet because the detective who visited us said 'don't say anything until the other people have been told'. And we have kept it quiet until now. But I can't cope with this all on my own. There's somebody else out there suffering like I am. Somebody should be standing up and saying they have done this. We were never ever told anything had been kept from John. In fact, after the Alder Hey scandal my daughter wrote to the authorities to find out if anything from his body had been kept and she was told no. She did that for me. I don't believe in cremation [Mrs Culshaw is a Roman Catholic]. We're now going to have another burial on Thursday and put those remains in his grave.[6]

The Culshaw family went back to the original grave plot at Westwood Cemetery, Ince, in Wigan and held a second burial service, some twenty-four years after they had interred John Culshaw.

This story is emotive because it has a history of emotions and oral history context. For that reason, it gets to the heart of many of the core themes of this book. First, it alerts us to the multilayered material pathways, networks and thresholds that dead bodies once broken up did not simply travel along – from supplier to medical research facility – but also occupied for some considerable period, often forgotten time, in cold storage. Second, because this pathology system had to be confidential to secure convictions in court, it could also be secretive about everything that was being done and retained out of interest by pathologists. Third, this meant that spaces were created in which time stood still as harvested human material was held in refrigerated suspension for far longer than the general public expected to happen, notwithstanding the legal imperative of a pending prosecution. Fourth, the personalised history of each body (organs, parts, tissues and brain) may have faded from public view, but the identify of each did not dissolve altogether. That which was dissected and disaggregated could be – with a great deal of detailed detective work by the police – reassembled and re-identified when public tastes changed. Fifth, that outcome shows that bio-commons could have been documented by post-mortem passports in the first instance; if it was possible to reactivate human identities, it was equally possible to keep track of them inside forensic path-ology facilities. It was therefore not impossible (as historically many inside the system claimed) to monitor working methods and paperwork protocols. Sixth, this finding represented a major public relations challenge for pathologists trained clinically to conduct their expertise because the feelings of families were a human checking mechanism that had never been a direct part of their standard workload allocations. As a result, the challenge for a historian of the body when assessing what was done and why is to rebalance hidden histories of the dead in these clinical settings with experiential perspectives after public exposure. Our approach is therefore that introduced in the conclusion of Chapter 3, namely, to build on Paul Thompson's seminal book about the value of oral history, *The Voice of the Past* (2000).

Thompson argues that there needs to be a reconstruction of the written and spoken historical record because it 'can give back to the people who made and experienced history, through their own words, a central place'.[7] To do so, we must keep in mind Julianne Nyhan and Andrew Flinn's important observation that it is essential to keep asking of oral histories whether or not they were or are 'fatally compromised by the biases and uncertainties introduced by the inter-view process'.[8] In other words, what we are going to do in this chapter is to subject the evidence base that came to light since 2000 to a 'rigorous cross-checking with other sources, arguing for the general accuracy of memory and its suitability as a source of historical evidence'. For as Alessandro Portelli reminds us, oral histories when combined with histories of emotion can provide new perspectives often hidden from public view. Indeed, he is praiseworthy of what he called 'the peculiarities of oral history' and their subjectivity precisely because they are 'not just about what people did, but [what] they wanted to do, what they believed they were doing, and what they now think they did'.[9] This conceptual approach is pivotal to this chapter's method of listening to both sides – the clinical (by pathologists) and emotional (by the families) – to arrive at a consensus about what the balance of the evidence is telling us. For as William Reddy points out, the advantage of exploring the navigation of feelings is that historians of emotions can appraise the extent to which giving voice to a set of difficult experiences gives those involved a greater awareness of their fragility in trauma, or an ability to cope in a difficult personal crisis. Often it provides the chance to reconcile difficult circumstances which can produce a more philosophical outlook and thus a positive set of outcomes from something that was imposed but can be accommodated by the person or people involved.[10] In other words, we can assess did people feel worse, about the same, or much better than they thought they might once hidden histories of the dead and their missed body disputes about brain harvesting were revealed for the first time. And what do those discoveries tell us about the changing shape of cultural attitudes to the body and its material afterlives in a Genome era? It is exactly this set of human scenarios that we will encounter as we appraise the Culshaw story with others like it, and encounter those spoken by pathologists at the time, too. For the Culshaws' position (as was inferred in the oral history evidence) was not unique.

It soon came to light in the national press that: 'the Police Service of Northern Ireland kept the most samples with 71 items, West Midlands kept 30, Metropolitan Police 39, Merseyside 37, Cambridgeshire 35 and West Yorkshire 31'.[11] These had been located after an investigation was ordered following the discovery that 'many criminal investigations failed to record accurately why human material had been kept'. In response to the public furore in the media about this finding in 2017, all the families involved stated they would have wanted to have been kept informed about material retentions, whether in the past, present or future. The majority spoke to journalists about the emotional 'bolt out of the blue', 'the shock of not knowing', and 'the knock at the door telling us we did not know what had really happened' after so many years.[12] Those who learned their dead child was part of the 'sample size' were understandably very upset indeed. In the cases of body parts retained from '90 children' often involving their brains, it was being misinformed that bereaved parents objected to the most. Hannah Cheevers was one bereaved parent. She told BBC Radio 4's *Today Programme* how after her baby son died of heart failure, she and her husband assumed they had buried him. Then one day a police officer came and told them: 'totally out of the blue. . . . We had his funeral, we got on with our lives as you have to and 13 years later we have a knock on the door from the Dorset police to inform us that his brain has been retained at Southampton hospital.'[13] There were no suspicious circumstances surrounding their child's death and therefore his brain retention had no legal justification or the family's consent for over thirteen years. Hannah, like Jenny Culshaw, was not against donation. It was the lack of consultation which was objectionable. Now she too was involved in a missed dispute. She felt this outcome was very sad, since: 'We had absolutely no idea that they had kept his brain.' Indeed, the Cheevers family, despite the controversy, 'decided to donate his brain to hospital research, rather than have it destroyed or reburied after another funeral'. Hannah told BBC News that the family decided they 'did not want to disturb his human remains again', even though they were very heart-broken by the hidden history of what had happened.

These symbolic but not unrepresentative cases attest both to the emotive nature of not being informed and to the almost universal feelings of revulsion felt by most people when missed disputes were exposed to public enquiry. Since these missed disputes often involved brain retentions, we need to engage with two practical factors before we encounter more human stories and engage with their historical lessons in hidden histories of the dead. First, why was medical death so confusing after WWII, and how did that context shaped *brain banking* and *brain collecting* that led to so many missed disputes? Part I now outlines that pivotal medical landscape, before Part II takes up their human stories again.

Part I

Medical Death's Dead-End?

> Contrary to perception, death is not a specific moment but a potentially reversible process that occurs after any severe illness or accident causes the heart, lungs and brain to cease functioning. If attempts are made to reverse this process, it is referred to as 'cardiac arrest'; however, if these attempts do not succeed it is called 'death' [Sam Parnia, Professor of Critical Care Medicine and Director of Resuscitation Research at the State University of New York at Stony Brook, USA, 2014].[14]

In April 2016, *National Geographic* opened with a lead article that posed a thought-provoking medical question: 'Is Science Redefining the Boundaries of Life and Death?'.[15] The answer was a resounding yes, thanks to new, sophisticated technology. An investigative journalist explained that once soci-ety accepted that death was a physical set of processes (based on a growing body of empirical evidence in emergency room medicine), the boundaries of when that occurred in medico-scientific parlance were always going to shift. This new status quo had prompted a Harvard University panel of experts in 1968 to look at the two ways death had been defined since the eighteenth century: 'the traditional way, by cardiopulmonary criteria, and a new way, by neurological ones'.[16] Their conclusions led to a new recognition that death in the brain mattered just as much as death in the heart and lungs. Evidence showed how, unaided and without extra oxygen, the brain could still survive for about three minutes even after the heart had stopped and the lungs had ceased to inflate. Consequently, 'brain death' in medico-legal circles now had 'three cardinal benchmarks'. These included: 'coma or unresponsiveness, apnea or the inability to breath without a ventilator, and the absence of brainstem reflexes'; these have tended to be 'measured by bedside exams such as flushing the ears with cold water to see if the eyes move, poking the nail bed to see if the face grimaces, or swabbing the throat and suctioning the bronchia to try to stimulate a cough'. Therefore, death acts like a dimmer switch in the body; it can be turned down in trauma, but that does not mean that the light of life has expired in the brain or vital organs. Quoting Dr Sam Parnia (who opened this section), the article observed:

Death is 'a process, not a moment', writes critical-care physician Sam Parnia in his book *Erasing Death*. It's a whole-body stroke, in which the heart stops beating but the organs don't die immediately. In fact, he writes, they might hang on intact for quite a while, which means that 'for a significant period of time after death, death is in fact fully reversible'. ... He says 'CPR works better than people realize and that under proper conditions – when the body temperature is lowered, chest compression is regulated for depth and tempo, and oxygen is reintroduced slowly to avoid injuring tissue – some patients can be brought back from the dead after hours without a heartbeat, often with no long-term consequences'. Now he's investigating one of the most mysterious aspects of crossing over: why so many people in cardiac arrest report out-of-body or near-death experiences, and what those sensations might reveal about the nature of this limbo zone and about death itself.[17]

Yet, the interesting thing about this storyline was the reaction to the online newsfeed by regular readers of *National Geographic*. Some subscribers blogged that they thought the evidence presented of a number of cases in which patients had been brought back from the dead many hours after they seemed to expire in the emergency room was disturbing. Others dismissed the notion of a Near-Death Experience (hereafter NDE) calling it pseudo-science. Many more believed that this NDE grey zone proved life after death existed in some form and thus validated how many people had a spiritual faith in the global community. Few, however, expressed an opinion about the reporting of the history of resuscitation and whether 'the facts' as presented in the article were reliable or not. Although the reportage did not intend to mislead, it did not cover just what a long and disruptive issue medical death has been in the history of anatomy: an important context for this chapter's central focus on the role that medical death and brain research would play in creating missed disputes by the turn of the twenty-first century.

Recently, historical scholarship has established that English penal surgeons had been very troubled by when to call medical death since at least the mid-eighteenth century. As this author has argued extensively elsewhere, those medical men who were given the task of dissecting criminals convicted and hanged for murder on the gallows under the Murder Act (25 Geo. 2. c. 37: 1752) found that in the winter, cold corpses that should have been dead could be revived when cut down from the hangman's rope.[18] Hypothermia in the body protected the brain, heart and lungs from expiring, and when warmed up the deceased began to wake up in the dissection theatre. Since they were socially dead (having committed homicide), legally dead (being condemned in court and hanged in public) but not medically dead (still having life signs in the body), the only solution was to transport the convict for life to the Americas or Australia. Somewhere today there are the ancestors of condemned criminals who are living proof that the boundaries of life and death have always been fluid. This unforeseen outcome seldom features in standard historical accounts, so it is perhaps unsurprising that such findings have not informed modern debates concerning when death really occurs. In other words, from the eighteenth to the twentieth century medicine behind closed doors knew about the complexities of 'calling the time of death'. Indeed, one physical factor that eighteenth-century surgeons encountered regularly, which twenty-first-century consultants in emergency medicine know to be a physical fact, is that to keep the brain-stem alive, effective oxygenation of the bloodstream must be sustained in trauma. It is best to start oxygenating the blood at the point of injury, even before ambulance transfer. This is because biomedicine really does work best when it is as easy as breathing. That discovery has complicated today when exactly to call the time of death. For traditionally doctors used to call the time of death at twenty minutes in emergency rooms around the world. That was when they accepted the flatline of the heart as proof of medical death. There seemed little point in continuing to do compressions or jolt the heart with an electrical stimulus beyond the twenty-minute marker if the brain was beyond repair. The person in trauma would be in a vegetative state, functioning on a heart-lung machine but not capable of an independent quality of life. This customary practice, however, started to run counter to the new capabilities of medical technology. From the 1980s, it was feasible to monitor even the very faintest traces of life in the brain-stem. Sophisticated equipment began therefore to elongate the timing of medical death. In resuscitation medicine, the twenty-minute marker looked outdated. Thus, in the recent past, saving a life involved oxygenating the brain-stem and reviving patients thought dead. This discovery has redrawn the fine line we all will cross one day into our individual deadlines.

In other words, by the 1960s research facilities around the world reliant on brain material to advance neuroscience now faced new practicalities, and medical ethics had to respond in kind.

In 1968 (as we have seen) invited scientists, anaesthesiologists and experts working at the forefront of emergency medicine, as well as leading ethicists and a medical historian, convened at Harvard University. They styled themselves the Ad-Hoc Committee on Brain Death (hereafter AHCBD) and assembled at Harvard Medical School. Their remit was to review and make new policy recommendations concerning the changing ethics of 'irreversible coma' and shifting medico-legal definitions in a biotech world.[19] The AHCBD concluded that in a non-functioning brain, permanent death needed a clinical description of 'brain death', re-defined in three diagnostic ways:

1. *Unreceptivity and unresponsitivity* – patient shows total unawareness to external stimuli and unresponsiveness to painful stimuli
2. *No movements or breathing* – all spontaneous muscular movement, spontaneous respiration and response to stimuli are absent
3. *No reflexes* – fixed, dilated pupils; lack of eye movement even when hit or turned, or ice water is placed in the ear; lack of response to noxious stimuli; unelicitable tendon reflexes[20]

However, because there was also a considerable weight of medical evidence that some bodies in hypothermia or after drug intoxication could sometimes be revived in the brain-stem and still had a beating heart, a fourth checking mechanism was required, too. Each patient had to have an electroencephalogram (EEG) and two experts in resuscitation medicine to check the reading. They had to agree that the person was deceased and could potentially be part of an organ donation scheme, provided, that is, they met the new medico-legal protocol steps 1–3 plus EEG. A patient was only then essentially 'brain dead' and this diagnosis defined their end of life, rather than a non-beating heart. The hope was that this new diagnostic tool would separate out 'brain dead' patients from those in a 'persistent vegetative state': the latter can still physically experience cycles of sleep and wakefulness despite being in a deep unconscious state.[21] A priority was to protect transplant surgeons against accusations of killing patients during technical procedures when the heart had to be stopped to be transferred to a donor or a kidney was taken from a so-called 'living cadaver' on life support until the transplant was complete. In medico-legal circles ever since, the AHCBD meeting became renowned as a landmark ethical event.[22] It also stimulated considerable controversy.[23]

From the outset, critics observed the close links between the AHCBD report and organ donation schemes in Intensive Care Units (hereafter ICUs). Collected evidence from around the medical world seemed to indicate that the majority of 'brain dead' patients became 'solid organ' donors (heart, lungs, kidneys and liver). Harvesting of on average four donations per dead donor soon became the norm. Other 'donors' became 'tissue transplants' (eyes, bone grafts and general human material). Sceptics questioned therefore the degree to which 'the dead donor rule' was ethical. Did it effectively drive up donation rates? It looked like those involved in transplantation actor networks could have been motivated to improve biotechnology, rather than promoting medical altruism (in that order of priority). For this reason, the AHCBD report, whilst influential, did not create a global medical consensus about an agreed precise timing of 'brain death'. Consequently, the US government convened a President's Commission for the Study of Ethical Problems in Medicine and Biomedical and Behavioural Research in 1981. The aim was to look again at patients who seemed to be 'beyond coma'. This diagnostic emphasis stressed that it was ethical to explore when the 'whole of life' appeared to have ended in a patient in deep trauma. As Margaret Hayden, bioethicist, explains: 'The report's other reason for this new definition was equally pragmatic, stating that patients in irreversible comas (with beating hearts but irreversible brain damage) could place an undue burden on families and hospitals.'[24] The review group hence concluded that the holistic essence of life is in the brain. Hayden elaborates that in 1981 the President's Commission drew 'on both biological and philosophical premises' concluding that:

death is the moment at which the body's physiological system ceases to constitute an integrated whole. Even if life continues in individual cells or organs, life of the organism as a whole requires complex integration, and without the latter, a person cannot properly be regarded as alive.[25]

In other words, brain research and advances in emergency medicine were dealing with a new reality – death's door stayed open for longer than many skilled medics cared to admit in public – and on its threshold were the living-dead which required new protocols. Soon, the 1981 President's Commission findings were being enacted across America.

Forty-five US states adopted a definition of 'total brain failure' under new legislation known as the Uniform Determination of Death Act (1981) (hereafter UDDA). Again, however, critics like Hayden point out: 'Much of the clinical guidance is designed to mitigate and mask the ambiguity between what a brain dead individual looks like (well-perfused, warm skin, with a beating heart) and how we expect a dead body to appear (grey, "lifeless," with no heartbeat or pulse).'[26] Often ICU staff reported on families feeling upset and confused about being informed their relative was 'technically alive' and not knowing what exactly this meant clinically. Thus, the UDDA had provided a useful working-protocol, but families trusted their instincts too and this led to a cultural stand-off, sometimes culminating in body disputes. What further complicated the separation of life from death by the Millennium were new clinical findings highlighted by Dr Caroline M. Quill, the lead author of a disquieting study into ICU practices across the USA. These were co-ordinated by the Pearlman School of Medicine at the University of Pennsylvania. As *NBC News* explained in May 2013: 'If you land in an intensive care unit sick enough for doctors to consider withdrawing life support, be warned – Whether and when to pull the plug may depend in large part on the practices and culture of the ICU itself ...'

Quill and her team analysed records of more than 269,000 patients treated in 153 ICUs in the United States between 2001 and 2009. Overall, nearly 12 percent of patients had a decision made to go from a 'full code' – an all-out effort to save lives – to some kind of limit on care. That could have included: a DNR or do-not-resuscitate order; an order to withhold CPR or cardio-pulmonary resuscitation plus removing mechanical ventilation; dialysis or other life-saving treatments; or simply an order to provide only comfort measures or hospice care. About 59 percent of the patients died in the ICU and another 41 percent survived to discharge, the study found. Particular patient characteristics accounted for most of the variability in decisions to withdraw life support, Quill acknowledged. But even after age, illness, functional status and other factors were analysed the variation among ICUs to authorize a DFLST – decision to forgo life-sustaining therapy – was striking.[27]

Dr Douglas White, an Associate Professor of Critical Care Medicine and Director of the Ethics of Critical Illness at the University of Pittsburgh, likewise pointed out that often 'decisions about whether and when to withdraw support are not scientific ones'. Hence, patients should be encouraged to talk much more openly about what they would want to happen in a critical situation at the end of life and leave a legal will stating their healthcare wishes. Yet, many in the recent past felt unable to do so; others put off the inevitable, or hoped their families would take over, often with mixed results, as an anonymous nurse working in ICU explained to *NBC News*:

Speaking as a registered nurse in a hospital myself, the choice to withdraw life support is one of the hardest decisions to make during the crisis. Often times what I see is not so much that the person in crisis isn't ready to go, it's usually the family isn't ready to let go. I once had a patient wheeled up to floor who looked me in the eye and said: 'I want to die'. He had stage 4 cancer with no chance of treatment, his body was starting to shut down little by little, he was confused but not THAT [*sic*] confused. So, because of the 'confusion' he had to depend on his family to withdraw life support. They didn't want to. So, instead of letting the man go with some dignity, he ended up tied to a bed for trying to pull his lines out, he ended up with an infection as his body had stopped fighting off invaders, his kidneys had stopped working properly so he gained water weight from all the IV antibiotics we gave him. A few days later he did eventually pass. I just remember thinking, instead of being able to die peacefully in his right mind, he had to beg every day to die, live through the torture of feeling his body shut down piece by piece, and what was accomplished? Nothing. People deserve to die with dignity and honour, and sometimes life support is a curse.[28]

Even so, a further complicating factor was advances in emergency medicine during the same period.

In April 2013, Sam Parnia expanded on his hands-on experiences of medical death. In *The Lazarus Effect*, he wrote about how after training in resuscitation medicine at Guy's and St. Thomas' hospitals in London and then becoming head of ICU at Stony Brook University Hospital in New York, he observed that:

The one thing that is certain about all of our lives ... is that we will all eventually experience a cardiac arrest. All our hearts will stop beating. What happens in the minutes and hours after that will potentially be the most significant moments of our biography. At present, the likelihood is, however, that in those crucial moments we will find ourselves in the medical environment of the 1960s or 1970s. The kind of CPR (cardiopulmonary resuscitation) that we are familiar with from medical dramas – the frenzied pumping of the chest – remains rooted ... in its serendipitous discovery in 1960. It remains a haphazard kind of procedure, often performed more in hope than anticipation. Partly, this is a question of personnel. Most doctors will do CPR for 20 minutes and then stop. ... The decision to stop is completely arbitrary but it is based on an instinct that after that time brain damage is very likely and you don't want to bring people back into a persistent vegetative state. But if you understand all the things that are going on in the brain in those minutes – as we now can – then you can minimise that possibility There are numerous studies that show that if you implement all the various resuscitation steps together you not only get a doubling of your survival rates but the people who come back are not brain damaged.[29]

In other words, the culture of ICU functioned with an out-of-date historical concept of life and death: as Parnia explained at the start of this chapter's Part I. Such basic findings reflect how much medicine has been about looking forward, not back: criticisms which echo those of George Steiner discussed in the Introduction. He highlighted that science's methodologies have a fundamental flaw. Discarding 'old knowledge' happens routinely with each new medical breakthrough. By contrast, the medical humanities seldom casts off accumulated human experiences or their arts forms, recognising instead that the potential remains for the revival of old ways of thinking in a future context.[30] Kwame Anthony Appiah (philosopher, cultural theorist and novelist) said the same thing during the recent Reith Lectures for the BBC. He observed once more: 'Although our ancestors are powerful in shaping our attitudes to the past' and we need to always be mindful of this, we equally 'should always be in active dialogue with the past' to stay engaged with what we have done and why.[31] In many respects, mapping hidden histories of the body is an important way to reveal the flaws in medico-scientific methodologies, as this book and others by this author have done for the first time.[32] They reiterate that an eighteenth-century surgeon and his twenty-first-century equivalent in ICU face the same ethical dilemmas. It is not therefore the case that ICU has been too respectful of historical concepts of life/death, as many claim today in resuscitation medicine and standard historical studies.[33] What has really happened is that ICU never engaged with its own past practices. They thus lost sight of the working protocols of their surgical predecessors dissecting in the Georgian period. Eighteenth-century criminal surgeons first discovered the extraordinary capacity for resuscitation in the brain, even after it sounded like the heart had stopped beating in the chest cavity of a hanged criminal. Sam Parnia has therefore returned to old medical questions with renewed biomedical capabilities. In so doing, he alerts us to two important factors on missed body disputes of the modern period – that the brain was the frontier of medical research and that we know less than we should have done of its harvesting networks. To appreciate the importance of this context for our human stories later, it is important to reflect briefly on the dominance of neuroscience in our biomedical world.

Brainstorming Neuroscience

We have a brain, and people without brains don't have thoughts. So the brain must do it. It's a huge problem to discover how it does it, but that will come. There's no alternative.[34] [Professor Colin Blakemore, Chair in Neuroscience, University of Oxford, quoted in 'Brain research's golden age', *BBC News Magazine*, 22 June 2011]

Few scientists would disagree with Professor Colin Blakemore that brain research has become *the* medical frontier in a biomedical age across the global community, and a timely one. As the Brain Research Trust highlighted in 2016, 'over 12.5 million are affected by neurological conditions in the UK (that's one in five)'.[35] The medical charity's online promotional video explains that: 'the brain is the most complex organ in our body – it weighs just 3 pounds – yet it controls our emotions, senses, and actions – it's how we process the world around us – so when it breaks down, we break down'. In a similar refrain, Carl Zimmer explained how in 2014 he surveyed the most innovative brain research for *National Geographic* across America:

Some neuroscientists are zooming in on the fine structure of individual nerve cells, or neurons. Others are charting the biochemistry of the brain, surveying how our billions of neurons produce and employ thousands of different kinds of proteins. Still others . . . are creating in unprecedented detail representations of the brain's wiring: the network of some 100,000 miles of nerve fibres, called white matter that connects the various components of the mind, giving rise to everything we think, feel, and perceive. The U.S. government is throwing its weight behind this research through the Brain Research Advancing Innovative Neuro-technologies (BRAIN) Initiative. In an announcement last spring, President Barack Obama said that the large-scale project aimed to speed up the mapping of our neural circuitry, 'giving scientists the tools they need to get a dynamic picture of the brain in action.'[36]

In many respects, new digital technology entrepreneurs and their personal computer revolution have also been leading the way globally, too. One such is the late Paul G. Allen, co-founder of Microsoft with Bill Gates. He created the Allen Institute for Brain Research in 2003 with a philanthropic donation of $100 million. Subsequently, Allen donated another $400 million to ensure that brain research remains an 'Open Science'. His window-on-the-world legacy is a data portal known as the Allen Brain Atlas – 'part of a 10-year plan launched in March 2012 to understand the neural code—how activity in the brain's cortex leads to perception, decision making, and ultimately action'. His foundation thus promises: 'We will be focusing our understanding through simultaneous study of the brain's components, computation and cognition.'[37] Allen, before his untimely death (he died of septic shock related to a terminal cancer diagnosis), was the personification of an *Idea Man* (the fitting title of his 2012 memoir), for he has taken up the anatomical legacy of the past and pushed it forward into a neurological future he often described in his public speeches as *'What if'*. It is a motto penal surgeons working on the dark science of the brain were once very familiar with in the past, too. They punished the 'dangerous dead' in popular culture and found that around 25 per cent of criminals hanged came back to life on the dissection table across England between 1752 and 1832.[38] Continually, the boundaries of life and death shifted in the anatomy theatre. They proved to be more fluid than conventional European science traditionally thought over the next two centuries. So much so, that with the advent of biotechnology and the rise of neuroscience, the boundaries of life and death came into even sharper clinical and research focus, revealing differential power relations depending on claims of scientific expertise. And even though this remarkable work on the brain looked like it was robust, this was not necessarily the case. One example stands in for many at the time, and it explains why the general public started to become more sceptical about missed body disputes involving brain retentions once they came to public attention in modern Britain.

On 6 July 2016, *Forbes* magazine asked its readers to think the unthinkable – 'Could Brain Research from the Past 15 years Really Be Wrong?' The lead article, penned by Bruce Lee (Assistant Professor of International Health at Johns Hopkins University Bloomberg School of Public Health) highlighted how three researchers from Linköping University in Sweden had published a startling neurological study in the *Journal of the Proceedings of the National Academy of Sciences of the United States of America*.[39] It explored the use of Functional Magnetic Resonance Imaging (fMRI) in brain research. This was a twenty-five-year old piece of technology and surprisingly few researchers have ever asked: Does it actually work properly, and have its research results been reliable? Essentially, the Swedish research team found a flaw in the operation of software used to detect brain activity, tracked under fMRI scans. As Lee explained:

Anders Eklund, Thomas E. Nichols and Hans Knutsson examined fMRI data from 499 healthy patients and found that the software (i.e., SPM, FSL and AFNI) used to generate the fMRI images often showed parts of the brain lighting up when it shouldn't have, in some cases up to 70% of the time (i.e., a false positive rate of up to 70%). These software packages had bugs or glitches in them that were leading to faulty images and may have existed for 15 years until they were recently found and corrected. This means that up to around 40,000 fMRI studies published in the scientific literature over this period could have shown incorrect results.[40]

Soon Lee's article made medical news around the world because as he asked: 'Why wasn't this software glitch caught earlier?' There were 'Several Reasons', he explained –

First, there is not enough research being done on the software used for medical research and how to improve or develop new software. Secondly, scientific journals often will not publish studies that try to recreate already-published studies. At the same time, funders may not support research that tries to recreate other people's research. This means that once a study is published, others may have no incentive to check or re-do the study. Instead, we need to change the system to encourage people to test and re-test scientific hypotheses and findings. Like a new fashion, scientific ideas are sexiest when they are first demonstrated, and then the scientific community quickly loses interest afterwards. But the first person to find or study something is not always right.[41]

In other words, in brain studies leading researchers had taken their own working histories for granted. *Science Alert* likewise highlighted that although scientists thought they were measuring brain function using fMRI, what they had really been doing was interpreting data produced by a machine, not the actual human brain. In other words, 'Software, rather than humans . . . scans the voxels looking for clusters [of brain activity]. . . .When you see a claim that *"Scientists know when you're about to move an arm: these images prove it,"* they're interpreting what they're told by the statistical software' – an important data distinction.[42]

The particular computer software bug that the Swedish study identified was located and repaired in May 2015. Even so, it had skewed the results in some 40,000 published papers since the 1970s. As the Swedish team explained: 'One of the biggest obstacles has been the astronomical cost of using these [fMRI] machines – around US$600 per hour'. Thus, 'studies have been limited to very small sample sizes of up to 30 or so participants, and very few organisations have the funds to run repeat experiments to see if they can replicate the results.'[43] An added problem had been 'that because software is the thing that's actually interpreting the data from the fMRI scans, your results are only as good as your computer, and programs used to validate the results have been prohibitively slow'. Debates and disputes should have been happening on a more regular basis inside the medical research community about the status of the science involved in brain work, and what this might have meant for public relations in terms of brain bequests. But this was not the case. To appreciate that context, and why it would later give rise to missed disputes, it is necessary to focus on the advent of *brain banking* because this provided the backdrop for future NHS scandals over retentions.

Cambridge University in the 1970s was the centre of new directions in neurosciences. In particular, it started to attract talented researchers interested in neurodegenerative disorders such as Huntington's disease. By 1975, a consortium of these researchers had come together to form what became known as the Cambridge Brain Bank. Not only was this one of the first research facilities in the UK, but one of only four in the world at that time. Its nearest geographic rival was an early brain collection set up by Professor John (Nick) Corsellis (1915–1994) at Runwell Hospital in Essex during the 1950s which contained over 6,000 specimens from patients suffering from psychiatric illnesses, as well as neuro-degenerative diseases. However, although Corsellis shared brains with other leading researchers from time to time, his main research focus was *brain collecting* for his own use, rather than *brain banking* (in the latter, brain tissue is shared routinely for distribution amongst the research community). What made *brain banking* a new trend at Cambridge, and elsewhere, from the 1970s was the discovery that enzymes in brain tissue could be studied chemically post-mortem. So, for instance, in the case of dementia it was feasible after death to still study the enzymes active in brain tissue and reach meaningful results to potentially make better drug treatments. At a recent Witness Seminar run by the Wellcome Trust in London, Professor Gavin Reynolds described what it was like to be a young researcher and to acquire brain material at Cambridge in the 1970s:

... we were often seen, I think, as sort of eccentric scavengers. In Cambridge I, or my technician, used to go downstairs to the mortuary and negotiate over brains. This was, of course, in the days when this sort of thing was rather more possible. We could discuss the opportunity that we might be able to provide some pathological feedback in exchange for having these brains that we could then bank and formally provide for those who in the future wished to withdraw. But it was very much a sort of negotiated process, wasn't it?[44]

Likewise, Professor David Mann elaborated on how a *brain bank* was set up in Manchester too and for what research reasons. Although lengthy, his explanation is worthwhile quoting in full, as it sets the scene for the *Isaacs Report* that we will be encountering later in this chapter. This was the typical sort of research pathway and actor network in pathology and new neuroscience that we have been rediscovering throughout this book:

We wanted really to follow this up in a large number of cases, and getting cell biopsies and the right amount of material from cell biopsy was really not easy to achieve. So we looked and said: 'How can we use post mortem material to answer that question?' In Manchester we set up a system whereby we obtained pre-mortem consent to brain recovery with the relatives fully involved when the whole situation was explained to them. They gave their agreement that we could obtain the brain tissues as soon as the patient died, so we weren't hidebound by this 'green form' paraphernalia that so besets us nowadays. And the net effect of that was that I would make journeys across Manchester at 2 o'clock in the morning to Prestwich Hospital, a big psychiatric hospital at the time, where many of the patients were resident. There, I would meet the local mortician and we would extract the contents of the head from these individuals who had kindly agreed to donate the tissues for research, and I would hot foot, literally, across Manchester back to the University of Manchester laboratories, where we would dissect the brain and put it into these wonderful containers that David and Paul had devised, which contained preservative fluids. The next day the brain would find its way, courtesy of British Rail, down to Queen Square, and Paul will love to tell the tale that I would ring him up at some unearthly time in the day or night and say in my best Yorkshire voice: 'Hello Paul. There's a brain on a train for you.' [Laughter] And really, as Paul says, it was the chemistry that drove the need not only to collect brains, but to collect brains of better quality than those you could simply get hold of from pathological archives, where everything had just been stuck willy-nilly into preservative. It was a rather surreal experience carrying really warm brains across a city at 2 o'clock in the morning.[45]

Mann was pressed for his views on what he believed the general public thought about this sort of brain research at the time. He replied: 'I think actually it was not in the public perception until the Alder Hey story broke and then the stuff really did hit the fan at that time. That really did impact upon brain collections and brain donations.' It was his perspective as a young researcher that: 'I think, by and large, people had an understanding of why it was necessary to collect brains and were happy to participate in that process, but with the Alder Hey scandal, the whole notion of pathologists became people who kept things in cellars and dark rooms. We were tarnished badly by the whole business.'[46]

Other participants at the same oral history event spoke up for the first time concerning their personal feelings about Alder Hey. As Professor Margaret Esiri explained: 'I felt very, very undermined by it. I felt the media portrayed it in the wrong way.'[47] She elaborated that:

I felt we were the victims of a system that involved particularly coroners' post mortems, which had nothing to do with the hospital system, where we had what we called medical interest post mortems and that often contributed to the brain banking as well. That was completely different to the coroner system where the problem was, I think, that the coroners never really explicitly said what you should do with an organ after you'd examined it for their purposes, which was to find the cause of death.[48]

These ethical issues were exacerbated, she explained, by a lack of communication. There were too many overlapping agencies involved. As a consequence,

missed disputes occurred routinely in what was a fundamentally flawed cor-
oner/pathologists' set of procedures: 'So [hospital] departments ended up with
a lot of organs that they'd taken from coroners' cases, and they didn't know
what to do with those organs afterwards.' This was the complex cultural
context that the Culshaw family experienced, too, in this chapter's opening
story. In order, however, to assess the historical value of these oral histories
taken from a pathology perspective, and engage with the navigation of their
feelings too, to balance the evidence of clinical and family lived experiences, it
is necessary to understand a little bit more about the history of brain banking. In
particular, we are going to focus in on the detailed activities of the Cambridge
Brain Bank because it was pivotal to the actor networks of pathologists across
the country and set new research standards that came in for significant public
criticism involving many potential missed disputes after WWII.

Brain Banking

In 2003, the Department of Health (DofH) decided to investigate the controversial issue of brain retention in the post-war era. The research focus soon fell
on the Cambridge Brain Bank because it was of national importance. Civil
servants examined its paperwork processes and pathology records. The results
of their findings are summarised in Table 6.1. In total, '2,547 . . . whole brains'
were banked for research purposes between 1980 and 2001, something that can
be confirmed by cross-matching to Addenbrooke's Hospital pathology records.
The DofH report concluded that: 'The Cambridge brain bank evolved from
research undertaken by Dr. Bird in the Neurochemical Pharmacology Unit in
the early 1970s. The first research was into Huntington's Chorea (now referred
to as Huntington's disease).' Having explained that context briefly, the report
went on to state its broad findings from the DofH audit in 2003 (Tables 6.1
and 6.2). There were several important observations that would create
a growing climate of mistrust in medical research, culminating in HTA2004.
The first was that pathologists did not maintain proper post-mortem records.
The DofH had a great deal of difficulty locating the incomplete paperwork trail.
This meant that the figures they were able to ascertain were probably very
conservative about the extent of unauthorised retentions. Anatomists, as we
saw in Chapter 5, faced the same audit trail problem. They had been under-
staffed, had not done their paperwork efficiently in the 1980s and 1990s and
thus had failed to get all their cremation work signed off officially by the DHSS
once they had completed their teaching and research work on the dead. They
looked guilty of holding on to human material for much longer than they
actually did. In the case of pathologists, there was so little paperwork that it
was difficult to assess for audit purposes whether the system was at fault
because of similar low staffing issues or whether everyone preferred to operate

Table 6.1 *Cambridge Brain Bank: an analysis of the brains collected, c.1980 to c. 2001*

Category	Number of brains received	Earliest date	Most recent date
Prader-Willi syndrome (B)	3	21.01.1997	24.02.2001
Normal control (C)	557	05.01.1980	08.10.2001
Dementia: long PM delay (D)	172	10.01.1980	02.03.1993
Epilepsy (E)	39	10.05.1983	28.12.1988
Dementia: short PM delay (FD)	272	21.11.1985	23.04.2001
CC75C (L)	206	22.06.1989	29.11.2001
Huntington's disease (H)	707	17.02.1980	10.12.2001
Fronto-temporal dementia (JH)	102	20.01.1992	16.01.2002
Down's syndrome (M)	16	04.03.1981	19.10.1998
Multiple sclerosis (MS)	2	12.03.1995	22.05.1997
Parkinson's disease (P)	62	01.02.1980	02.09.1992
CFAS (RH)	86	14.05.1993	21.12.2001
Schizophrenia (S)	182	04.01.1980	22.09.1994
Spinal cord (SC)	2	Unknown	Unknown
Progressive supranuclear palsy (SR)	1	07.09.1979	-
Depression (X)	66	01.02.1983	23.12.1992
Suicide (Y)	43	18.02.1983	13.03.1989
Tissue held for Oxford CFAS	29	In one batch, sometime mid 90s	
TOTALS	2547		

Source: TNA, *Isaacs Report*, 'The Cambridge Brain Bank', section 4, chapter 26, 'Recent analysis of brains collected by the bank', archived on behalf of the Department of Health, accessed 1/6/2017 at: http://webarchive.nationalarchives.gov.uk/+/www.dh.gov.uk/en/publicationsandstatistics/publications/publicationspolicyandguidance/browsable/DH_4889626

with a lack of efficiency and transparency. One outcome, though, was certain. The DofH report concluded that a significant amount of paperwork involving the Cambridge Brain Back was destroyed, misfiled or never created in the first place from the 1970s onwards.

The auditors concluded that although they lacked accurate figures for the 1970s–1980s period, the surviving but scattered figures they had located for the 1990s probably reflected general working protocols. The DofH auditor thus explained that:

The post mortem reports sent to the Coroner listed any tissue samples or other investigations made by the pathologist that could have a bearing on the cause of death. The reports did not mention that brains had been retained for the brain bank. All the post mortem reports on the 43 suicide victims whose brains had

Table 6.2 *Cambridge Brain Bank: audit report (2003–2004)*

I.	The Huntington's disease study had the active support of relatives and of COMBAT (the voluntary organization formed to support families of those with Huntington's disease). Consent was obtained for brain removal in these cases.
II.	Further programmes developed and in 1985 the MRC received a proposal to support the brain bank as a service facility to support research teams undertaking neurochemical and other investigations that required brain tissue.
III.	'Control' brains from 'normal' subjects were collected. Consent from the relatives was not sought or obtained.
IV.	The Department of Pathology of the University provided diseased brains and 'control' brains.
V.	No distinction was made between hospital and Coroners' cases when brains were obtained.
VI.	There is no record that the collection of 'control' brains was ever considered by an Ethical Committee before 1985.
VII.	The 1985 application to the MRC was ambiguous on the question of consent. One section, referring to collection of index cases, underlined the need for consent by the relatives. Elsewhere the requirement for 'control' brains is set out with no linkage to consent of the relatives.
VIII.	During the 1980s the brain bank technician would review the list of post mortems scheduled each day and identify brains that would be of interest to the brain bank.
IX.	In 1987 the funding basis of the bank changed. From that date it was to focus on individual projects rather than provide a 'banking' facility.
X.	In 1988 the bank became involved in a multi-centre prospective epidemiological study of dementing diseases of the elderly (the CFAS programme). This study received Ethical Committee approval.
XI.	For the CFAS programme, full consent for brain retention had been routinely obtained from the relatives.
XII.	Collection of brains from Coroners' cases as 'controls' and for the suicides study continued in parallel with the large prospective dementia study.
XIII.	The post mortem reports to the Coroners failed to record when brains were retained for use by the brain bank.
XIV.	In 1991 Mr Smith, the Coroner for Cambridge City, discovered that brains were being removed from Coroners' cases. He ordered that no brains or other organs from Coroners' cases were to be retained for research without the consent of the relatives. Organ retention was permitted only for diagnostic purposes.
XV.	The brain bank continues to collect brains, with consent, from hospital cases.
XVI.	As earlier chapters have indicated, the Cambridge brain bank was regarded as a model for other brain research routes to follow, and the methods of obtaining 'controls' from Coroners' cases appear to have been copied.

Source: TNA, *Isaacs Report*, 'The Cambridge Brain Bank', section 4, chapter 26, 'Recent analysis of brains collected by the bank', archived on behalf of the Department of Health, accessed 1/6/2017 at: http://webarchive.nationalarchives.gov.uk/+/www.dh.gov.uk/en/publicationsandstatistics/publi cations/publicationspolicyandguidance/browsable/DH_4889626

been obtained for the bank were examined. The records of the brain bank confirm that these brains were retained but none of the post mortem reports mentions brain retention. These reports were made to the Coroners for Cambridge City, South Cambridgeshire and Huntingdon Districts. A number of post mortem reports on cases where the brain had been retained as a control were also cross checked against the brain bank records. Again, the post mortem reports were silent about brain retention for the bank. In this respect these post mortem reports were deficient as they did not alert the Coroners to what was going on.[49]

There was therefore a sustained culture of a lack of informed consent for families. In other words, although the figures available were incomplete, it was reasonable to conclude that there had been many different sorts of missed disputes generated inside the brain research community. Leading brain researchers did not necessarily know everything on the supply side about the activities of coroners and their pathologists or morticians. However, they also did not choose to look in any greater detail. As a result, it is only the recent oral histories (introduced above and elaborated below) which confirm that there was a lack of persistent questioning, notably from the pathologists on duty. The system was peopled by caring staff, but it was equally careless in its working practices, and this was the chief cause of different sorts of missed disputes by the late 1990s. It seemed thus that many people felt tarnished by a lack of others' transparency. To better understand that wider context, we need now to turn our attention to the controversial *Isaacs Report* (2003), first introduced briefly in Chapter 2. It is a historical prism of what was happening on a regular basis inside hidden histories of the brain dead and outlines how paperwork was disguised, and crucial information withheld, to create missed disputes. Part II of this chapter is thus all about engaging with the human stories that people medical death and its neuroscience context.

Part II

The Isaacs Controversy

In April 2000, Mrs Elaine Isaacs discovered the retention of the brain of her deceased husband for post-mortem and further research purposes in Manchester.[50] She was very upset by this because the revelation came 13 years into widowhood under traumatic circumstances. On 26 February 1987, Mr Cyril Isaacs committed suicide. Aged 54 years, he had been suffering from episodes of mental ill health and had tried to take his own life on several occasions. His detailed medical case notes explain that during 1986–1987: 'In the five months before his untimely death, Mr Isaacs had experienced depressive mental illness and had been under the care of both private and NHS doctors.' In this state of mind: 'He had taken three overdoses, two of these in the same weekend within one month of his death.' Subsequently, it also reported that: 'Mr Isaacs had received in-patient psychiatric care as a voluntary patient. He had been prescribed medication at the time of his death and was due to see his general practitioner Dr Rosenburg' on the day he took his own life. In the evening, Mrs Isaacs and a relative named Mr Clive Lingard discovered Mr Isaacs dead at home. They made an emergency call to the police on Thursday evening, 26 February 1987. Mr Isaacs had hanged himself from a hatch in the loft. A duty police surgeon attended the suicide scene and pronounced death at 7.50 p.m. As the circumstances surrounding the unnatural death were unclear, it was essential to involve the coroner. This was when Mrs Isaacs lost control of the material fate of her dead husband, as Chapter 2 introduced, and a missed body dispute occurred that will be elaborated in detail here.

The Isaacs family were devout Jews. Their traditional faith required them to bury Mr Isaacs's body within twenty-four hours of death. It must be 'whole': according to religious rites, it must not be cut extensively, and the organs must not be removed. They argued that as the cause of death was obvious, there were witnesses to verify its sad circumstances, and medical notes would confirm a recent case-history of depression, no post-mortem should take place. The coroner had the option to do just an autopsy. In this way, the family could adhere to their deeply felt culture of laying out the body at home, saying prayers for the dead over it and burying it according to orthodox Jewish rites. It was therefore very distressing for Mrs Isaacs and her son to discover that Mr Isaacs's body was taken from the family home in preparation for a full post-mortem scheduled for Monday, 2 March 1987. An undertaker transported the body by arrangement with the local police. They issued instructions to deliver it to the mortuary at Prestwich Hospital, where the local coroner according to standard practice commissioned a full pathology report. The dead body arrived at 20.45 p.m. on 26 February 1987, just 55 minutes after the police surgeon on duty pronounced death. In material terms, it was a very fresh cadaver. The body, refrigerated overnight, would be in a good condition for pathology. It was also potentially ready for further medical research.

There were, according to the official records, two people present at the subsequent post-mortem – Dr R J Farrand (pathologist) and Mr Dennis Walkden (mortician) – both were acting for the coroner. They did bring forward the date of the post-mortem in recognition of the Jewish family's burial rites. A written record confirms the removal of Mr Isaacs's brain at 11.15 a.m. on Friday, 27 February 1987 by the conclusion of the post-mortem. In accordance with standard practice, those on duty telephoned the coroner, confirming that the cause of death was suicide. There was no evidence of foul play. The North Manchester's Coronial Office released the body for burial to the family's Jewish undertakers. Nobody informed them of the brain retention. Nor did it form part of the evidence presented at a reconvened Inquest conducted by Mr Bryan North, coroner for the area in which Mr Isaacs had died. As the verdict of suicide was unopposed, the coroner had the official capacity to declare it a 'paper inquest' (like the 'non-jury' cases of the past). This meant that various written documents (police report, GP statement, post-mortem evidence and so on) were enough to pass a verdict and establish there were no suspicious circumstances. Crime scene photographs were taken, but it was never officially explained why they did not form part of the Inquest evidence reviewed by the coroner (forensic teams in the event of an unexplained suicide take digital images as a matter of course). Mrs Isaacs did have an opportunity to attend the Inquest. She was supported by a solicitor and barrister arranged by the elders in the Jewish community. What upset the family the most was the final verdict of 'Suicide ... Hanging ... Cyril Mark Isaacs died of the aforesaid at his home. He was found hanging from the loft by an electric flex' [sic].[51] In the Jewish community, the taking of life is taboo and there had been no official reference to Mr Isaacs's accumulated history of mental ill health at the Inquest. The family felt that as it stood, the verdict could bring them cultural shame in their community since the exonerating circumstances did not form part of the official reporting.

Mrs Isaacs remained very troubled about her husband's death and the removal of his body from their home for a post-mortem without her consent. She wrote many letters to the coroner, Mr Brian North, between 1987 and 1991 to query the verdict because it seemed to her to reflect a lack of cultural and human understanding. Each time, the coroner informed her that it was his duty to base his verdict on the written evidence presented by the police, witnesses and pathologist assigned to the case; their medico-legal verdict was prescribed in regulations and could not be adjusted retrospectively. Eventually, Mrs Isaacs managed to get official access to Mr Isaacs's medical records still held by his general practitioner in April 2000. She was anxious to read these to see if they would exonerate in any way the stark verdict of suicide. What she found amongst her dead husband's medical papers was surprising and upsetting. A letter to Mr Isaacs's general practitioner, Dr Rosenburg, explained that the Department of Psychiatry at Manchester University 'had collected samples from Mr Isaacs' brain' and the research team were anxious to frame their research study by reference to his history of mental ill-health and medication for depression administered prior to death. The coroner permitted this hidden history to be used for research purposes, but he did not reconsider the humanity of the suicide verdict. A dead husband's brain was fresh, a research opportunity, and thus formed part of a large mental ill-health project. At the time of death, Mrs Isaacs had explained her religious convictions to the police, a coroner and her husband's general practitioner. It was self-evident she had been ignored. There was a clear breach of medical ethics, resulting in a missed body parts dispute. Mrs Isaacs's son thus wrote to the Secretary for Health, Hon. Alan Milburn MP, demanding a full investigation into the original circumstances surrounding the death, post-mortem, retention and disposal of Mr Cyril Isaacs's brain. Events revealed a pathology and medical research cover-up.

On 29 July 2001, Her Majesties Inspector of Anatomy, Mr Jeremy Metters, conducted a formal investigation on behalf of the government into the controversial *Isaacs Case*. Over the next two years, his enquiries were extensive and exhaustive. He found that there was a 'joint research team' involved in brain study comprising members of the physiology and psychiatry departments at Manchester University. Their main research focus was neuropathology and in particular mental ill-health conditions (broadly defined). North Manchester Coronial service from 1985 to 1997 had routinely permitted the retention of brains for further research purposes at Manchester University without the knowledge of the families involved: a common practice amongst many pathologists employed by coroners across the country. In addition, GMP were criticised for their officious conduct in relation to Mrs Elaine Isaacs (a theme we will be returning to later in this chapter since such criticisms have re-emerged with renewed force recently, as we saw in our opening story of the Culshaws in this chapter). Essentially, the *Isaacs Report* (2003) highlighted:

7. **The report shows, among other things, that relatives were not aware that:**
   - ➤ Organs would be removed as part of a coroner's post mortem examination;
   - ➤ Organs removed might not be returned to the body after the post mortem examination;
   - ➤ Organs could be retained legally by the coroner without their permission in connection with establishing the cause of death; and
   - ➤ Organs might be retained for other purposes, such as research, without their consent and thus without legal authority.

8. **Relatives were not given:**
   - ➤ Information about the coroners' post mortem process;
   - ➤ Information about the options for the ultimate disposal of any organs removed;
   - ➤ Support, advice or counselling; or
   - ➤ Suitable consideration of religious or cultural beliefs.[52]

Jeremy Metters provided a national census of all brain material held in research repositories across England and Wales (see Table 6.3). Mr Cyril

Table 6.3 *Nature of retentions in pathology stores, which had been accumulated since 1970, and were present at the National Census Point, c. 2001–2003*

Organ	Number of organs	Percentage of total retentions
Brains	23 900	44%
Hearts	9 400	17%
Lungs	6 900	13%
Other Organs	6 100	11%
Body Parts	3 700	7%
Stillbirths/Fetuses	2 900	5%
Not Specified	1 400	3%
Total(s)	**54 300**	**100%**

Source: Isaacs Report Response, written by the Department of Health, Home Office and Department for Education and Skills (London: HMSO, 2003), p. 25 [ISBN 011322611X] – see also, www.doh.gov.uk/cmo/isaacsreport/response

Isaacs's brain was one of 23,900 deposits that had been stored since the 1970s for further research purposes. Pathologists generated these on behalf of coroners across the UK. In Manchester, several morticians co-operated at Prestwich Hospital with this 'supply mechanism of donation' for a reported fee of '£10 per brain'. Although one particular coroner denied he knew the specifics of what was taking place, Metters concluded that this was 'hardly credible' under the circumstances. It appeared that 'brain collections' rather than 'brain banking' had constituted the majority of 'retentions-without-consent'; it was difficult to retrace the individual research thresholds inside the supply system because the paperwork trail was either never created in the first place, had been destroyed subsequently or was ambiguous at best. The media and patients' groups who took this as confirmation of a culture of duplicity queried the extent to which the official figures were a true picture of pathologists' covert working practices and their corporate culture of denial.

Metters concluded that his figures were the best indication of the scale of brain retentions, and he distributed them into three research categories: *Brain Accumulation* (generally created by coroners' cases via hospital mortuaries and commissioning pathology reports for post-mortem purposes); *Brain Collection* (held by pathology departments initially for diagnosis, but also for further teaching and research use); and *Brain Banking* (linked to pathology departments and university research centres), often working with relatives who have given consent to further specialised research into specific conditions like Creutzfeldt–Jakob Disease (hereafter CJD), Huntington's or Alzheimer's neuro-degenerative diseases. Metter decided that it was *Brain Accumulations* and *Brain Collections* that were ethically questionable. Pathologists had been working their way around the law to facilitate brain research.[53] Effectively, they colluded in a system of supply that ignored codes of practice on informed consent. In turn, these should have been defined properly under HTA1961 and Coroners Rules (see Chapters 2 and 5), but were not. The paternalism of the past had been exposed to public scrutiny and found wanting in a biomedical era. It was this culture of concealment which would result in HTA2004. Yet, like all new legislation, it would take time for ingrained attitudes to change. In other words, the medical research community that had relied on hidden histories of the dead for so long neglected to appreciate the range of disputes they had generated for the future. They did operate within the legal requirements of their time, but this also meant that medical ethics remain fixed in an era when biotechnology was fast changing. As a result, only by blending the numerous historical and hidden ethical issues created can we begin to appreciate their cultural ramifications, including, importantly, notions of trust and expertise, the problem of piecemeal legislation and the ambiguities of consent, which went undetected from the 1960s to 2000. This proved to be a public relations mistake, exposing differential power relations in an era of full democratic representation when everyone had a taxpayer stake in the NHS. There were many gains from the new era of medical research for the general public in this historical process, but equally the bereaved expressed how excluded they felt in terms of the role of memory, the changing boundaries of life and death and the scale of the Information State's lack of accountability in their medical lives. To better appreciate how pathologists defended their position in response, we need to trace a representative sample of oral histories that document typical reactions to the public outcry for HTA2004 because of the scale of the missed disputes being rediscovered.

Once HTA2004 became law, many pathologists in the UK resented the position they were placed in. Most felt hounded by the media, made a scapegoat for the degree to which the Coronial service relied on their expertise. The Pathological Society of Great Britain and Ireland hence took the decision in 2008 to commission a new book by Sue Armstrong called *A Matter of Life and Death: Conversations with Pathologists*,[54] based on extensive interviews with practicing pathologists. An important theme of the oral histories assembled was the Alder Hey scandal in the NHS and its aftermath. There was uniform agreement amongst participants that it was 'a dark hour for pathology' across the British Isles and Ireland. As Professor James Ironside – an expert on the neuropathology of CJD and member of the new Human Tissue Authority set up in 2005 – explained:

What happened in Alder Hey was terrible. It opened up the whole question of autopsies – retention of tissues and organs, how much relatives knew, how much relatives had been consulted – and had some terrible messages for all concerned. It was a dark hour for pathology, no doubt about it. Not helped, I must say, by the media. You were made to feel that not only had you examined a baby that had died from cot death or something, you'd actually gone out and killed it beforehand. Just terrible! And also I think that we were not best supported by the Minister of Health at the time, Alan Milburn. He just opted to go 'belly up' and do anything to satisfy the various pressure groups that had emerged from the media, and I think a more measured response would have been better. Some of the first attempts at the legislation were just completely unworkable. And through pressure from a whole range of groups, the legislation was changed in the UK. It's still not perfect, but it's better than it was.[55]

Professor David Levison (now retired), former Chair in Pathology at Dundee University, reflected with a slightly different emphasis:

I don't think that Alder Hey and Bristol were scandals. They're only scandals because the media say they were scandals. . . . I know of quite a few people who have given up being paediatric pathologists because of this – because they couldn't stand the kind of pressures they were being put under, the phone calls, and the abuse they were getting as they walked home, and this sort of thing. It has done a lot of harm to some people, and I mean it has really kicked paediatric pathology in the teeth. . . . I know of studies that have not been done because it's just not worth the effort of going through the ethical hoops. . . . It really does slow things up.[56]

Others such as Professor Sebastian Lucas, Chair in Clinical Histopathology at Guy's, King's and St Thomas' hospitals, pointed out that from a pathology point of view by 2008:

In a way things haven't got all that much better [since Alder Hey]. They've got more bureaucratic, but there's still a huge grey area in tissue retention across the consented to coronial autopsy spectrum, and it's not very clear. Or it's very clear what to do if you want to stay absolutely within the letter of the law, be squeaky clean. You do nothing! But the point is, to be good and to be useful for public health you need to do a bit more than that, and that's where the grey areas come in.[57]

Most argued that it was poor communication that was at the heart of recent biomedical debates and the public exposure of pathology's inner working practices. Irene Scheimberg, Consultant Paediatric and Perinatal Pathologist at the London Hospital, thus took the view that:

At one point during the Alder Hey crisis I said, 'I am going to go and talk to the Liverpool parents so that they realise that not all pathologists have horns and are horrible'. At the beginning they were all very confrontational – there were lots of them – and I said, 'I do understand what it is to lose people, to experience the untimely death of people' [as someone from the Jewish community who needed political asylum, she lost many friends and family to war and conflict]. And I told them my story –

because they were so immersed in their grief that they didn't realise other people might have had a traumatic history as well. They were surprised because I was crying. One of them came up and hugged me afterwards, and said: 'I never thought I'd ever hug a pathologist.'[58]

Scheimberg suggested that it was better for people when grieving to keep looking forward, an attitude of mind she had learned from the long history of being political refugees in her Jewish family of Russian extraction. Her personal motto was: 'Memory is very wise – you don't remember what you cannot live with.' She did respect the fact that learning later that information had been withheld about human harvesting could be shocking for families. Consequently she explained how:

In coroners' cases I write a personal letter to the families. I use the name of the child, and I explain to families why I'm asking them if we can keep blocks and slides. In the first place because it's important for their sakes in case there is a problem or something later. Then, so that we can use them for teaching and training. Because someone has to carry on with the work when I'm no longer here; the knowledge has to be passed on. And then I explain why we need them for research, and what type of research we're talking about – because it's important for them to know that it's research that will benefit them personally, but we can't do it unless we have specific consent.[59]

In this selection of oral history material we have therefore an important opportunity to elaborate on the conceptual approach of Alessandro Portelli, who reminded us at the start of this chapter about the importance of 'the peculiarities of oral history' and their subjectivity precisely because they are 'not just about what people did, but [what] they wanted to do, what they believed they were doing, and what they now think they did'.[60] Thus, it is apparent that some pathologists operated on a need-to-know basis because they felt it was better to keep pressing ahead with their research agendas, and unkind to tell the general public everything about brain research when they were grieving. Others did not accept that the organ donation and pathology retentions in the NHS around 2000 were a scandal but a media-generated medical outrage designed to sell newspapers. Most had been as open and engaging in their working-lives as they could be under difficult circumstances, committed to communicating the importance of their work and legacy of human material retentions. Pathologists were thus complex actors, shaped by social, cultural, political, economic and administrative circumstances. Like all human beings, they could fail, and some did so in terms of public relations; for there was a general recognition by HTA2004 that pathology's paternalism and patriarchy were past their clinical sell-by-date. Its actor network had to leave behind the ethics of conviction of the past and embrace the ethics of responsibility for tomorrow. Against this backdrop, the Royal College of Pathologists (hereafter RCP) have been working extensively to try to resolve these experiential issues, and they recognise the need for consensual medical ethics: a trend that has increased in the past ten years or so. There has been an official recognition that pathologists had taken a 'proprietorial' view of the body rather than a 'custodial' one: a theme that has run throughout all the chapters of this book.[61] At the same time, in the intervening years since HTA2004, common themes have emerged in conversations with pathologists: as we saw above and touch on below, too.[62] Ingrained attitudes have been of long duration, and some pathologists have refused to make the clinical adjustments, retiring early. There has continued to be ambivalence felt by many RCP members about the extent of public accountability required by new statutes, mushrooming bureaucracy and the media.

Today the RCP publishes widely its latest research and innovations, engaging the public with stories of how pathology into common cancers, for instance, saves lives every day in the NHS. It has also been keen to promote new solutions for old pathology problems. One innovation it has been eager to publicise is digital autopsies in cases where the probable causes of death are known in Coronial cases in England and Wales. RCP now recognises that CT scanning techniques could provide a cultural and practical solution for families like the Isaacs who would not consent to the cutting of the body and the removal of human material on religious grounds but would be amenable to a CT scan instead because it is non-invasive, replacing a post-mortem. The way it works is that the deceased can undergo a CT scan to confirm 'unnatural death' with a minimal amount of interference with the dead body. A new study published in the *Lancet*, co-ordinated by Professors Guy Rutty and Bruno Morgan at the University of Leicester, thus showed recently that in a sample size of 241 cases in which an adult had died of unexpected outcomes that were not necessarily suspicious, some 92 per cent of these coroners' cases (where n=222) could be established from digital CT solutions.[63] Currently, the cost is £500 per case, paid for by the family in question, raising ethical issues about fair access to the technology for everyone, especially in communities of high-density ethnicity and poverty patterns. Nevertheless, as the RCP press office told the *Guardian* newspaper in May 2017: 'The College fully supports further research in this area while reinforcing the need for thorough and robust governance in this emerging field.'[64] Evidently, the *Isaacs Report* was an important catalyst for cultural change in medical research around the Millennium in Britain. It has resulted in an emphasis on informed consent in brain research and finding new solutions to complex human dilemmas over the ownership and use of bodies and body parts. Even so, in interviews given off the record for this book, many pathologists have made it clear why they left the profession in the past five years or so. Most felt their job description 'was now too restrictive', 'there's just too much bureaucracy' and 'it's taken away my sense of professional standing ... I mean who wants to deal with all the hassle'.[65] So rather than reform from within, what has tended to happen since HTA2004 is that the numbers of qualified RCP members have thinned out. There is unquestionably a lot less hands-on experience than there once was inside the Coronial system. To balance this sense of a loss of professional expertise, the final section of this chapter thus returns to the human impact of pathologists' workload, particularly involving those who have just retired or resigned from office. In this way, we can engage with a wider cross section of lived experiences of missed disputes, similar to the storyline of the Culshaw family which opened this chapter. For the events described test public trust in pathology work since HTA2004, which was supposed to have been changed fundamentally the national conversation about harvesting brains and human tissue retentions.

'Hospital Stored Dead Children's Brains in Jars': *Southampton Hospital under Public Scrutiny*[66]

In 2012, the Association of Chief Police Officers (hereafter ACPO) faced an ethical dilemma. They had to inform the Human Tissue Authority that a large number of organ and tissue retentions had gone unnoticed at the time of HTA2004. This was because the police had special powers concerning human material retention up until 2006. They were exempt under Section 39 of the HTA2004, as follows:

Section 39 of Human Tissue Act

(1) Subject to subsection (2), nothing in section 14(1) or 16(2) applies to anything done for purposes related to—

(a) the prevention or detection of crime, or
(b) the conduct of a prosecution.

(2) Subsection (1) does not except from section 14(1) or 16(2) the carrying-out of a post-mortem examination for purposes of functions of a coroner.

Forensic PM examinations

If a person dies in circumstances considered to be 'suspicious' or where homicide is suspected, HM Coroner after consultation with the police can authorise a Home Office Registered Forensic Pathologist to perform a forensic PM examination to—

• Ascertain the identity of the deceased
• The cause/surrounding circumstances of death
• To allow collection of evidence from the body [67]

The Human Tissue Authority also issued a public statement clarifying that there were three statutes that authorised the police to hold human material. These were: the Coroners and Criminal Justice Act (Eliz. 2 c. 25: 2009), the Police and Criminal Evidence Act (Eliz. 2 c. 60: 1984, especially sections 19 &

22) and the Criminal Procedure and Investigation Act (Eliz. 2 c. 25: 1996). Together they permitted an investigating officer to be present at a post-mortem, which they had authorised by virtue of asking forensic scientists and Home Office pathologists to lawfully enter premises and seize whatever material evidence was necessary to bring a criminal act to justice. They also had extra powers under English Common Law of seizure for physical items or human material found elsewhere that were not on the premises of a specific crime in the locality where it was committed. Since these procedures had overlapping regulations, there was not a coherent national policy in the police force of how to seize, record, evaluate evidence, present in court and return human material after a conviction or court hearing. The Murder Manual (2006, especially Section 11) did try to give clear pathology guidelines, but this too resulted in disparity amongst actual police forces in England and Wales, with individual senior officers taking a pragmatic view of their particular medico-legal position. The ACPO thus conceded in 2012 that many police forces did not actually know what their responsibilities were in respect of human material retentions. Most thought this problem of a lack of uniformity was delegated to coroners and their pathologists to monitor and resolve, given the former's historic powers of discretionary justice (a theme we encountered in Chapter 5).

In 2012 a central government commissioned ACPO audit grew out of the National Gold Group established alongside the National Police Improvement Agency (later to be renamed the Home Office Pathology Unit). These policing bodies were granted permission to take proper legal advice from suitably qualified barristers during the national audit process, which was concerned with three categories of material infringement:

Category 1 – Material taken at PM examination which would not generally be considered part of the body e.g. scrapings, fingernails, hair, stomach contents
Category 2 – Samples of human tissue which are not a significant part of the body e.g. small tissue samples, blocks, slides & so on
Category 3 – Samples of human tissue that incorporate a significant part of the body e.g. organs, limbs & so on [68]

Category 3 formed the central focus of the ACPO audit, in liaison with the Human Tissue Authority. Together they found that '492 organs' or what was described as '*significant* [sic] body parts [brains] were held on police premises or other establishments. These related to historical cases going back to the 1960s.' To try to reassure the public that this did not repeat Alder Hey, the Human Tissue Authority issued a press release confirming that 'between 1960 and 2010 there had been 6.2 million PM [post-mortem] examinations' conducted in England and Wales. Of these 6.2 million, just 2.45 per cent, or 151,900, resulted in the need for a forensic examination in which the police became involved. Of the 151,900 cases, only 0.33 per cent, or 50,633, related to potential organ retentions or *significant* body parts kept by the police and their Home Office pathologists.[69] Yet, this statistical statement still did not provide enough reassurance to the families involved, because even a basic calculation underscored that in a 50-year period, on average there were not less than 1,000 cases a year that could potentially have resulted in missed body disputes. It was (again) media testimony of those who were misled that would prove to be a powerful reminder of the need to remain vigilant in a biomedical era.

At first, ACPO tried to counter any negative publicity by stressing the expertise of those that retained the human material and the important legal reasons for doing so. Thus, it was explained that under police powers, a selection of NHS hospital premises were designated as regional autopsy units. Here coroners and their pathologists on behalf of the Home Office had stored human material pending a court case. The Home Office expressed regret that human material had been kept without informing families, but the police tried to reassure the media that it was done in the best interests of criminal justice. One such location was Southampton Hospital in Dorset, a regional autopsy unit for the West Country. The families involved were told on a case-by-case basis that their loved one's remains were still in cold storage. It did not help that as this slow process was just getting under way, a civil servant at the Home Office was despatched to tell the press that: 'It is down to individual forces to decide ... whether the material is needed or not. In some cases the retention period may have been longer than necessary.' This was a classic case of official understatement, as events subsequently proved in the press.

On 14 August 2012, the *Sun* newspaper led with a headline – 'They took brains from our boys too ... WHY?' Their investigative journalist, John Coles, spoke to Hannah Cheevers, whose baby son had died of a heart defect aged 2 days old in 1998, and Melanie Galton, whose infant son died aged 1 of sudden infant death syndrome in 1997. Each was told that there would be a post-mortem, but neither was informed that their offspring's brain had been retained and kept for 15 years by pathologists on behalf of the police. Melanie explained:

They turned up just before Christmas and told me, 'We've found Ricky's brain at the hospital'. I was stunned, I couldn't believe what I was hearing. ... I asked them 'Why have you kept it so long?' and all they could say was something like it had 'got lost in the system' and they were now chasing everything up. ... They gave me a letter and leaflet explaining the situation – but instead of 'son' the letter refers to him in one place as 'mother' and 'father' in another. ... I'm disgusted and angry as well as upset. I'm not going to let this drop. ... They had a post mortem which found the cause of death as sudden infant death syndrome, so why did they need to keep his brain? I imagine it's been forgotten about on the back of a shelf somewhere. I want to have another funeral – it will probably be just me by his grave – because I want it returned to his body where it should be. I don't want it to go *missing* [author's emphasis] for another 15 years.[70]

In a similar refrain, Hannah Cheevers and her partner, Martin Lovell, from Wimborne Dorset were shocked to be in an equivalent missed body part dispute. Hannah recounted:

They told us tissues from Rhys had been retained – I thought they meant a sliver of tissue on a slide. Then they said it was his whole brain. I was shocked. I was never told about this and if they'd asked my permission I would have said 'no'. They wouldn't tell me why it had been kept and they said that nothing had been done to it. It was dreadful – I had a new baby in my arms and it brought it all back. . . . If they'd kept Rhys's heart I might have understood, but there was no reason to keep his brain. When he died they offered us a post mortem to find out what had happened and we agreed because we wanted to know. So he was taken from Poole Hospital to Southampton Hospital, but we had no idea they would keep his brain. It's absolutely disgusting what has happened. I remember the Alder Hey scandal, and I said to my mum at the time that I was glad it wasn't Southampton. There really needs to be an inquiry into this.[71]

Each mother recalled having to go through a harrowing series of police enquiries at the time of their child's death to make sure that it was not suspicious – it felt as though old and very painful memories were being re-opened again. Indeed, one of the most poignant press stories to appear was that of Ryan Franklin who 'was killed by his dad, aged two in 2002'. A case of manslaughter was secured in court based on medical evidence that the child had been battered to death. His mother then explained what happened a decade later. She was told by Southampton Hospital that her dead baby's brain, eyes and spinal cord had been retained. Like the other mothers affected, she had known it was necessary to have a post-mortem but she claimed that she had said 'no to donating his organs', telling doctors in 2002: 'He came into this world full and I want him to go out full – don't touch him.'[72] Around the time of the Alder Hey scandal, she began to suspect that she may have been misinformed. This uneasy sense of a missed dispute re-emerged in 2012: 'When I heard about this review police are carrying out I hoped they would have got in touch with me. I would like someone to come forward and tell me what's happened to his organs so I can have closure.' Catherine Franklin 'discovered that some of Ryan's organs had been taken. His eyes went to a hospital in Sheffield for research – but no one knew what happened to the rest.' The newspaper reporter explained how she had gone on to have 'another son, Benjamin, eight'. Nonetheless Catherine stressed: 'Every time I try to find out what happened I hit a brick wall. I hope now police are doing their audit I'll finally get the truth' about what really happened. In fact, it soon emerged that there were forty cases in Southampton all relating to young dead children whose brains had been removed and stored.[73] In the majority of cases, it appeared that any fears of suspicious deaths were cleared up quickly and no physical evidence for the criminal court was necessary to secure a conviction. Each was a tragic tale of child bereavement. The mothers, according to their own testimony, all found the pain of loss almost unbearable to experience again after ten years had elapsed.

Personal spoken and reported histories like these representative cases provide thought-provoking testimony concerning the conduct of the medical research community in a biomedical era. Their discourse reiterates Alessandro Portelli's inciteful comments (encountered earlier in this chapter's introduction) about the value of the 'the peculiarities of oral history' in the medical humanities. Their subjectivity again reveals 'not just about what people did, but [what] they wanted to do, what they believed they were doing, and what they now think they did'.[74] To many pathologists, it had seemed that the press has been responsible for stirring up emotive stories and putting the spin of scandal on the editorial byline to sell more newspapers about the recent ACPO audit findings. Yet, it is undeniable that the same sorts of experiential histories were often repeated, and verbatim by those families involved. Indeed, as Philip Cheung has recently pointed out, it is impossible to deny how much the twice-bereaved have needed each other for support when missed body parts disputes recur, exemplified by the number of support groups that have been set up and continue to flourish today. There is:

NACOR (The National Committee Relating to Organ Donation), and PITY II (Parents who have Interred their Young Twice) … Respect for Leicester, Stolen Hearts in Birmingham, Bristol Heart Children's Action Group, Cambridge Area Support Network, Derbyshire Organ Retention Support Group, South Yorkshire/North Derbyshire Support Group for Post-Mortems Retention Parents and Relatives, NERO North East Organ Retentions Group), Storm in Manchester, Our Children, REGAIN groups in Nottingham, Legacy Faborio, PORSH in Plymouth, and so on.[75]

Cheung points out that there is 'a danger that' such support groups will 'be seen by scientists and medical researchers as anti-science and anti-research'.[76] Many scientists do not believe in an afterlife or appreciate that the physical remains can have a powerful meaning in the grieving process of the bereaved, even though there is ample evidence that the GMP failed not only the Isaacs family in 2002, but the Culshaws and others more recently. Too often, points out Cheung, such families who express strong natural emotions are 'perceived in the same light as animal research campaigners'. He thus argues that the medical research community need to accept 'the challenge of shaping ideas and attitudes' to their work and its importance by meeting those bereaved with genuine humanity to bridge the recent past to a better biomedical future for everybody. It is therefore informative and important how the journal *Science* reported on 7 April 2017 that: 'the Rules of Memory are being *beautifully rewritten*'.[77] Because such perspectives have the potential to reshape how historians evaluate oral histories on the sensitive topic of missed disputes too.

It is often said in the global media that the British have a character trait that is admired around the world. They are renowned for being stoic, exemplifying the stiff upper lip in times of adversity. It was a national trait that was said to have brought the country through two world wars, associated food rationing and many millions of deaths. As, however, public tastes changed during the 1960s with the liberalisation of British society, the old values of a wartime generation were refashioned. It became culturally less acceptable to button-up emotions, and instead many more people began to speak about issues of mental health and well-being. Today, it is a popular topic of national conversation in Britain. At the same time as this process of promoting more compassion and understanding of mental and physical well-being was happening, neuroscience was also contributing to debates about the relationship between the brain and emotions. Recently, evidence has come to light that the way we thought the brain absorbed and accommodated trauma has been misleading. In the past, a medical assumption was made that the best way to help people to get over a very traumatic episode in their life was never to talk about it again – the stoic approach. Then this changed from the 1960s with qualified therapists encouraging those suffering from mental ill-health to come to terms with a dramatic experience by talking it through – the compartmentalising approach. Each medical intervention was about reviewing negative experiences and helping the patient to move on in a more positive direction. However, new scientific studies in Japan and the USA have challenged the neuroscience of this type of trauma management, and the results of these recent scientific findings are very important for assessing the emotional reactions of families to the missed disputes of the ACPO audit in 2017. The key to understanding what the bereaved were going through has been to better appreciate that the way we thought we handled and remembered trauma has been scientifically incorrect.

The brain is clever. It seeks to protect us in trauma. To do this, it does not ask us to be exclusively stoic or to compartmentalise what is happening when confronted by extreme stress. Instead, new scientific studies in Japan and the USA have found ground-breaking evidence that all painful memories are absorbed in two ways. First, the brain will store short-term recollections when we are in shock. Then, at the same time, it begins a neurological process of transferring the memories of that initial trauma from the hippocampus of the brain. Slowly, the brain has a neurological mechanism that converts short-term experiences into long-term memories in the cerebral cortex where they are 'banked' for life. In this way, the brain 'doubles up' its memory system. It creates two simultaneous memories that mirror each other every time we experience something out of the ordinary as human beings.[78] This neurological balancing act is unconscious in the mind. The function of this doubling up is to help us as human beings to live with what has happened. We cope by assimilating together physical reactions (short-term shock, hippocampus) and their emotional impact (long-term feelings, cerebral cortex) of trauma. This works well neurologically, provided that the balancing mechanism is not disturbed. If, many years after a shocking event, it revived in an unexpected manner, then that would have the effect of unbalancing the brain's trauma survival mechanism. So, we can be stoic and we can compartmentalise, precisely because of the amazing balancing mechanism in our brains, and this is what scientists mean when they say that 'the Rules of Memory are being *beautifully rewritten*'.[79] In 2017, the families involved in the findings of the ACPO audit experienced what happens when this newly discovered neurological balancing system was disturbed by reviving painful memories.

When we encounter oral histories and the navigation of their feelings in a history of emotions, it is important in the medical humanities not simply to dismiss their testimony of trauma as too subjective. In fact, what people recount is telling us that we need to fully consider the latest neurological perspectives of what is happening in the brains of the bereaved. The ACPO families experienced what it was like to go through a missed dispute about withheld information. This destabilised the short-term and long-term neurological centres of memory formation and unbalanced the maintenance of their well-being. Those involved thus found it mentally very hard to cope, and this is verifiable by the neuroscience of memory formation and maintenance. Effectively, some experienced a neurological U-turn that triggered a very stressful episode in the mind's emotional centres. Importantly, the implications for this book's study into missed disputes and how people emotionally react (hippocampus, short-term shock) and learn to live with the unpalatable facts (cortex assimilation, very painful emotions) are profound. If medically correct, Mrs Jean Culshaw and others like her were not being duplicitous or exaggerating when they said they were 'suffering' mental upheaval in March 2017. In neurological terms, their minds were, literally, disturbed, as they had to again go through very painful memories from 1993. Thus, in a history of emotions, scholars, such as William Reddy, are correct to emphasise how talking about feelings is essentially the only way that a person can then rebalance if forced to revisit something so painful.[80] Ironically, science, which has long stressed its dispassionate and secular purpose (laudable aims), has itself discovered that the brain has a '*beautiful*' medical function that is all about re-balancing the rational and the instinctive when missed disputes occur. It works with human nature holistically, and this is a significant finding for the medical humanities, echoing what George Steiner the moral philosopher suggested in this book's Part I. The brain does not discard 'old' information for 'new' memories – instead, it runs these lived experiences 'in parallel' because life is like that, and this is what keeps us creative as human beings. In other words, those involved in missed disputes could cope well, provided communication was very good and trust existed between all those involved in the network of actors when a crisis point involving the death of a loved one had to be revisited. To illustrate that there could be more positive outcomes in this more transparent process for pathologists too, we end with the sort of brain story that seldom features in oral histories or the press on this sensitive topic.

In 2000, Sean and Sarah Luff became new parents. Tragically, soon after birth, their 3-day-old baby died because of medical negligence in Southampton Hospital. Mistakenly, staff on duty gave him a morphine overdose – '100 times the proper dose of painkillers' – in an attempt to save his young life.[81] At a subsequent Inquest, the medical evidence established that their son would have died in any case, such were the fatal complications in this sad case. This did not excuse the medical errors, but the hope was that the forensic findings would alleviate the Luffs' concerns that their baby was not in pain when he died. However, the family was shocked when Dorset police informed them in 2012 that Southampton Hospital had retained their baby son's brain in a jar without their consent in 2000. Sean Luff asked: 'How many times can one family, and one little baby, be betrayed by the authorities?' He questioned in the press: 'How much more heartache can they inflict on us?' There was, even so, to be a twist to this news story, and one that exemplifies the Janus-like nature of pathology expertise today. In February 2012, Sean Luff received a diagnosis of myeloid leukaemia. This happened just several months after Dorset police informed him about his dead son's brain retention. Sean became very ill and had to endure 'three gruelling sessions of chemotherapy and a bone marrow transplant'.[82] Unfortunately, this series of life-saving treatments compromised his immune system, and he caught pneumonia just before the Christmas holidays in 2013. Because Sean was unable to fight the serious infection in his lungs, doctors judged it best to place him in a medically induced coma. It would take eight months of intensive care before Sean was stabilised and able to go home. Yet, the medical team that had saved his life three times in those eight months was based at Southampton Hospital, where his baby son had died under exceptionally stressful and medically culpable circumstances, twelve years earlier. Even so, the Luff extended family were grateful for Sean's recent medical interventions. They hence decided to raise money for more medical research at Southampton Hospital in August 2013. The Luffs were happy to publicise the good work of medical staff in the local press. There was self-evidently a pathology paradox in this case, and a poignant one. Sean Ruff was kept alive by the same expertise that had once retained his baby son's brain without his consent. The latter's successful outcome did not justify the lack of medical ethics in the former case-history. Yet, it did make for a thought-provoking parallel in what have too often been hidden histories of the brain.

For it left open the unanswered question: How much more could have been achieved if brain research and retentions had been a more open and engaging research partnership with the bereaved across Britain after WWII?

Conclusion

In 2010, a consortium of scholars convened at the University of Manchester to explore 'forensic cultures' in contemporary society prompted by the fact that coroners, pathologists and DNA specialists 'now have an unprecedented level of visibility' across the UK, not least because of 'true crime' drama on television.[83] The conference concluded that 'forensics is best understood as a historically-shifting material and social entity but also as mediated through a cultural grid of forms, languages and resources, through which credibility is built up, negotiated and contested'. Simon Cole, one thoughtful contributor, 'questioned the idealised image of a scientific culture as a unified entity governed by a clear and stable set of rules which produce and guarantee a single form of knowledge'. This was essentially the case in many types of missed disputes in brain research, too, of the modern era. Recently, Paul Roberts has hence helpfully pointed out that histories of forensic science and pathology cannot simply be pieced together to produce a harmonious picture that does not reflect local realities or public sensibilities. Indeed, he has been critical of a strong confirmation bias in histories of science covering laboratory studies that elevate the positive and ignore the negative aspects of secretive working cultures (themes the Introduction and Chapter 1 highlighted). Thus, the Manchester conference concluded that there is more

value of attending to the complex interrelationships, cultural specificities, and diverse and shifting identities of forensic practitioners, the institutions within which they work, the techniques they deploy to produce and display forensic truths, and how these truths are transformed in public as forensic cultures engage the worlds in and for which they act.[84]

One of the main difficulties with researching the nature of pathology and neuroscience in the modern era has been the culture of the closed door. Not only was recording of brain retentions insubstantial but those records that survive in archive collections are often sealed under the 100-year rule. General statistics are obtainable under special written request according to the provisions of the Freedom of Information Act (Eliz. 2 c. 26: 2000) in the UK. Even so, there are many legal barriers erected to complicate better open and transparent research in the medical humanities. In protecting the past, pathology has often looked guilty of maintaining a culture of denial and subterfuge, and this has unquestionably damaged its reputation. When, moreover, new evidence emerges of past failings, like the GMP revelations recently after the ACPO audit, those conducting the conversations with relatives came across as insincere. Occasionally, named pathologists were revealed, but most remained hidden behind an anonymous title or official jurisdiction disclosed in the most general terms to families left confused and upset – angry about the faceless mandarins of a Home Office firewall. The corporate-speak which was often repeated by the police force about holding 'open and honest conversations' with relatives informed of brain retentions, sounded more like a publicity campaign for the press than a genuine attempt to engage with how the twice-bereaved felt. Jenny Culshaw and others felt understandably that their emotional well-being was being devalued and undermined. Indeed, it is noteworthy just how many shocked parents in the same situation repeated their shared understandings, using the same phrases and words to describe common predicaments and feelings of distress. In tragic circumstances, they had to re-open painful memories to gain concrete information. That neuroscience itself has discovered the 'Rules of Memory are being *beautifully rewritten*' in order to explain the double memory and its careful balancing mechanism we all create in the brain to deal with traumatic events in our lives is informative.[85] The Culshaw and Isaacs families were not, it turns out, being excessive, overdramatic or unreasonable in their reactions, but rather their neurological response was functioning in a normal manner. In a history of emotions, it has always been essential to talk about such feelings to rebalance traumatic experiences reopened by time delays, misinformation, and half-truths.[86] As all good historians know, careful attention should, likewise, be paid to what is not said, just as much as to what is. For the history of these missed disputes is like a dry-stone wall – in its research gaps are the future human solutions to consensual medical ethics. First we have to locate them, and then we must look that past honestly in the face to ensure we provide better access for professional researchers to evaluate those gaps in a measured manner.

In an ageing population around the world, brain research has a powerful role to play wherever we live in our community settings. With approximately one in five people in Britain now suffering from neuro-degenerative disorders, healthcare practitioners need the co-operation and co-creation of the public to make new medical breakthroughs. This cannot, though, be achieved in cultural isolation – the consent of the silent majority being taken for granted is no longer the modus operandi of pathologists, post–Alder Hey. Most recognise this and are working together to promote the sort of expertise in histopathology that we all need. Others resent the levels of bureaucracy and have retired or resigned from the profession, bruised by the public criticisms, which they still believe is excessive. That this will be a lost research opportunity in some respect, curtailing individual career paths in the short term, is undeniable. Yet, it is equally irrefutable that such a status quo had been created by closing ranks and not engaging with the public enough in the recent past. The responsibility, therefore, first and foremost, for this cultural stand-off, rests with pathologists and not society as a whole. The history of missed body disputes and disputed body ethics brought together in this chapter shows clearly that some pathologists acted as though they owned the human body, its parts, organs and tissue. In the 1950s, those entering the medical profession spoke of a vocation, a calling, a sense of purpose that this was the job they were meant to do. Some were arrogant about their expertise; others genuinely thought that they were working hard for the greater good. Medical science too has become an endeavour concerned with career progression, enhancing one's scientific reputation and making headlines promoting the latest drug therapy. Those with a vocation did and do still people the system, yet the consensual and custodial only very slowly – too slowly, in many cases of missed disputes – gained ascendancy over proprietorial approaches to bodies and body ethics. Thus, missed disputes in brain research are a function of, and embody, slow and partial processes of cultural change in the post-war era. Yet even as medicine and the medical sciences have learned to talk *with*, rather than *at*, their patients, the expanding frontiers of the possible in terms of the cure and the extension of life made possible through precision medicine introduce a new potential for body disputes and a much more complex landscape of body ethics. It is to this matter that we turn, finally, in Chapter 7, the conclusion to this book, when we reflect on the question of scientific eternities of material afterlives in a Genome era.

Notes

1. BBC News, 'John Culshaw: mum's anger over son's organs stored in police lab', 15 March 2017, accessed 4/4/2017 at: www.bbc.co.uk/news/uk-england-manchester-39274707
2. Ibid.
3. John Scheerout, 'My murdered son's body parts were stored in secret – the human remains scandal revealed', *Manchester Evening News*, 13 March 2017, accessed 4/4/2017, at: http://www.manchestereveningnews.co.uk/news/greater-manchester-news/my-murdered-sons-body-parts-12734965
4. Ibid.
5. Scheerout, 'My murdered son's body parts', 13 March 2017.
6. Ibid.
7. Paul Thompson, *The Voice of the Past, Oral History*, 3rd ed. (Oxford: Oxford University Press), quote at p. 3.
8. Julianne Nyhan and Andrew Flinn, *Computation and the Humanities: Towards an Oral History of the Digital Humanities* (Basingstoke: Palgrave, 2016), see notably, chapter 'Why oral history?', pp. 21–36, quote at p. 26.
9. Alessandro Portelli, 'The peculiarities of oral history', *History Workshop Journal*, 12 (1981): 96–107, quote at pp. 99–100.

10. See, notably, William Reddy, *The Navigation of Feeling: A Framework for the History of Emotions* (Cambridge: Cambridge University Press, 2001). Refer also, Fay Bound Alberti, *Matters of the Heart: History, Medicine and Emotion* (Oxford: Oxford University Press, 2010); Jan Plamper, *The History of Emotions: An Introduction* (Oxford: Oxford University Press, 2017); Dolores Martin Moruno and Beatriz Pichel, *Emotional Bodies (The History of Emotions): The Historical Performativity of Emotions* (Champaign: University of Illinois Press, 2019)

11. BBC News, 'Almost 500 body parts kept by police', 21 May 2012, accessed 4/4/ 2017 at: http://www.bbc.co.uk/news/uk-england-18122332. The Association of Chief Police Officers (APOC) audit covered England, Wales and Northern Ireland, as they operate under an English legal system of justice in cases of homicide and unexplained fatalities that came to the criminal court.

12. Rowena Mason, 'Police secretly kept body parts of 90 children and babies', *Daily Telegraph*, 22 February 2013, accessed 4/4/2017 at: http://www.telegraph.co.uk/n ews/uknews/law-and-order/9887514/Police-secretly-kept-body-parts-of-90-chil dren-and-babies.html

13. BBC News, 'Children's body parts were kept by police', 22 February 2013, accessed 7/6/2017 at: http://www.bbc.co.uk/news/uk-england-bristol-21521872

14. See, Sam Parnia et al., 'AWAreness [*sic*] during REsuscitation [*sic*] – a prospective study', *Resuscitation, Official Journal of the European Resuscitation Council*, 85 (December 2014), 12: 1799–1805; and Parnia, University of Southampton, 'Results of world's largest Near-Death Experiences study: interview with Dr Sam Parnia', *Research Bulletin* (7 October 2014), accessed 7/4/2017 at: http://www.southamp ton.ac.uk/news/2014/10/07-worlds-largest-near-death-experiences-study.page

15. Robin Marantz Henig, 'Crossing over: how science is redefining life and death', *National Geographic*, April 2016, pp. 30–41, accessed 10/4/2017 at: http://www .nationalgeographic.com/magazine/2016/04/dying-death-brain-dead-body-con sciousness-science/

16. The two defining Anglo-American statements in the 1960s and 1970s were: [Anon], 'A definition of irreversible coma: report of the Ad Hoc Committee of the Harvard Medical School to Examine the Definition of Brain Death', *Journal of the American Medical Association* (1968) 205: 337–403 and [Anon], 'Diagnosis of brain death. Statement issued by the honorary secretary of the Conference of Medical Royal Colleges and their faculties in the United Kingdom on 11 October 1976', *British Medical Journal* (1976), 13: 1187–1188.

17. Henig, 'Crossing over', pp. 30–41.

18. E. T. Hurren, *Dissecting the Criminal Corpse: Staging Post-Execution Punishment in Early Modern England* (Basingstoke: Palgrave Macmillan, 2016), chapter 2, 'Becoming *really dead* takes time', pp. 33–68.

19. See, footnote 14 and 16 above; [Anon], 'A definition of irreversible coma: report of the Ad Hoc Committee of the Harvard Medical School to examine the definition of brain death', pp. 337–360.

20. See, Harvard Ad Hoc Committee on Brain Death, Resources for Researchers website, accessed 16 May 2017 at: http://euthanasia.procon.org/sourcefiles/Harva rd_ad_hoc_brain_death.pdf

21. Refer, notably, US State Department, President's Commission for the Study of Ethical Problems in Medicine and Biomedical and Behavioral Research, *Defining Death: A Report on the Medical, Legal and Ethical Issues in the Determination of Death* (Washington, D.C.: US Government Printing Office, 1981).

22. It was, for instance, reprinted as Anon [Editorial], 'Landmark article' by the *Journal of the American Medical Association*, 252 (3 August 1984), 5: 677–679.

23. See, for instance, Mia Giacomini, 'A change of heart and a change of mind? Technology and the redefinition of death in 1968', *Social Science of Medicine*, 44 (1997), 10: 1465–1482; Robert Truong, 'Is it time to abandon brain death?' *The Hastings Center Report*, 27 (1997), 1: 29–37; M. S. Pernick, 'Brain death in a cultural context: the reconstruction of death 1967–1981', in S. J. Youngner, R. M. Arnold and R. Schapiro (eds.), *The Definition of Death: Contemporary Controversies* (Baltimore: Johns Hopkins University Press, 1999), pp. 3–33; Eelco F. M. Wijdicks, 'The neurologist and Harvard criteria for death', *Neurology*, 61 (October 2003): 970–976; Leonard S. D. Baron, Jeannie Teitelbaum Shemie and Christopher James Doig, 'History, concept and controversies in the neurological determination of death', *Canadian Journal of Anesthesiology*, 53 (2006), 6: 602–608.

24. Margaret Hayden, 'No ambiguities in life and death' (30 May 2016), pp. 2–3, published online and accessed 25/9/2019 at: http://bioethics.hms.harvard.edu/sites/g/files/mcu336/f/Hayden_Beecher.pdf

25. *Defining Death*, p. 33.

26. Hayden, 'No ambiguities in life and death', pp. 2–3.

27. *NBC News*, 'Pulling the plug: ICU "culture" key to life or death decision', 21 May 2013, accessed 16/5/2017 at: http://vitals.nbcnews.com/_news/2013/05/21/18382297-pulling-the-plug-icu-culture-key-to-life-or-death-decision

28. Ibid. The registered nurse disguised their identity in a newsfeed blog as 'Flower in Bloom', response 16 to the news article.

29. Tim Adams, 'Sam Parnia – the man who could bring you back from the dead', Health section, *Observer*, 6 April 2013, p. 1.

30. See notably, George Steiner, *Grammars of Creation* (London & New York: Faber and Faber, 2001).

31. Professor Kwame Anthony Appiah, Chair of Philosophy and Law at New York University, Lecture 1, 'Creed', *Mistaken Identities*, BBC Reith Lectures (2016), at: www.bbc.co.uk/programmes/articles/2sM4D6LTTVlFZhbMpmfYmx6/kwame-anthony-appiah. See, also, Gillian Reynolds, 'How this year's Reith lecturer broke new ground', *Daily Telegraph*, 19 October 2016, p. 32, column 1.

32. Hurren, *Dissecting the Criminal Corpse*, especially chapter 2, pp. 33–68.

33. It has been claimed, erroneously, that medical death is a historical phenomenon that can be dated to the 1960s in, for instance, Helen MacDonald, 'Guarding the public interest: England's coroners and organ transplants, 1960–1975', *Journal of British Studies*, 54 (October 2015) 4: 926–946.

34. Tom Fielden, 'Brain research's golden age', Science Correspondent, *BBC News Magazine*, 22 June 2011, accessed 1/6/2017 at: http://www.bbc.co.uk/news/science-environment-13874585

35. The Brain Research Trust website, accessed 1/6/217 at: https://www.brt.org.uk/

36. Carl Zimmer, 'Brain science: secrets of the brain', *National Geographic*, February 2014, accessed 1/6/2017 at: http://ngm.nationalgeographic.com/2014/02 /brain/zimmer-text

37. See, Allen Brain Atlas Data Portal, accessed 1/6/2017 at: http://www.brain-map.org /overview/index.html

38. Hurren, *Dissecting the Criminal Corpse*, chapter 5, pp. 171–216.

39. Anders Eklund, Thomas E. Nichols and Hans Knutsson, 'Cluster failure: why fMRI inferences for spatial extent have inflated false-positive rates', *Journal of the Proceedings of the National Academy of Sciences of the United States of America*, 113 (12 July 2016) 28: 7900–7905.

40. Bruce Y. Lee, 'Could brain research from the past 15 years really be wrong?' *Forbes*, 6 July 2016, pp. 1–2, accessed 1/6/2017 at: https://www.forbes.com/sites/ brucelee/2016/07/06/could-brain-research-for-the-past-15-years-be-wrong /#347861622ed0

41. Ibid., p. 2.

42. Bec Crew, 'A bug in fMRI software could invalidate 15 years of brain research', *Science Alert* (6 July 2016), accessed 1/6/2017 at: http://www.sciencealert.com/a-bug-in-fmri-software-could-invalidate-decades-of-brain-research-scientists-discover

43. Ibid.

44. Wellcome Trust Library, GC/253, 'The history of Modern Biomedicine Research Group', publications prepared by C. Overy and E. M. Tansey (eds.), *The Development of Brain Banks in the UK c.1970 – c.2010, Wellcome Witnesses to Contemporary Medicine*, Volume 53 (London: Queen Mary University, 2015) – evidence by Professor Gavin Reynolds, pp. 19–20.

45. Wellcome Trust Library, GC/253 – evidence by Professor David Mann, p. 23.

46. Ibid., Mann, p. 24.

47. Wellcome Trust Library, GC/253 – evidence by Professor Margaret Esiri DM, Emeritus Professor of Neuropathology at Oxford University, p. 29.

48. Ibid.

49. The National Archives [hereafter TNA], *Isaacs Report*, 'The Cambridge Brain Bank', section 4, chapter 26, 'Recent analysis of brains collected by the bank', archived on behalf of the Department of Health, accessed 1/6/2017 at: http://webarchive.nationalarchives.gov.uk/+/www.dh.gov.uk/en/publicationsand statistics/publications/publicationspolicyandguidance/browsable/DH_4889626.

50. All quotations in respect of the Isaacs family case-history are taken from TNA, *Isaacs Report*, archived on behalf of the Department of Health, accessed 1/6/217 at: http://webarchive.nationalarchives.gov.uk/+/www.dh.gov.uk/en/publicationsand statistics/publications/publicationspolicyandguidance/browsable/DH_4889626

51. Ibid.

52. *Isaacs Report Response*, written by the Department of Health, Home Office and Department for Education and Skills (London: HMSO, 2003), p. 10 [ISBN 011322611X] – see also, www.doh.gov.uk/cmo/isaacsreport/response

53. A point argued convincingly, and reiterated throughout this book, by Marie-Andree Jacob, *Contemporary Ethnography: Matching Organs to Donors, Legalising and Kinship in Transplants* (Philadelphia: University of Pennsylvania Press, 2012), p. 8.

54. Sue Armstrong, *A Matter of Life and Death: Conversations with Pathologists* (Dundee: University of Dundee Press, 2008).
55. All quotations are on open access at the oral history digital community portal 'Conversations with pathologists', accessed 7/6/2016 at: https://www.pathsoc.org /conversations/.
56. Ibid.
57. 'Conversations with pathologists', accessed 7/6/2016.
58. Ibid.
59. 'Conversations with Pathologists', accessed 7/6/2016.
60. Portelli, 'The peculiarities of oral history', quote at pp. 99–100.
61. A point explored convincingly in Prue Vines, 'The sacred and the profane: the role of property concepts in disputes about post-mortem examination', *Sydney Law Review*, 29 (2007): 235–261. This also featured in our discussion in the Introduction, all chapters in Part II and will be revisited in Chapter 7, the conclusion, too.
62. Refer, The Royal College of Pathologists, accessed 7/6/2017 at: https://www .rcpath.org/
63. G. N. Rutty, B. Morgan, C. Robinson, et al., 'Diagnostic accuracy of post-mortem CT with targeted coronary angiography versus autopsy for coroner-requested post-mortem investigations: a prospective, masked, comparison study', *Lancet*, 390 (May 27, 2017), 10090: 145–154.
64. Nicola Davis, 'Digital autopsies should be standard for probable nature deaths, study says', *Guardian*, Health News section, Thursday, 25 May 2017, accessed 7/6/ 2017 at: https://www.theguardian.com/science/2017/may/25/digital-autopsies-should-be-standard-for-probable-natural-deaths-says-study
65. This author is grateful to all those pathologists who agreed to speak personally about their career experiences off the record. Many have since retired from the profession. Interviews were given on the basis of guaranteed anonymity in perpetuity because of public sensibilities.
66. '"*Hospital stored dead children's brains in jars*": Southampton Hospital under public scrutiny', BBC News, 16 February 2012 at: https://www.bbc.co.uk/news/uk-england-17959183
67. *Human Tissue Authority Report*, Pravat Battaacharyya, 'Police processes and the HTA', 18 March 2015, pp. 1–18.
68. Ibid.
69. *Human Tissue Authority Report*, pp. 1–18.
70. John Coles, 'They took the brains from our boys too – WHY?' *The Sun*, 14 January 2012, accessed 8/6/216 at: https://www.thesun.co.uk/archives/news/30 3995/they-took-the-brains-from-our-boys-too-why/
71. Ibid.
72. Coles, 'They took the brains'.
73. See, for example, Harriet Marsh, 'Organ scandal: parents' anger as authorities refuse to reveal numbers', *Bournemouth Daily Echo*, 26 January 2012, accessed 8/6/2017 at: http://www.bournemouthecho.co.uk/news/9494702.Organ _scandal__Parents__anger_as_authorities_refuse_to_reveal_numbers/
74. Portelli, 'The peculiarities of oral history', pp. 99–100.
75. Philip Cheung, *Public Trust in Medical Research? Ethics, Law and Accountability* (Oxford: Radcliffe Publishing Ltd, 2007), p. 138.

76. Ibid., p. 139.
77. Takashi Kitamura, Sachie K. Ogawa, Dheeraj S. Roy, et al., 'Engrams and circuits crucial for systems consolidation of a memory', *Science*, 356 (7 April 2017), 6333: 73–78.
78. BBC News, James Gallagher, Science Correspondent, 'Rules of Memory being *beautifully* rewritten', 7 April 2017, accessed 30/6/2017 at: http://www.bbc.co.uk/news/health-39518580
79. Kitamura et al., 'Engrams and circuits', pp. 73–78.
80. See, selectively, William Reddy, 'Against constructionism: the historical ethnography of emotions', *Current Anthropology*, 38 (1997): 327–351; Reddy, 'Emotional liberty: history and politics in the anthropology of emotions', *Cultural Anthropology*, 14 (1998): 256–288; Reddy, 'Sentimentalism and its erasure: the role of emotions in the era of the French Revolution', *Journal of Modern History*, 72 (2000): 109–152; Reddy, *The Navigation of Feeling*; Reddy, 'Historical Research on the Self and Emotions', *Emotion Review*, 1 (2009): 302–315.
81. See, Will Frampton, 'Hospital saved my life three times, so fundraising is my way of saying thank you – says Sean Luff', *Bournemouth Daily Echo*, 22 August 2013, accessed 7/6/2017 at: http://www.bournemouthecho.co.uk/news/10629093
82. Ibid.
83. Ian Burney, David A. Kirby and Neil Pemberton, 'Introducing "forensic cultures"', *Studies in History and Philosophy of Biological and Biomedical Sciences*, 44 (March 2013), 1: 1–3.
84. Ibid., p. 3.
85. Gallagher, 'Rules of memory'.
86. See, footnote 80 above.

Part III

Death Sentences Delayed

For death betimes is comfort, not dismay.

And who can rightly die, needs no delay [Petrarch]

7 Conclusion

Flesh Is a Dead Format? – Remapping the 'Human Atlas'

We began this book by asking a series of sensitive ethical questions about hidden histories of the dead of the sort that tended to be sidestepped or concealed from public view inside the British scientific community of the twentieth century. This new approach has not sought to detract from the many collective achievements of the medical sciences, which have been profound for us all as patients of more advanced healthcare systems in a global community. Rather, it is asking us to reflect on a historical context which has had many missing pieces of a complex medical humanities jigsaw. For the recycling of human research material was a subject that few people knew much about, and the management systems for which tended to be taken for granted. Often, they were opaque, hidden from public view. Even those working inside the system thought that older statutes covered their monitoring of medical ethics, but they did not. Few audit processes kept pace with the development of biotechnologies after WWII. As a result, body disputes started to highlight for public scrutiny discrepancies that had occurred inside NHS hospitals or involved even reputable UK research establishments. At first, these were judged exceptional, and then gradually there was a recognition in medical circles that some abuses and discrepancies were normal. This came about because one aspect of medical confidentiality involved the objectification of human research material. This created a bio-commons which had, and has, been necessary to push the boundaries of medical knowledge.

In the historical archives, a related missing human perspective is how exactly and for what research purposes bio-commons was disaggregated from the 1950s. The extent of the removal of personal identity from body and body part 'donations' likewise raised, and raises, questions of dignity in death. De-identifying human material may have fulfilled the medical obligation of discretion, but it equally left undocumented the nature of potential body disputes involving the public. There similarly seemed to be a lack of maintenance of humanisation inside modern research cultures. The degree to which we could remap actor networks and their research threshold points was thus an important historical endeavour since that missing information could reveal the logistical costs, timings and staffing resources that shaped the material realities of medical ethics in post-war Britain. Exploring these neglected histories of the dead has shown that the 'work of the dead' always matters to the living in some respect, especially for those that have benefitted from an extension of the deadlines of life after 1945.[1]

In the course of this book, ethicists and moral philosophers, sociologists, economists, transplant surgeons, hospice staff, experts in resuscitation medicine, neuroscientists and the public have each played a part in ongoing ethical debates about the need to adopt a 'custodial' rather than 'proprietorial' view of the body today.[2] This was played out against a transition from an older *ethics of conviction* (patriarchal medical experts, authoritarian and inward looking, prioritising their exclusive research agendas) to a new *ethics of responsibility* (reflecting much more medicine's impact on society as a whole, economically, culturally and politically). Whilst HTA2004 tried to bridge this ideological gap, it never resolved some fundamental differences of opinion. Historically, there is often a time lag between the passing of legislation and genuine cultural change. There thus remain considerable levels of scepticism amongst some professional experts about whether or not to open up and share medical science's inner working practices with everybody. That debate is healthy and reflects that science has a curiosity-driven and enquiring nature, but it also highlights how for too long there has been a cultural gap between the working practices of science (open, enquiring, debating and disputing to disprove hypotheses) and the ways in which it has interacted with ordinary patients and their relatives (denying body disputes; controlling information flows; being evasive, furtive and paternalistic, as well as often caring but overprotective). At a time when precision medicine is just around the next historical corner, the medical sciences are facing some fundamental ethical choices because of the legacy of hidden histories of the dead. They need to embrace a world in which DNA coding will democratise how we see and interact with a newly visible self. At this research frontier, the old death sentences of the past are being delayed and we stand on the threshold of new scientific eternities that challenge our historical imaginations and patient-practitioner working relationships.

Henceforth with each new biomedical step we take, close monitoring of our medical ethics is going to be very necessary; otherwise, we could find that we arrive at new healthcare solutions but are ill informed about their human costs because we neglected perspectives of hidden histories of the dead. Such ethical questions matter because the bedrock of our medical philosophy is public support. Often science has neglected how much this is in a constant cultural process of negotiation and re-negotiation, as we are seeing in the media with the current pandemic, Covid-19. Social media too is a force for change, but it would be a mistake to think that its public engagement reach was triggered by recent technological development alone. In many respects, scientific reticence about clandestine medical research cultures after WWII created the preconditions for more vocal and visible patient-led perspectives to start to reshape public opinion from the 1960s in Britain, and beyond its shores. The substantial data employed in this volume has allowed us to explore existing historiographical agendas, and to set new ones. Thus, a recent case in the Family Division of the High Court in London personifies the medical possibilities that have been created, as well as the potential body disputes that do still arise as we continue to remap the human atlas.

Remapping the 'Human Atlas'

In 1972, the Alcor Life Extension Foundation (hereafter ALCOR) founded a new not-for-profit nanotechnology venture in the USA. It promised to explore the medico-scientific potential of cryonics research, hoping that a future technology known as transhumanism (patients integrated with machines) would have the facility to revive human material frozen with nitrogen. In many respects, ALCOR was a logical development of the transplantation era, copying the technique of freezing 'solid' organs and human eggs for future use. ALCOR today stresses that 'it is not an interment or mortuary practice'. It maintains that medical death is a more liminal state than conventional medicine currently understands.[3] Thus, it seeks to preserve the brain 'as soon as possible after legal death' so as to 'prevent the loss of information within the brain that encodes memory and personal identity, which is the true boundary between life and death'. The ALCOR staff stress that: 'cryonics is an extension of critical medical care ... if cryonics patients are preserved well enough ... they might *someday* [sic] be resuscitated ... then they aren't dead: they are cryopreserved'. In 2015, the promise of this biotechnology to push the boundaries of life and death attracted the attention of a British teenage girl dying of cancer. She thought it offered her the promise of a scientific eternity – part of the legacy of hidden histories of the body – stimulating new conversations in the scientific community today.

'JS' (her name was anonymised to disguise her identity in the press) thus applied to the Family Division of the High Court in London to be cryopreserved. In a letter to the adjudicating Judge, she wrote:

> *I have been asked to explain why I want this unusual thing done.*
> *I am only 14 years old and I don't want to die, but know I am going to die.*
> *I think that being cyro-preserved gives me a chance to be cured and woken*
>   *up – even in hundreds of years' time.*
> *I don't want to be buried underground.*
> *I want to live longer and I think that in the future they may find a cure for my*
>   *cancer and wake me up.*
> *I want to have this chance.*
> *This is my wish [sic].*[4]

The judge was concerned that the case 'did give rise to serious legal and ethical questions for hospitals'. However, he exceptionally agreed to the dying request. On 17 October 2016, JS went into hospital for the final time in London. Her post-mortem wishes were respected, but not without controversy. JS became simultaneously an implicit, explicit and missed body dispute.

JS believed in a medical technology that was implied and unproven. She placed her secular faith in the promise of a medical scientific eternity – that there would be a future cure for her cancer. Her resuscitated brain, she thought, would survive medical death by cryopreservation, until humans and machines could function together to maintain life. Yet media commentators and family members questioned whether this reasoning was ethical and rational or simply science fiction. What was implied may not be deliverable: a potential implicit dispute sometime in the future. Her estranged father did not agree with his teenage daughter's decision, generating an explicit body dispute. Although JS's parents had separated acrimoniously in 2002 when she was aged 6, and there had been no contact with her biological father since 2007, he still felt responsible for the unverified medical procedure she wanted.[5] In the absence of a robust scientific study, he thought that his daughter 'had been "brainwashed" into thinking she could cheat death'.[6] Meanwhile, JS's mother and grandparents became involved in a missed dispute. In court, they supported the teenager's request to be frozen. The grandparents paid ALCOR a fee of '£37,000'. Yet, as events soon proved, the mishandling of her body attracted widespread negative publicity and revealed the close family's misunderstanding of what was about to happen next.

Cryonics UK clashed with the medical team on site, due to concerns about a lack of dignity in death. The cryopreservation personnel appeared to be 'under-equipped and disorganised' after an ambulance, due to collect JS's body, broke down and was replaced by a volunteer's van.[7] Procedures were hasty and haphazard, and had to be moved to a hospital morgue where there was a 'rush to replace JS's blood with anti-freeze to cool her body to – 70°C'.[8] Disquiet amongst doctors and the mortuary staff resulted in a case referral to the Human Tissue Authority (who were in fact powerless to act retrospectively). JS's mother's focus had been to carry out her daughter's dying wishes, but the procedures she was promised, and those the court had consented to, were questionable. According to a detailed report in the *Daily Telegraph*, 'a cousin' of the child's mother admitted 'there had also been misgivings on that side [maternal] of the family' about what had taken place and family members would have objected had they known what was about to happen.[9] This missed dispute resulted in JS's body being 'stored upside down in a vat of liquid nitrogen at –196°C ... a week after her death, her body, packed in dry ice, [was] flown to Michigan in the US' for safe storage with '100 other "patients" awaiting revival' in the Cryonic Institute in

Detroit.[10] What everyone involved in the case would now do was to query the inside story of JS's deadline of life and the biomedical promise of scientific eternity.

Matthew Parris, writing in *The Times* on 19 November 2016, queried 'JS's sad case'. As he put it: 'Snap-freezing yourself into immortality is surely a medical dead-end?'[11] He did not doubt that in the future a cure for many types of cancers would be made by biomedicine, but that did not excuse sidestepping the really big ethical questions facing us now – 'When does "life" in any meaningful sense, end? When should it? How much room is there on our planet for contemporaneous human lives – and could we – should society – reach a shared understanding about the limits?' What the JS case had shown was that life expectancy has 'a sliding scale' – many people can be in a situation of a living death – what if this young girl were to wake up in 200 years or so and find she is only '*partly* alive'? If her brain was not damaged, then she would in theory lead a '*useful* [sic] life'. But if semi-damaged, she could be condemned to a life-support machine. What would her quality of life be when adjusting to such a different concept of a normal life that might be beyond her powers of comprehension as a human being? As Yuval Noah Harari puts it: 'Trans-humanism seeks to upgrade the human mind and give us access to unknown experiences and unfamiliar states of consciousness.' As a global community we need, however, to think a lot more carefully about how 'revamping the human mind is a complex and dangerous undertaking'.[12] It is possible, he points out, that: 'We may successfully upgrade our bodies and our brains, while losing our minds in the process.'[13] For, this legacy of hidden histories of the body of the modern era is not far-fetched. It has very recently led us in new mind-altering research directions that moral philosophers in the 1950s warned could happen.

The Royal Society in September 2019 issued a press release to the BBC warning of the future dangers of technologies with the facility to brain hack. Their spokesperson explained: 'Devices that merge machines with the human brain need to be investigated . . . gadgets, either implanted in the body or worn externally, that stimulate activity in either the brain or nervous system' are groundbreaking, but they raise serious ethical issues too.[14] Whilst spinal cord stimulators, cochlear ear implants, electrodes planted into patients with paralysis, deep brain electrical stimulus of those with Parkinson's disease, artificial pancreases, wireless heart monitors and so on are promising innovations, equally there are three 'future possibilities of neural technology' that require more ethical monitoring:

- the ability to beam a 'neural postcard' to someone so they could see what you see even if they are not there
- people being able to converse without speaking through access to each other's thoughts
- people being able to simply download new skills[15]

Keeping the peace in this brave new world of biotechnology and AI robotics might necessarily involve 'the narrow interests of governments, armies and corporations' creating the need to downgrade humans to better control their transhuman revolution.[16] As Dr Tim Constandinou, Director of the Next Generation Neural Interfaces (NGNI) laboratory at Imperial College London and co-chair of the recent Royal Society–sponsored report, warned:

By 2040 neural interfaces are likely to be an established option to enable people to walk after paralysis and tackle treatment-resistant depression, they may even have made treating Alzheimer's disease a reality. While advances like seamless brain-to-computer communication seem a much more distant possibility, we should act now to ensure our ethical and regulatory safeguards are flexible enough for any future development. In this way we can guarantee these emerging technologies are implemented safely and for the benefit of humanity.[17]

The fine line between far thinking and being far-fetched really depends on where you sit in the cryopreservation pool of public opinion. Yet, anatomists have always known that: 'The brain – the mind – is the manifestation of the liminal spaces into which doctors' plunge. It is 'where personhood resides, of ourselves and our loved ones' and we should, therefore, go gently in a Genome era.[18]

Dissection teaches us that in all centuries, 'anatomy takes a nasty turn once we go above the neck – not only does the information increase in detail like crazy (the skull is amazing in its intricacy – seemingly endless numbers of holes, indentations, seams, processes)' but 'the force necessary' to know more can 'feel barbarous' too – something that we also saw in Chapters 3 and 6. As one medical student conceded recently – 'I am still fascinated by what is revealed' in brain dissections 'but hate the push and tug necessary for revelation'.[19] It is a sentiment at the heart of the JS case and one awaiting us around the next historical corner. Professor George Santayana thus observed that we would remain 'infantile' in our medical ethics if we did not resolve the paternalism of the past together, forever 'condemned to repeat mistakes'.[20] If, then, JS embodies the key research themes of this book (implicit, explicit and missed disputes), and highlights how these research thresholds are not necessarily sequential but can in fact happen in combination too, what challenges await us and how might we confront them?

Remapping and Remodelling the Dead-End of Life

There are first numerous hidden histories of the dead-end of life. Broadly speaking, the New Poor Law helped to establish medical education's research base in the late-Victorian period. This publicity-shy anatomical teaching and research culture carried forward into the 1930s economic depression. After wartime, it emerged under the new NHS as public healthcare was reorganised in 1948. Thereafter, it flourished in the fast-moving climate of medical enterprise during the 1950s. There was consequently a privileging of certain research cultures to cement professional status and secure grant funding from successive central governments of all political persuasions. This created the context for a burgeoning bureaucracy that was confusing and convoluted, and authorised the ambitious in their chosen career paths to 'go around the law *while* going through the legal processes'. This, as the ethnographer Marie Andree Jacob puts it, 'is how legality is experienced' in modern medical research cultures.[21] This material fact in hidden histories of the body also came about because of medical science's insistence on the 'global' over the 'local'. As Jacob explains, bio-commons acted as a buffer to proper public accountability. The task of the historian is to 'privilege the microscope over the telescope': to trace actor networks and their research threshold points in body and body part disputes, which were the central focus of Part II.[22] Chapters 4–6 have thus demonstrated the historical research reach of quantitative and qualitative research methods. Figure 7.1 is therefore a template applicable to all such studies in the future, whether on a national or international basis. It illustrates the multilayered material pathways that facilitated research networks and those threshold points that the dead passed through as bodies were broken up in a complex but secretive chain of supply mechanisms. This raises important ethical questions because it provides an opportunity to engage with a more personalised history of the body at the end of life and to consider how historical longevity might still be shaping our world today. We have glimpsed part of this

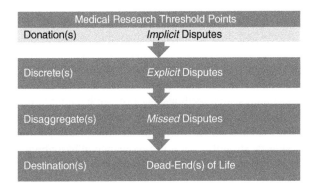

Figure 7.1 New paradigm of medical research threshold points in Britain, c. 1945–2015 (author designed)
Source: Author designed from core themes embedded in Part II (refer also, Figure 1.1).

medical mosaic of progress, but we need to know much more since it is the foundational story of biomedical research now and in the near future.

Until we can remap in their entirety the human atlas and its research components, we will never know just how much modern medical research became a breakers-yard business of the body. Nor will it be feasible in biomedicine to identify why some medical breakthroughs within actor networks were deemed profitable for public healthcare, and others not. What we still do not know is what healthcare interventions were missed or mislaid because the system of accountability was so secretive (due either to carelessness or because those involved were caring but over-cautious). We also cannot tell what funding decisions were taken for political reasons. Nobody can therefore say for certain whether crucial medical information may still be awaiting our rediscovery. How sad it would be if human beings had suffered more in the meantime from painful conditions. As Donna Dickenson highlights, it remains all too common that a patient consents to bequest their human tissue, but then discovers it is recycled for someone's career or commercial gain. Too often, it is still very difficult to define the sharing of knowledge or profits generated.[23] In other words, as Dickenson emphasises: 'Researchers, biotechnology companies and funding bodies certainly don't think the gift relationship is irrelevant: they do their very best to promote donors' belief in it, although it is a one-way gift-relationship.'[24] That is the real ethical danger of consignments at the dead-end of life.

To name the dead still matters and remains an important endeavour of medical ethics. It is necessary to be dispassionate about medical research, but equally the medical humanities need the balancing mechanism of human stories that test whether progress has ethical probity. Although these are concepts under constant negotiation in popular culture, they require everyone in society to stay engaged. In the immediate post-war world, the opposite happened. Science's self-defence position was that to name bio-commons was an impossible task. Certainly, it was logistically difficult and complex, but not unachievable. It would be more historically accurate to say that the balance of the evidence in this book points to the medical sciences seldom trying to humanise its research methods. As a research community, those that staffed systems had little idea of whether it was an insurmountable task or not, since so few checked its feasibility in the first place. The evidence in Parts I and II suggests, strongly, that it is a fundamental basic human impulse that material afterlives merit an acknowledgement of some description, one embodying the ethics of the 'gift relationship'.[25] Tracking human material has considerable merit today. For the future, giving it a named post-mortem passport and making it part of a transcript of forthcoming transplant treatments would more transparently connect the 'gift' to new healing cultures. Too few medical research studies did this in the post-war biomedical community. It is strictly speaking legally correct that they were not expected to do so at that time.[26] Yet, that status quo does not excuse those who made conscious choices to be evasive and not engage with the changing world around them at the time. For the NHS is state financed, but much medical research remains embedded in private-sector funding contexts with investment targets to meet. Given that context, it was, and is, reasonable of the general public to suppose that just as medicine has embraced new scientific breakthroughs on the basis that these would benefit humankind, equally it should have devoted as much energy, money and time to being forward thinking in its research ethics too.

Medical Elisions

Contemporary critics of the medical sciences argue persuasively that what we are currently living through is a data explosion of personal information. It is becoming available in multiple online formats and requires responsive medical ethics as well as constant vigilance.[27] This book's second major finding, however, presents a much more multilayered historical picture than this. Medical science has been all about positioning itself centre stage as a profession in Western society. It tells us that we must 'follow the science' and trust in its data collection methods that help us all to make better healthcare decisions. But there is often little public discussion about the sheer amount of data collection this requires, how confusing and complex its results can be, and the ways in which scientists often disagree with each other concerning their findings and modelling of disease patterns: cultural trends we are witnessing during the Covid-19 pandemic. An added complication has been that the data the general public thought was the basis of our collective decision-making in medical ethics has been insubstantial and therefore akin to standing on scientific quicksand. Chapters 4–6 have shown that bureaucracy was used to hide what was really going on with personal data and patient case records. Typically, this happened by filling in a general form to pass a body from hospital ward to mortuary attendant – then to coroner and their pathologist – before putting a brake on that bureaucracy to elongate the time spent with the corpse for teaching and research purposes. In this way, official death certification often did not happen for up to two months after medical death. In the meantime, in law the dead did not exist. They were technically '*abandoned*' and therefore their bereaved relatives could not have traced them, even if they had known what was really happening inside the system of so-called bequests. The symbolic cases of the dead war-hero in Chapter 1, a deceased young child in Chapter 4 and the sad demise of Mr Isaacs in Chapter 6 show this very well. Medical science has therefore been all about creating what this book has identified as the extra time of the dead, and this has been the basis of what some critics are now calling the 'Data Religion' of our biomedical world.[28]

The new evidence presented establishes that medical science is a major time player in Western society. Often its significant medical breakthroughs have been presented in the media as edited highlights – as the 'chosen moment' of a success story. This use of elision may have had a narrative efficiency in science and far-reaching medical benefits, but it also relied on there being many hidden histories of the dead in medical research and considerable public ignorance. A lot of medical information that was being collected was partially disclosed, often destroyed and certainly de-commissioned (involving many sorts of valuable research archives), without thinking through future timescales or potential ethical lessons. It is one of the reasons that patient groups and their online medical communities exist in such proliferation today; its storytellers have been sceptical about the use of medical elision in the recent past. Balancing such views, scientists are complex actors in their own right; they are shaped by cultural, political, economic and administrative circumstances. Yet, as this book has shown, they do not stand outside narratives of popular culture.

On a case-by-case basis – and there were some 10,000 cases reconstructed for this book – what one often engages with is the material fact that: 'Dataism adopts a strictly functional approach to humanity, appraising the value of human experience according to their functioning in data-processing mechanisms.'[29] As commentators like Harari point out: 'If we develop an algorithm that fulfils the same function better, human experiences will lose their value.' This is not as far-fetched as it might seem. In Chapter 2, we encountered the current concerns of the Royal Society of Medicine (hereafter RSM) membership, which reflected in 2016 on 'the good, the bad and the ugly' of HTA2004.[30] They have foreseen a major ethical issue around dead human bodies disaggregated into bio-property. International patent law currently protects the medical sciences against litigation in the civil court for claims of a share of profits generated from re-engineering in biotechnology (altruistic, financial, patent or otherwise). Even so, as a keynote spokesperson, Hugh Whittall, Director of the Nuffield Council on Bioethics, said to the RSM: 'The long-term challenge is the issue of tissue banking.' What happens to 'the huge amount of data . . . once you put it through any kind of biochemical or genetic analysis'?[31] HTA2004 is not set up to monitor this, and once an algorithm has turned it into a data pattern there is no statute that can protect what happens next on the super-connective internet highway. Thus, critics like Harari highlight how: 'Dataism undermines our main source of authority and meaning, and heralds a tremendous religious revolution, the like of which has not been seen since the eighteenth century.'[32]

The findings of this book suggest that 'dataism' certainly has the potential to 'sideline humans'. Taking a longer trajectory, we can see that from 1752 to 1832 (phase 1) the body was studied as a reflection of the divine. From the 1790s that 'old anatomy' (the study of creation) gave way gradually to 'new anatomy', the study of the science of the body. From 1832 to 1929 (phase 2) Christian beliefs continued to dominate in dissection spaces – what historians call deo-centric, namely, God-centred belief systems. Nonetheless, from the 1930s to 1945 (phase 3) with the shift to more secular values in society, a homo-centric emphasis gained cultural ascendancy. Between 1945 and 2000 (phase 4) popular culture embraced the moral value of medical ethics and distanced itself from the religious tenets of the past. Finally, there was another noteworthy shift again around the time of HTA2004 when the deo-centric and homo-centric tipped in favour of a data-centric world. We did not, however, necessarily take forward the historical lessons from body phases 1–4, because until now they have been undocumented. This complex phased-in process is illustrated in Figure 7.2.[33]

Looking to the near future, DNA coders and systems biologists disagree fundamentally over what all the current genetic data generated really tells us about the basis of human existence. We are mapping the proteins of life at a 'selfish-gene' level, but individuals do not function in bits and pieces. As Denis Noble, the eminent systems biologist, explains, 'the logic of life' is to integrate, collaborate and work together to co-create what we often call the quality of life. That individual genes can undermine this living process is not disputed, but there is a holistic aspect to 'the systems-level [organs, for instance] interactions of proteins'. In other words:

We have become transfixed by the great success in explaining sequences in terms of encoded DNA sequences. This is a great achievement, one of the most important successes of twenty-first-century biology. But we sometimes seem to have forgotten that the original question in genetics was not what makes a protein, but rather what 'makes a dog a dog, a man [woman], a man [woman]'. It is the phenotype that stands in need of explanation. It is not just a soup of proteins [sic].[34]

Many hidden histories of the dead came about because anatomists, coroners and pathologists lost sight of their data. It was dispersed along all sorts of complex research pathways and the more it was distributed, the more difficult it became to keep track of the bigger picture of science. Historically, the evidence base confirms it became a breakers-yard business. The relatively recent recognition that brain death is very complex is a timely warning that 'the self' has been broken down too much in the past: after all, neuroscience has learned that only a *whole* person can function cognitively as a human being with a reasonable quality of life. Ironically, in embracing genomics, there is the very real possibility that we will repeat the same medical error of breaking the

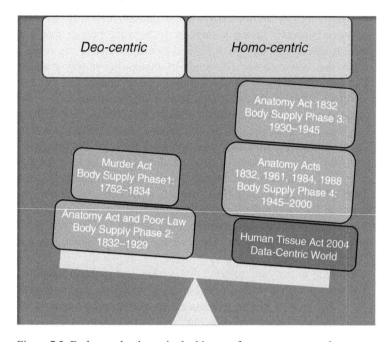

Figure 7.2 Body supply phases in the history of anatomy – mapped onto changing cultural concepts of the body modelled by Yuval Noah Harari
Sources: Harari, *Homo Deus: A Brief History of Tomorrow*, p. 388, a trend verified in three books by this author: E. T. Hurren, *Dissecting the Criminal Corpse: Staging Post-Execution Punishment in Early Modern England* (Basingstoke: Palgrave Macmillan, 2016) covering the 1752 to 1834 period, *Dying for Victorian Medicine: English Anatomy and Its Trade in the Dead Poor, c. 1834–1929* (Basingstoke: Palgrave Macmillan, 2012) and this book detailing the 1945 to 2000 era.

holistic circle that has peopled so many research threshold points in the post-war era. It is difficult not to arrive at the conclusion that we might need to unlearn what we think we knew because we only ever collected such a partial view of this past medical history. In the future, this acknowledgement could involve standing back and asking what sort of medical mosaic we let the medical sciences create for us in the first place.[35]

When Is Medical Death?

Humanity is in a mess – it has always been in a material mess and, thankfully, it will always be so until our last breath. Because we are such a muddle inside, we

stay alive – being cleaned up, constantly excreting things surplus to requirements, forever shedding and spilling, dripping and squeezing, shaving and
purging ourselves. Learning about this in a history of anatomy has revealed
that defining medical death has been a significant medical conundrum. Today it
is still common to read in the historical literature that brain death was redefined
by medical science in 1968 at Harvard University.[36] Yet, in Britain, anatomists
re-defined medical death under the Murder Act of 1752. They discovered the
possibility of reviving bodies in the winter cold after deliveries of the 'dangerous dead' to the dissection theatre from the public gallows. In a previous book
by this author, it was established that brain death is a scientific realisation that
can be dated to 1812 and it applied to one quarter of those executed for
homicide that survived the hangman's rope in England from 1752 to 1834.[37]
This book has built upon the foundation stone of that finding by identifying just
how much this central dilemma in modern medicine was often hidden from
public view. Because so much was secretive in the past, it is remains difficult to
take the long view of brain death. Essentially, what happened is that by 1945,
there had developed a 'mind the gap' in medical ethics. It can be located to the
working definitions of *peri-mortem* (at or close to the point of death) and *post-
mortem* (being in death). The assumption was that a liminal space resulted from
the advancement of new technologies, with the ability to monitor even the
faintest traces of life, and indeed better machinery did play a significant part in
this historical process. Yet, it would be a mistake to presume that it was
a specifically twentieth-century phenomenon.

It was the remarkable recent research of Professor Sam Parnia into near-
death experiences that has questioned the tradition of calling medical death at
a twenty-minute mark in emergency rooms in the USA.[38] And it is
a perspective today that surgeons who once received bodies from the gallows
in Georgian England would have recognised. They had to make pro-life
choices or break the Hippocratic Oath and commit human vivisection. In
turn, because we did not share death's dilemmas transparently as a Western
society, we have neglected to engage with, and improve how we die. Medicine
often employs euphemism to avoid speaking about the subject of death because
doctors are powerless to stop it at some time in all our lives – '*They have passed
on*' – '*S/he is no longer with us*' – '*Your relative has gone before their time*' –
gone where – passed on, to whom – whose timing do you mean? Because
medicine handled the dying so clumsily, what happened to the dead followed
suit. Intensive Care Units (ICUs) became in many respects the locations where
the medical ethics of the living and the dead were developed but not necessarily
with a transparent discussion about quality of life debates or material afterlives
being created, as we have seen throughout Parts I and II. Moreover, researching
this sensitive research area reveals that ICU cultures do differ between countries:
a factor that the Covid-19 pandemic throws daily into sharp relief. This matters

because we need to better appreciate whether what happened to the dead *post-mortem* was shaped by what was happening to the dying at the end of life when *peri-mortem*.

Public Policy and Engagement

In rediscovering archival material, we have encountered why neglected material realities in the recent past matter today and can stimulate new debates to better inform future public policy directions and their potential public engagement. We have seen that the data generated by anatomy departments in England from 1954 to 2000 shows that women have been the main source of body bequests since WWII. Neglecting this material fact has public policy ramifications when it comes to improving organ donation rates in Britain.[39] Public health campaigns to increase organ donation have tended to target young people since the 1980s. The assumption has been that teenagers and those in their 20s are more forward looking than their parents and grandparents. Indeed, NHS2020 strategy to increase organ donation rates is designed to get the whole family involved so that medical science can 'increase family consent rates to 80% by 2020'.[40] In the midst of the pandemic, however, the NHS2020 impact on these figures has yet to be calculated. Nonetheless, to get to an 80 per cent level, the NHS2020 team concedes that there will have to be a major cultural change in British society. Young people, it is predicated, will need to talk in advance to their families and set out their dying wishes verbally and in print. The problem with this public engagement approach is twofold: first, few young people think to talk about death, and second, they seldom talk about something so unpalatable or write down their dying wishes. Most people need to be prompted to do so by someone close to them whom they respect and love enough to converse with. Historically, mothers and grandmothers tend to be the chief source of communication in families. That being the case, why is the NHS2020 strategy not working more closely with women – the sort of females who are good at getting loved ones talking and who have been so prepared to body bequest in the recent past? When we neglect hidden histories, it can have very real consequences for a patient on a long waiting list desperate for an organ transplant. It is time to work with the demographic realities of the female principle of gifting presented in this book.

The generic issue of compulsory organ donation likewise raises another important public engagement point that we have explored throughout Parts I and II. This book has argued that medical paternalism has been defined for too long by 'proprietorial' rather than 'custodial' property rights over the dead body.[41] And in the most recent debates in 2017 around the need to introduce an opt-out of organ donation system in England, we see this out-of-date language emerge again. The law change means all adults are considered to have agreed to be an organ donor when they die unless they have recorded a decision not to donate or are in an excluded group. Yet, however needed the scheme, what this new policy reflects is how medicine tends to revert to its traditional default position when confronted with an undersupply of human material; it simply presses government to reintroduce past practices. This brings us to an important question – how does medicine advance, resolve long waiting lists for transplantation and balance the rights of all patients to respect their cultural and religious viewpoints? One of the implications of the work done for this book is the urgent need for a National Ethics Trust in Britain.[42] Patients self-evidently want more say in medical treatment. They also need ethical safety-nets, especially as they approach the most difficult end-of-life decisions. The solution is a National Ethics Trust – a medical safety-*NET* for the near future. It has to be an organisation patients can trust to give their research profiles to – to help others to resolve pandemics on our behalf but also to help them make the most difficult decisions.[43] If a *NET* were established, patients could decide to donate in life their health profiles to it. To secure public trust, it needs to be set up independent of government, politicians and the medical lobby. Just then as a patient can donate their body in death, why do we not as a society provide a mechanism for everyone to bequest their health profile whilst living?

Medical researchers could apply to a *NET* for access to NHS profiles, provided they in return use post-mortem passports and advertise future treatments detailing how many *NET* donors helped to make a medical breakthrough. There would be a list of those living bequests made public on an annual basis. Imagine being treated on the NHS and reading down the details of those that helped you to heal. That would be a very powerful 'custodial' expression of medical ethics for everybody. If a *NET* had existed in the recent high-profile cases of the young children Charlie Gard and Alfie Evans, in both of which there were legal challenges to the withdrawal of life support, then there would have been no need for the parents involved to crowdfund on the Internet due to a lack of legal aid, seek a public debate on social media or clash with doctors in court over medical evidence.[44] An independent *NET* with the powers to call on relevant expertise could have been their impartial advocate. The *NET* could have consulted with medical ethicists, doctors and lawyers, as appropriate, to help each family make difficult end-of-life choices for their dying children. Although Charlie Gard's parents have succeeded in getting a private members bill called Charlie's Law passed in Parliament to set up a better medical advocacy scheme outside the law courts, there is no reason why this type of advocacy role could not be extended to everybody via a *NET* initiative.[45] It would demonstrate that medical science has shifted culturally from an *ethics of conviction* to an *ethics of responsibility* – of international importance for everyone.

Pollution

Stop what you are reading – take a deep breath – pause for a moment – and think about just how lucky you are that your lungs filled up with air that was of good quality. Often life expectancy is about biological luck, but it is also about pollution levels where you live and work. The data generated over this author's career on anatomy supply-lines now forms a research base that stretches from 1752 to 2000. One remarkable new finding is that no matter where those dissected and sent for medical research lived and died in Britain in the past 265 years, the majority all died from lung complaints (broadly defined). Such complaints (historically and in the present) have multiple causations. Thus, from 1752 to 1930, they were associated in the records used for this book (and two others that have preceded it) with substandard housing conditions, coal smog in cities and polluted river systems cleaned up by public health schemes laid down by the Victorian Information State. After WWII, central government nonetheless recognised that pollution in various forms was a growing cause of lung diseases and thus an urgent healthcare priority was to pass a series of Clean Air Acts, notably in 1952. Yet, instead of pollution diminishing as a major cause of death, one urban healthcare problem replaced another. Coal fires gave way to car smog. Consequently, asthma levels remained high and blighted major cities in the UK. They still do. At the same time, the cover-up story of pathology meant that coroners' death certificates that should have been a treasure trove of epidemiological information had illegible handwriting. Most were filed and forgotten. There were also ongoing discrepancies in the design of the official death certification scheme in England and Wales. It has continually prioritised proximate cause of death and understated underlying co-morbidity complications: as Chapters 4 and 6 set in their proper historical context. This has been an enormous wasted opportunity for public health at the dead-end of life.

In January 2017 the leading journal *Science* reported that a prominent feature of modern biomedicine is 'The Polluted Brain'.[46] Globally there is a strong case to be made that car pollution may be one of the biggest factors in the growth of Alzheimer's disease. As its lead article writer explained: 'Some of the health risks of inhaling fine and ultrafine particles are well-established, such as asthma, lung cancer, and, most recently, heart disease. But a growing body of evidence suggests that exposure can also harm the brain, accelerating cognitive aging, and may even increase risk of Alzheimer's disease and other forms of dementia.' Although this is a young field of biomedical research, nevertheless there appear to be worrying epidemiological trends associated with greater car pollution levels in community medicine globally.[47]

One persistent problem often highlighted is a lack of historical, comparable, reliable data generated in the UK and Europe. The *Guardian* newspaper thus led with a startling headline in January 2017 that '1 in 10' people tracked from '6.6 million' participants who lived near traffic and its heavy road congestion appeared to be at a higher risk of dementia.[48] More robust research was called for on 'the impact of air pollution on public health'. In many respects, however, as this book has shown, the solution to this knowledge gap has been an obvious one. Multi-user data-sets from contemporary anatomy records assembled specifically for the chapters in Part II fill in the demography picture. Those who appear in dissection records prior to 1954 died below the threshold of relative to absolute poverty. This means that we can say with confidence that they contain important medical information of lives lived amidst the worst extremes of pollution. Combining those with modern record sets after 1955 when the Clean Air Act came into force then balances that historical picture by showing that even when fresh water supplies, better nutritional standards and free medical care under the NHS started to redress perennial Victorian social problems, pollution levels never abated. The automobile may yet prove conclusively to be the biggest cause of degenerate brain diseases, provided we stop losing sight of the importance of hidden histories of the dead and their long-term health profiles. Sometimes, in filling our lungs with air, it is the thing we cannot see that can make the biggest contribution to humanity.

A Historical Lesson for the Near Future

All books have their critics and this one will be no exception, but in concluding there is one final point to be made that unifies the human condition. If there is a central, undeviating narrative thread that runs throughout this research, it is that in not a single case study that has been examined, covering over half a million archive entries, has this author ever discovered an anatomist that did not respect the human capacity for dignity and love at the dead-end of life. Even what little was left after dissection was buried or cremated, eventually, with moral respect and full religious rites in Britain. There were no shortcuts, though there was ample reason to do so in a history of the marginalised and forgotten. It is a remarkable historical finding – perhaps the most notable of all in hidden histories of the dead, which we neglect at our peril. It is also a keen reminder of the old Tuscan saying that once inspired Leonardo da Vinci to quest for a knowledge that was more complete. Like all anatomists, he searched for the secret of the creation of life in the womb, dissecting at night to discover the beauty and wonder of our capacity for anatomical awe and embodied revelation. Even so, da Vinci never lost sight of the homespun wisdom of his Italian birthplace, where the old women that were midwives whispered to each new mother, *'There is not love, only proof of love'*.[49] It is a moral philosophy, which in so many respects has gone on shaping human experience everywhere for everybody. It also happens to be the basis of all religious beliefs, every secular creed, as well as the entire history of medical ethics that stretches from ancient Greece to the present day.

For everyone wants to be loved completely in their lifetime. It might be the hand of a doctor that stretches out when we are ill, the smile of a nurse that comforts us in pain or the person close to us who hugs us to the end. The essence of oral histories and their histories of emotion – whether penned before or during a pandemic that has alerted us all to the power of medical events to take over our lives – continue to express words worth repeating at this finish-line that were first penned by Hippocrates – '*Wherever the Art of Medicine is loved, there is also a love for Humanity*'.[50] In the medical humanities, empathy is seldom '*proof of love*' until compassion is exchanged between two people. For this reason this book did not dissect stories of those dissected, offering the reader just a short summary; instead, it reassembled them with their emotional subtexts and material contributions because both perspectives are together intrinsic to the sort of narrative medicine that features in improved medical education today. If we meanwhile commercialise the Human Genome, then patients' voices, motivated by this most basic and most important of human impulses, will step in and take back control from medicine. We underestimate, to our collective cost, the capacity for compassion and healing that one human being can feel for another. Precision medicine promises much but it cannot co-create in cultural isolation – this is our historical lesson for the near future too. The beauty of medicine at the bedside is a two-way conversation, and one valued by all of humanity. And because on this there is universal agreement in a global community, we therefore approach the inside stories of our scientific eternity on this historical horizon with perhaps the greatest challenge of all in biomedicine. Namely, never to put aside or dismiss offhand the undeviating central narrative of medicine that '*what will survive of us is love*', because in a history of anatomy it has always done so and there is thankfully every expectation that it will go on doing so.[51]

Notes

1. Thomas Laqueur, *The Work of the Dead: A Cultural History of Mortal Remains* (Princeton: Princeton University Press, 2015).
2. Prue Vines, 'The sacred and the profane: the role of property concepts in disputes about post-mortem examination', *Sydney Law Review*, 29 (2007): 235–261.
3. See, ALCOR website, accessed 22/8/2017 at: http://www.alcor.org/
4. Josh White, Colin Fernandez and Ben Wilkinson, 'British cancer girl, 14, frozen – in hope she'll be brought back from dead', *Daily Mail*, Friday, 18 November 2016, p. 5.
5. Lexi Finnigan and Gordon Rayner, 'Frozen girl's father: "I wasn't allowed to say goodbye"', *Daily Telegraph*, News section, Saturday, 10 November 2016, p. 8.
6. 'Sorrow of girl's father in cryogenic case', *Daily Telegraph*, Front page feature, 20 November 2016, p. 1.

7. See, criticisms raised in: 'The ambulance was kaput so her body went in the back of my van', *Sunday Times*, News section, 20 November 2016, pp. 8–9; 'Father tells of his grief over cryonic girl's death', *Times*, 19 November 2016, p. 10; 'Desperate for another chance at life', *Daily Telegraph*, 19 November 2016, pp. 23–24.

8. 'Frozen and flown to US by a bunch of amateurs', *Daily Mail*, News Review and Features section, Saturday, 19 November 2016, p. 8.

9. 'Frozen girl's father: I wasn't allowed to say goodbye', *Daily Telegraph*, News section, 19 November 2016, p. 8 and column, 'How it might work – the theory of cryogenics', p. 8.

10. As reported in David Brown, Chief News Correspondent, 'Judge backs dying child's bid to have body frozen: cancer victim, 14, preserved after legal first', *Times*, Front page feature, Friday, 18 November 2016, p. 1.

11. Matthew Parris, 'Sometimes it's wrong to choose life over death', *Times*, Comment section, Saturday, 19 November 2016, p. 25.

12. Yuval Noah Harari, *Homo Deus: A Brief History of Tomorrow* (London: Harvill Secker, 2016), p. 353.

13. Ibid., p. 363.

14. Jane Wakefield, Technology reporter, 'Brain hack devices must be scrutinised, says top scientists', BBC News, 10 September 2019, p. 1, accessed 11/9/2019 at: https://www.bbc.co.uk/news/technology-49606027

15. Ibid.

16. Harari, *Homo Deus*, p. 364.

17. Wakefield, 'Brain hack devices must be scrutinised', p. 1.

18. A point made in Christine Montross, *Body of Work: Meditations on Mortality from the Human Anatomy Lab* (New York: Penguin Press, 2007), p. 255.

19. Ibid.

20. George Santayana, *Winds of Doctrine: Studies in Contemporary Opinion* (New York & London: Scribner's & Dent, 1913), p. 199.

21. Marie-Andree Jacob, *Contemporary Ethnography: Matching Organs to Donors, Legalising and Kinship in Transplants* (Philadelphia: University of Pennsylvania Press, 2012), p. 8.

22. Ibid., p. 10.

23. Donna Dickenson, *Body Shopping: The Economy Fuelled by Flesh and Blood* (Oxford: One World Books, 2008), pp. 42–43.

24. Ibid., p. 43.

25. Rowan Williams, 'Thinking Anglicans: Easter sermon', Canterbury Cathedral, 11 April 2004, accessed 17/01/2017 at: http://www.thinkinganglicans.org.uk/archives/000556.html

26. See, for instance, this standard defence in, Duncan Wilson, *The Making of Bioethics* (Manchester: Manchester University Press, 2014).

27. Refer, notably, Harari, *Homo Deus*, pp. 367–397.

28. Ibid.

29. Harari, *Homo Deus*, p. 388.

30. See, Royal Society of Medicine, 'The Human Tissue Act 12 years on, the good, the bad and the ugly', Pathology section, 23 June 2016, accessed 11/9/2019 at: https://www.rsm.ac.uk/events/ptg03.

31. Ann McGauran, World Report section, 'Regulation of human tissue in the UK', *Lancet*, 388 (17–23 September 2016), 10050: e-4–e-5.
32. Harari, *Homo Deus*, p. 388.
33. Ibid., p. 388.
34. Denis Noble, *The Music of Life: Biology Beyond Genes* (Oxford: Oxford University Press, 2006), p. 17.
35. Themes in, Haider Warraich, *Modern Death: How Medicine Changed the End of Life* (London: Duckworth Overlook, 2017).
36. There is a vast literature on this topic – see, for example, a useful summary of basic misinformation in, David Hamilton, *A History of Organ Transplantation: Ancient Legends to Modern Practice* (Pittsburgh: University of Pittsburgh Press, 2012). A recent example of 'historical facts' being stated incorrectly without being verified with extensive record linkage work in the archives can be found in Helen MacDonald, 'Crossing the rubicon: death in the "Year of the Transplant"', *Medical History*, 6 (2017) 1: 107–127.
37. E. T. Hurren, *Dissecting the Criminal Corpse: Staging Post-Execution Punishment in Early Modern England* (Basingstoke: Palgrave Macmillan, 2016), figures in chapter 5.
38. Refer notably, Sam Parnia with Josh Young, *Erasing Death: The Science That Is Rewriting the Boundaries between Life and Death* (New York & London: HarperOne Books, 2013) and Sam Parnia, *What Happens When We Die?* (Carlsbad, Calif. & London: Hay House, 2005).
39. See, for instance, Sir Liam Donaldson interviewed by the *Daily Telegraph* on 17 July 2007 – 'Organ donation must be automatic', Health News, p. 1; and British Medical Association, 'Organ donation – soft opt-out option', 28 February 2017, accessed 30/8/2017 at: https://www.bma.org.uk/collective-voice/policy-and-research/ethics/organ-donation
40. 'A strategy for delivering a revolution in public behaviour in relation to organ donation', prepared by 23red for NHS Blood & Transplant, pp. 1–63, available as a PDF, accessed 6/12/2016 at: https://nhsbtdbe.blob.core.windows.net/umbraco-assets-corp/4254/nhsbt_organ_donation_public_behaviour_change_strategy-2.pdf
41. A point explored convincingly in, Prue Vines, 'The sacred and the profane', pp. 235–261.
42. A national bioethical trust was proposed in Britain in the 1960s. It was dropped as a public policy by the 1990s. This was because it was too closely associated with a partnership with the British Medical Association. Patients' groups distrusted the medical profession to act impartially in medical research. The proposal in this book is therefore a very different conceptual one. Regarding previous policy failures, refer, Wilson, *The Making of Bioethics*, chapter 6, p. 220.
43. George Steiner, *Grammars of Creation* (New Haven: Yale University Press; London & New York, Faber and Faber, 2001), preface.
44. See, for instance, 'Charlie Gard and Alfie Evans legal fees cost NHS £400K', BBC Radio Manchester, 25 April 2018, at: https://www.bbc.co.uk/news/uk-england-merseyside-45855029
45. 'Charlie Gard's parents: new law will help others avoid "court hell"', BBC News, 6 February 2020, at: https://www.bbc.co.uk/news/av/uk-51403395/charlie-gard-s-parents-new-law-will-help-others-avoid-court-hell

46. Emily Underwood, 'The polluted brain: evidence builds that dirty air causes Alzheimer's disease', *Science*, Lead article, 26 January 2017, p. 2.
47. Ibid., p. 3.
48. Hannah Devlin, Science Correspondent, 'Living near heavy traffic increases risk of dementia, says scientists', *Guardian*, Health section, 5 January 2017, p. 1.
49. I am grateful to Robin Sellick for making me the gift of *Leonardo's Collected Works* in his will in 2016 from which this quotation is taken. I hope this final paragraph is a tribute to the trust he placed in me before his death.
50. Elizabeth. T. Hurren, *Dying for Victorian Medicine: English Anatomy and Its Trade in the Dead Poor, c. 1834–1929* (Basingstoke: Palgrave Macmillan, 2012), chapter 7, for a discussion of the importance of this central aspect of Hippocrates' writings.
51. See, 'Christopher Hitchens – last public appearance with Richard Dawkins', at the 2011 Free Thought Convention Texas, accessed 11/8/2018 at: https://www.youtube.com/watch?v=B06tiTwAuvg

Bibliography

Primary Sources

Journals and Newspapers

American Journal of Nursing
Barts and the London Chronicle
BBC Listener
Bournemouth Daily Echo
British Medical Journal
Daily Mail
Daily Telegraph
Esquire Magazine
Evening Standard
Financial Times Weekend Magazine
Forbes
Global Affairs
Guardian
Household Words
Independent on Sunday
Lancet
Leicester Mercury
Live Science
London Review of Books
Los Angeles Times
Manchester Evening News
National Geographic
Nature
New Scientist
New York Times
Observer
Punch
Science
Science Alert
Stoke Sentinel
Sun
Sunday Times

Sutton and Croydon Guardian
The Sentinel
Times
Vanity Fair
Vogue
Washington Post
Woman's Herald
Women's Penny Paper

Articles and Books (pre-1900)

Carroll, Lewis *Alice in Wonderland* (London: Macmillan, 1877)
Dickens, Charles *Little Dorrit* (London: Bradbury and Evans Publisher, 1857)
Editorial, 'Various & lemon feature, Mark [Editor] facts for foreigners', *Punch, or the London Charivari*, XXXVIII (18 February 1860), p. 71
Hook, Theodore Edward, *Maxwell: A Novel* (London: R. Betley & Co, 1834)

Ancestry

'Mr Herbert Thomas Jones', '£7, 241 14 s[hillings] to his widow', 15 February 1963 at Winchester Probate Division, National Probate Calendar (1963), Index of Wills and Administration, p. 159

British Parliamentary Papers and Hansard

Hansard, HC, vol. 753, cc. 334W, 6 November 1967
A complete PDF copy of *British Parliamentary Papers, Coroners (Amendment) Act* (16 & 17 Geo. 5 c. 59: 1926), was consulted on 20/10/2016 and can be accessed online at: www.legislation.gov.uk/ukpga/1926/59/pdfs/ukpga_19260059_en.pdf
Hansard, HC, vol. 980. cols. 488-491, 5 March 1980, 'Human Organs (Anonymity of Donors)', brought forward by Mr. John Farr, Rt. Hon. Member for the Market Harborough division
Hansard, HC, Volume 416, column 995, 2.31pm speech, 15 January 2004, 'Sir Mark Wolpert (and others), evidence on behalf of the Royal College of Surgeons and Wellcome Trust to the House of Commons reading on the Human Tissue Bill' – with evidence by Mr Andrew Landsley (Conservative Member of Parliament, South Cambridgeshire), accessed 17/01/17 at: www.publications.parliament.uk/pa/c m200304/cmhansrd/vo040115/debtext/40115–16.htm
Statement by HHJ Peter Thornton QC, Chief Coroner for England and Wales, on 'Reforming the Inquest' to the All-Party Penal Affairs Parliamentary Group held on 5th November 2013 at the House of Commons, Minutes reported verbatim by the Prison Reform Trust website, accessed 4/4/2017 at: www.prisonreformtrust.org.uk/ PressPolicy/Parliament/AllPartyParliamentaryPenalAffairsGroup/ Nov2013ReformingtheCoronerService

Cambridge University Library

University Archives collection, Anatomy Department Records, ANAT, 1/4 – 1955–1999
ANAT 2/3 – 2 volumes, 1959–1073, 1972–3, Accounts of the Department of Anatomy
Papers relating to the rare book collection of West Suffolk Hospital Trust transferred from the Anatomy Department Library to the University Library in 1999

High Court of Justice (Family Division) London [Courts & Tribunals Judiciary]

Case No: FD17P00103, Neutral Citation Number: [2017] EWHC 1909 (Fam.), *In the High Court of Justice Family Division, before The Honourable Mr Justice Francis between Great Ormond Street Hospital [Applicant] and (1) Constance Yates (2) Christopher Gard (3) Charlie Gard (by his Guardian) [Respondents], Hearing dates 10, 13, 14, 21 and 24 July 2017,* Approved Judgement dated 24 July 2017. Counsel in the case being, Ms K Gollop QC (instructed by GOSH Legal services) for the Applicant, Mr G Armstrong and Mr G Rothschild (instructed by Harris da Silva Solicitors) for the Respondents, and Ms. V. Butler-Cole (instructed by CAFCASS) for the *Guardian*
Case No: FD16P00526 [2016] EWHC 2859 (Fam.), 10 November 2016, *The Honourable Mr Justice Peter Jackson between 'JS' applicant versus 'M' 1st Respondent and 'F' 2nd Respondent [parents of 'JS']* Counsel in the case being, Frances Judd QC & Dr Rob George (instructed by Dawson Cornwell) for the Applicant, Stephen Crispin (instructed by Bindmans) for the 1st Respondent, Helen Khan (instructed by Kilic and Kilic Solicitors) for the 2nd Respondent, William Tyler QC & Kate Tomkins (instructed by CAFCASS Legal) as Advocate to the Court, Christina Helden (Hempsons Solicitors) for the Hospital Trust – Hearing dates: 26 September, 4 October, 6 October 2016 Judgment date: 10 November 2016 – JUDGMENT: Re JS (Disposal of Body) – Reporting Restrictions applied to the Case in perpetuity

London Metropolitan Archives

Health & Coronial records, Harperbury Hospital, 1930–1960
Civil Registration Death Index, 1 December 1952 for St. Albans Hertfordshire
Electoral Registers for Harrow North West Ward 1945–1965
Kelly's Directory for Hertfordshire and St. Albans (1937)

National Health Service

'A strategy for delivering a revolution in public behaviour in relation to organ donation', prepared by 23red for NHS Blood & Transplant, pp. 1–63, accessed 6/12/2016 at: https://

nhsbtdbe.blob.core.windows.net/umbraco-assets-corp/4254/nhsbt_organ_donation_pu
blic_behaviour_change_strategy-2.pdf

National Portrait Gallery

Bauhaus Photographic Collection, 'Ellen Maurice (Nelly) Heath' available at: www
.npg.org.uk/collections/search/portraitLarge/mw185159/Ellen-Maurice-Nellie-Heath)

Northwestern University Library, USA

Garnett Family Papers, acquired by Northwestern University Library, USA in 2008,
and deposited in the Charles Deering McCormick Library of Special Collections with
an online catalogue at: http://findingaids.library.northwestern.edu/catalog/inu-ead-
spec-archon-1489

Nuffield Trust

Nuffield Trust Official Report on Human Tissue: Ethical and Legal Issues, 'Ethical
Principles: Respect for Human Lives and Human Bodies', produced by Bioethics
Division; to download a PDF copy, see, https://www.nuffieldbioethics.org/publica
tions/human-tissue

Royal Court of Justice

Royal Court of Justice, Queen's Bench Division, Lord Justice Leggatt and Mr Justice
Nicol, [2018] EWHC 1955 (Admin), Case No: CO/367/2018

Royal Institute of British Architects

©Royal Institute of British Architects Archive, 'Photographic Image of St. Bartholomew's
Medical School, lecture room of the anatomy department, used in the modern era'

Royal London Hospital Records

GB 0387 PP/KNU, Holland, Sydney, 2nd Viscount Knutsford (1855–1931)
PP/KNU/1 – Speeches and notes, 1897–1931
PP/KNU/2 – Correspondence, 1898–1929
PP/KNU/3 – Publications, 1910–1925
PP/KNU/5 – Photographs, [c. 1904]–1931
PP/KNU/6 – Miscellaneous Items, 1897–[c. 1931]

Royal Society of Medicine

Royal Society of Medicine, 'The Human Tissue Act 12 years on, the good, the bad and the ugly', Pathology section, 23 June 2016, at: www.rsm.ac.uk/events/ptg03

St Bartholomew's Hospital Archives

© St Bartholomew's Hospital Archives, Photographic Collection, 'Dissection Room, 1915', reproduced under (CC BY-NC-SA, 4.0), authorised for open access, and non-profit making for academic purposes only
St Bartholomew's Hospital Dissection registers MS81/5–81/6 (1930–1965)

Staffordshire Local History Archives

Memorial Inscriptions Freehay Staffordshire, St. Chad's Churchyard, Grave 0.60, 'Graham Alcock, Accidentally Killed, 12 December 1983, Aged 28, Husband of Jean and Father of Tracey and Joanne'

The National Archives

The National Census, 1911
The Ministry of Health Circular (No. 7/54), July 1954
Home Office, and Memorandum CRN/84 28/29/1, dated 19 February 1987, and annotated in pencil CC5/3/53, issued by R. B. Snow, HM Coroner, central London, as a newsletter to regional HM Coronial offices
HO375, Committee on Death Certification and Coroners (Broderick Committee) minutes and papers, 1964–71
JA 3/1, HM Anatomy Inspectorate Returns on Dissections, 1992–1998
Lucre Report (2003), HMSO, CM 5831, 'Death Certification and Investigation in England, Wales and Northern Ireland: The Report of a Fundamental Review' pp. 1–361, accessed 16/03/2017 at: http://webarchive.nationalarchives.gov.uk/2013120 5100653/http:/www.archive2.official-documents.co.uk/document/cm58/5831/5831 .pdf
Isaacs Report (2003), accessed 24/10/2016 at: http://image.guardian.co.uk/sys-files/S ociety/documents/2003/05/12/isaacs_report.pdf
Isaacs Report (2003), 'The Cambridge Brain Bank', section 4, chapter 26, 'Recent analysis of brains collected by the bank', archived on behalf of the Department of Health, accessed 1/6/2017 at: http://webarchive .nationalarchives.gov.uk/+/www.dh.gov.uk/en/publicationsandstatistics/publica tions/publicationspolicyandguidance/browsable/DH_4889626
Isaacs Report Response, written by the Department of Health, Home Office and Department for Education and Skills (London: HMSO, 2003), p. 10 [ISBN 011322611X] – see also, www.doh.gov.uk/cmo/isaacsreport/response

The Redfern Inquiry (16 November 2008), by Right Hon. Chris Huhne MP, Secretary of State for Energy & Climate Change, accessed 24/10/2016 at: http://webarchive .nationalarchives.gov.uk/20101214091701/http://www.theredferninquiry.co.uk/

Ministry of Justice: Draft Charter for the Bereaved Who Came into Contact with a Reformed Coroner System TSO (London: HM Stationary Office, 2008)

Human Tissue Authority Report, Pravat Battaacharyya, 'Police processes and the HTA', 18 March 2015, pp. 1–18

Coroners Statistics Annual 2015 England and Wales Ministry of Justice Statistics Bulletin (London: HMSO, Stationary Office, 12 May 2016)

United States, State Department Archives

Drug use and mental well-being in US states (2015–16) reports: at www.samhsa.gov/ – annual reports available on open access online

US State Department, President's Commission for the Study of Ethical Problems in Medicine and Biomedical and Behavioural Research, *Defining Death: A Report on the Medical, Legal and Ethical Issues in the Deteremination of Death* (Washington, D.C.: US Government Printing Office, 1981)

Wellcome Collection

Wellcome blog, 'Paris Morgue', 1 June 2015, accessed 18/01/2017 at: https://wellcomecollection.org/articles/paris-morgue/

©Wellcome Image, L0014980, 'Photograph of Newcastle Dissection room 1897', by J. B. Walters reproduced under (CC BY-NC-SA, 4.0), authorised for open access, and non-profit making for academic purposes only

©Wellcome Images, Reference Number V0010903, *A Juror Protesting that the subject of the Coroner's Inquest is alive; showing the dangers of blind faith in doctors when declaring medical death* – Coloured aquatint by Thomas McLean, 26 The Haymarket, London, c. 1826

©Wellcome Images, Reference Number L0062513, Watercolour drawing done by Leonard Portal Mark on 7 July 1894, depicting the face and chest of a man (unnamed) to show the appearance caused by rapid post-mortem decomposition. Sketched about twelve hours after death, during the hot weather of July 1894 at St Bartholomew's Hospital dissection room

©Wellcome Images, Reference Number L0029414, 'Royal Liverpool University Hospital: a pathologist cutting open a body in the mortuary', original drawing on site by Julia Midgley, Liverpool 1998, artwork dimensions 42 x 29.7cm

Wellcome Trust Library

Research Defence Society papers, 1908–1931

GC/253, 'The history of Modern Biomedicine Research Group', publications prepared by C. Overy and E. M. Tansey (eds.), *The Development of Brain Banks in the UK c.1970–c.2010, Wellcome Witnesses to Contemporary Medicine*, Volume 53 (London: Queen Mary University, 2015) – evidence by Professor Gavin Reynolds, pp. 19–20 – evidence by Professor David Mann, p. 23 – evidence by Professor Margaret Esiri DM, p. 29

Web – Primary Sources

Alcor Life Extension Foundation [ALCOR], accessed 22/8/2017 at: www.alcor.org/

Alfred, Lord Tennyson, 'Ulysses' (1833), see, his collection of papers and writing in the Hallam bequest, Trinity College, Cambridge, now located at Cambridge University library, accessed January 2019 at: https://cudl.lib.cam.ac.uk/collections/tennyson/1

Allen Brain Atlas Data Portal, accessed 1/6/2017 at: www.brain-map.org/overview/index.html

BBC Archive Collection, *Tomorrow's World Special*, 'Barnard faces his critics', televised 2 February 1968, 22/02/2017 at: www.bbc.co.uk/archive/tomorrows world/8006.shtml

BBC News Magazine, 22 June 2011, Tom Fielden, 'Brain research's golden age', Science Correspondent, accessed 1/6/2017 at: www.bbc.co.uk/news/science-environment-13874585

BBC News report, 8 February 2005, 'The impact of cancer diaries', by Jane Elliott, Health Reporter, accessed 11/0/2019 at: http://news.bbc.co.uk/1/hi/health/4243257.stm

BBC News report, 17 July 2007, 'Everyone should donate organs', accessed 24/10/2016 at: http://news.bbc.co.uk/1/hi/health/6902519.stm

BBC News report, 21 May 2012, 'Almost 500 body parts kept by police', accessed 4/4/2017 at: www.bbc.co.uk/news/uk-england-18122332

BBC News report, 22 February 2013, 'Children's body parts were kept by police', accessed 7/6/2017 at: www.bbc.co.uk/news/uk-england-bristol-21521872

BBC News report, 2 July 2013, 'Organ donation opt-out system given go-ahead in Wales', accessed 21/10/2016 at: www.bbc.co.uk/news/uk-wales-politics-23143236

BBC News report, 1 August 2016, 'Cancer: Thousands surviving in the UK decades after diagnosis', accessed 2/8/2016 at: www.bbc.co.uk/news/health-36925974

BBC News report, 2 December 2016, 'The fog-catcher', accessed 3/12/2016 at: www.bbc.co.uk/news/magazine-38175202

BBC News report, 15 February 2017, 'Air pollution "final warning" from the European Commission to the UK', accessed 20/02/2017 at: www.bbc.co.uk/news/uk-politics-38980510

BBC News report, 15 March 2017, 'John Culshaw: mum's anger over son's organs stored in police lab', accessed 4/4/2017 at: www.bbc.co.uk/news/uk-england-manchester-39274707

BBC News report, 7 April 2017, James Gallagher, Science Correspondent, 'Rules of Memory being *beautifully* rewritten', accessed 30/6/2017 at: www.bbc.co.uk/news/health-39518580

BBC News report, 27 July, 2017, 'The Charlie Gard case: the story of his parents' legal fight', accessed 22/8/2017 at: www.bbc.co.uk/news/health-40554462

BBC News report, 28 April 2018, 'Alfie Evans case reported on BBC News', accessed 29/8/2019 at: www.bbc.co.uk/news/uk-england-merseyside-43754949

BBC News report, 14 October 2018, 'Charlie Gard and Alfie Evans legal fees cost the NHS £400,000', accessed 11/9/2019 at: www.bbc.co.uk/news/uk-england-merseyside-45855029

BBC News report, 20 July 2019, 'NHS waste backlog: what are the rules on disposal?', accessed 24/7/2019 at: www.bbc.co.uk/news/health-45760576

BBC News report, 10 September 2019, 'Brain hack devices must be scrutinised, says top scientists', Jane Wakefield Technology reporter, accessed 11/9/2019 at: www.bbc.co.uk/news/technology-49606027

BBC News report, 6 February 2020, 'Charlie Gard's parents: new law will help others avoid "court hell"', accessed 7/2/2020 at: www.bbc.co.uk/news/av/uk-51403395/charlie-gard-s-parents-new-law-will-help-others-avoid-court-hell

BBC News report, 1 April 2020, 'Coronavirus: GP apology over 'do not resuscitate order', accessed 1/4/2020 at: www.bbc.co.uk/news/uk-wales-52117814

BBC Reith Lectures (2016), Professor Kwame Anthony Appiah, Chair of Philosophy and Law at New York University, *Mistaken Identities*, Lecture 1, 'Creed', accessed 20/11/2017 at: www.bbc.co.uk/programmes/articles/2sM4D6LTTVlFZhbMpmfYmx6/kwame-anthony-appiah

The Brain Research Trust website, accessed 1/6/217 at: www.brt.org.uk/

'Christopher Hitchens – last public appearance with Richard Dawkins', at the 2011 Free Thought Convention Texas, accessed 11/8/2018 at: www.youtube.com/watch?v=B06tiTwAuvg

Crew, Bec, 'A bug in fMRI software could invalidate 15 years of brain research', *Science Alert* (6 July 2016), accessed 1/6/2017 at: www.sciencealert.com/a-bug-in-fmri-software-could-invalidate-decades-of-brain-research-scientists-discover

Crown Prosecution Service, public information website, 'Coroners and their legal responsibilities', accessed 18/01/2017 at: www.cps.gov.uk/legal/a_to_c/coroners/

Douglas, Heather E., 'The moral responsibilities of scientists: tensions between autonomy and responsibility', *The American Philosophical Quarterly* (5 December 2012), accessed 13/10/2016 at: www.academia.edu/987446/The_moral_responsibilities_of_scientists_tensions_between_autonomy_and_responsibility

'The Hart Island Project', accessed 9/2/2017 at: www.hartisland.net/

Harvard Ad Hoc Committee on Brain Death, Resources for Researchers website, accessed 16/5/2017 at: http://euthanasia.procon.org/sourcefiles/Harvard_ad_hoc_brain_death.pdf

Hayden, Margaret, 'No ambiguities in life and death' (30 May 2016), pp. 2–3, accessed 25/8/2019 at: http://bioethics.hms.harvard.edu/sites/g/files/mcu336/f/Hayden_Beecher.pdf

Henig, Robin Marantz, 'Crossing over: how science is redefining life and death', *National Geographic*, April 2016, pp. 30–41

Hertfordshire and Middlesex Hospital Health authorities wartime schemes, accessed 15/11/2016 at: www.hertfordshire-genealogy.co.uk/data/topics/t070-long-stay-hospitals.htm

Human Tissue Act website, accessed 2/11/2016 at: www.hta.gov.uk/policies/human-tissue-act-2004

Hurren, E. T., 'Patients' rights: from Alder Hey to the Nuremberg Code', *History and Policy* (6 May 2002), accessed 3/11/2016 at: http://health-equity.pitt.edu/4042/1/pol icy-paper-03.html

Lee, Bruce Y., 'Could brain research from the past 15 years really be wrong?' *Forbes*, 6 July 2016, pp. 1–2, accessed 1/6/2017 at: www.forbes.com/sites/brucelee/2016/07/ 06/could-brain-research-for-the-past-15-years-be-wrong/#347861622ed0

Leicester Medical School, Body Donation Programme, Public Information Sources, accessed 10/1/2017 at: https://cms.le.ac.uk//medicine/about/body-donation-programme

Leicester University Medical Centre, ©University of Leicester – accessed 10/1/2017 at: https://www2.le.ac.uk/departments/medicine/resources-for-staff/clinical-teaching/i mages/students-in-dissecting-room/view, authorised for open access, and non-profit making, reproduced under (CC BY-NC-SA, 4.0), for academic purposes only

Lopez, Barry. US children's author, accessed 13/6/2017 at: www.barrylopez.com

'Lost Hospitals of London', accessed 6/12/2016 at: http://ezitis.myzen.co.uk/banstead .html

NBC News, 21 May 2013, 'Pulling the plug: ICU "culture" key to life or death decision', accessed 16/5/2017 at: http://vitals.nbcnews.com/_news/2013/05/21/18382297-pulling-the-plug-icu-culture-key-to-life-or-death-decision

NCEPOD 2006 Report (www.ncepod.ork.uk), pp. 1–176, accessed 26/6/2016 at: www .ncepod.org.uk/2006Report/Downloads/Coronial%20Autopsy%20Report%202006.pdf

Oral history digital community portal, 'Conversations with pathologists', accessed 7/6/ 2016 at: www.pathsoc.org/conversations

Papworth Hospital, 'Papworth heroes', public engagement webpages, 'Terence English', accessed 21/02/2017 at: www.papworthhospital.nhs.uk/papworthher oes/papworth-hero.php?hero=9

Parnia, Sam Research Group, accessed 24/9/2019 at: https://medicine .stonybrookmedicine.edu/medicine/sleep/resuscitation

Parnia, Sam, 'We'll soon be able to bring the dead back to life – Dr Sam Parnia', *Daily Mail*, 30 July 2013, accessed 3/8/2016 at: www.dailymail.co.uk/health/article-2381 442/Dr-Sam-Parnia-claims-corpses-soon-revived-24-hours-death.html

Parnia, Sam, University of Southampton, 'Results of world's largest Near-Death Experiences study: interview with Dr Sam Parnia', *Research Bulletin*, 7 October 2014, accessed 7/4/2017 at: www.southampton.ac.uk/news/2014/10/07-worlds-largest-near-death-experiences-study.page

The Pituitary Foundation, range of conditions and current treatments available online, accessed 25/9/2017 at: www.pituitary.org.uk/information/what-is-the-pituitary-gland

Rettner, Rachel, 'Cancer spreads from organ donor to 4 people in "extraordinary" case', *Live Science*, 15 September 2018, accessed 5/8/2019 at: www.livescience.com/635 96-organ-donation-transmitted-breast-cancer.html

The Royal College of Pathologists, accessed 7/6/2017 at: www.rcpath.org/

St. Joseph's Hospice: Our History, accessed 26/6/2016 at: www.stjh.org.uk/about-us/o ur-history

Social Care Institute for Excellence, 'Mental Capacity Act [MCA], Deprivation of Liberty Safeguards [DofL]', accessed 22/2/2017 at: www.scie.org.uk/publications/a taglance/ataglance43.asp

Society for Critical Care Medicine, accessed 30/11/2019 at: www.sccm.org/Communi cations/Critical-Care-Studies – critical care statistics in the US, 2000–2010

US Library of Medicine, Medline Information Resource, 'Pituitary disorders', accessed online 20/10/2016 at: https://medlineplus.gov/pituitarydisorders.html

Williams, Rowan, 'Thinking Anglicans: Easter sermon', Canterbury Cathedral, 11 April 2004, accessed 17/01/2017 at: www.thinkinganglicans.org.uk/archives/000 556.html

World Medical Association, Declaration of Helsinki, 'Ethical principles for medical research involving human subjects', *Journal of the American Medical Association*, 20 (27 November 2013), 10: 2191–2194, accessed 21/10/2016 at: DOI: 10.1001/ jama.2013.281053

Zimmer, Carl, 'Brain science: secrets of the brain', *National Geographic*, February 2014, accessed 1/6/2017 at: http://ngm.nationalgeographic.com/2014/02/b rain/zimmer-text

Secondary Sources

Alberti, Fay Bound, *Matters of the Heart: History, Medicine and Emotion* (Oxford: Oxford University Press, 2010)

Annema, C., S. Op den Dries, A. P. van den Berg, A. V. Rachor and R. J. Porte, 'Opinions of Dutch liver transplant recipients on anonymity of organ donation and direct contact with donors' families', *Transplantation Journal*, 99 (April 2015), 4: 879–894

[Anon], 'A definition of irreversible coma: report of the Ad Hoc Committee of the Harvard Medical School to examine the definition of brain death', *Journal of the American Medical Association* (1968) 205: 337–403

[Anon], 'Diagnosis of brain death. Statement issued by the honorary secretary of the Conference of Medical Royal Colleges and their faculties in the United Kingdom on 11 October 1976', *British Medical Journal* (1976), 13: 1187–1188

Anon [Editorial], 'Landmark article' by the *Journal of the American Medical Association*, 252 (3 August 1984), 5: 677–679

Anyanwu, Emeka G., Emmanuel N. Obikili and Augustine U. Agu, 'The dissection room experience: a factor in the choice of organ and whole body donation – a Nigerian survey', *Anatomical Sciences Education*, 7 (2014), 1: 56

Armstrong, Sue, *A Matter of Life and Death: Conversations with Pathologists* (Dundee: University of Dundee Press, 2008)

Azuri, P., and N. Tabak, 'The transplant team's role with regard to establishing contact between organ recipient and the family of a cadaver organ donor', *Journal of Clinical Nursing*, 21 (March 2012), 5–6: 888–896

Baron, Leonard S. D., Jeannie Teitelbaum Shemie and Christopher James Doig, 'History, concept and controversies in the neurological determination of death', *Canadian Journal of Anesthesiology*, 53 (2006), 6: 602–608

Bates, Victoria, 'Yesterday's doctors: the human aspects of medical education in Britain. 1957–1993', *Medical History*, 61 (2017), 1: 48–65

Bell, Michelle L., Davis L. Devra and Tony Fletcher, 'A retrospective assessment of mortality from the London smog episode of 1952: the role of influenza and pollution', *Environmental Health Perspectives*, 112 (January 2004), 1: 6

Belkin, George S., 'Moving beyond bioethics: history and the search for medical humanism', *Perspectives in Biology and Medicine*, 47 (2004), 3: 372–385

Blond, Antony, *Jew Made in England* (London: Timewell Press, 2004)

Boardman, A. P., A. H. Grimbaldeston, C. Handley, P. W Jones and S. Wimlott, 'The North Staffordshire Suicide Study: a case control of suicide in one health district', *Psychological Medicine*, 29 (January 1999), 1: 27–33

Borges, Jorge Luis, *The Aleph and Other Stories* (New York and London: Penguin Classic Books, 2004 edition, first published in 1949)

Boruch, Marianne, *Cadaver, Speak* (Port Townsend, Wash.: Copper Canyon Press, 2014)

Brandon, Sydney (Department of Psychiatry, Leicester Royal Infirmary), Letters to the Editor, *British Medical Journal*, 289 (1 September 1984): 558

Brazier, M. 'Organ retention and return: problems of consent – symposium on consent and confidentiality', *Journal of Medical Ethics*, 29 (2003): 30–33

Brennan, Michael (ed.), *Theorising the Popular* (Newcastle-up-Tyne: Cambridge Scholars Press, 2017)

Brimblecombe, P., 'The Clean Air Act after 50 years', *Weather*, 61 (2006), 11: 311–314

Brown, Kevin, *Harperbury Hospital from Colony to Closure, 1928–2001* (Hertfordshire: Harper House Publications, 2001)

Brown, Michael, 'Book review section', *History*, 98 (2013), 330: 302–304

Bruce, Robert, 'The laundry foetus; disposal of human remains, the Anatomy Act 1984 and the Human Tissue Act 2004', *Journal of Forensic and Legal Medicine*, 17 (2010): 229–231

Buklijas, Tatjana, 'Cultures of death and the politics of corpse supply: anatomy in Vienna, 1848–1914', *Bulletin of the History of Medicine*, 83 (2008), 3: 570–607

Burney, Ian, *Bodies of Evidence: Medicine and the Politics of the English Inquest 1830–1926* (Baltimore: John Hopkins Press, 2000)

Burney, Ian, David A. Kirby and Neil Pemberton, 'Introducing "forensic cultures"', *Studies in History and Philosophy of Biological and Biomedical Sciences*, 44 (March 2013), 1: 1–3

Burney, Ian, and Neil Pemberton, *Murder and the Making of the English CSI* (Baltimore: John Hopkins Press, 2016)

Burton, Antoinette and Tony Ballantyne, *World Histories from Below: Disruption and Dissent, 1750s to the Present* (London: Bloomsbury Academic Publishing, 2016)

Burton, Julian L. and Guy N. Rutty (eds.), *The Hospital Autopsy: A Manual of Fundamental Autopsy Practice*, 3rd ed. (London: Hodder Arnold, 2001)

Bynum, William and Linda Kalof (eds.), *A Cultural History of the Body: Volumes 1–6* (London: Bloomsbury, 2010)

Callon, Michel, John Law and Arn Rip, *Mapping the Dynamics of Science and Technology: Sociology of Science in the Real World* (Basingstoke: Macmillan, 1986)

Caplin, Arthur L., James J. McCartney and Daniel P. Reid, *Replacement Parts: The Ethics of Procuring and Replacing Organs in Humans* (Washington, D.C.: Georgetown University Press, 2015)

Carney, Scott, *The Red Market: On the Trail of the World's Organ Brokers, Bone Thieves, Blood Farmers, and Child Traffickers* (New York: William Morrow, 2011)

Carr, E. H., *What Is History?* (Cambridge: Cambridge University Press, 1961)

Chen, K., 'The coroner's necropsy – an epidemiological treasure trove', *Journal of Clinical Pathology*, 49 (1996): 698–699

Chesterton, G. K., *Alarms and Discursions* (London: Good Reads Ltd, 2016)

Cheung, Philip, *Public Trust in Medical Research? Ethics, Law and Accountability* (Oxford: Radcliffe Publishing Ltd, 2007)

Chisholm, Anne, *Frances Partridge: The Biography* (London: Weidenfeld & Nicolson, 2009)

Chisholm, Hugh (ed.), 'Craigie, Pearl Mary-Teresa', *Encyclopaedia Britannica*, 11th ed. (Cambridge: Cambridge University Press, 1911 edition), 12

Cowen, Veronica 'Feature article "coroner's update"', *Criminal Law and Justice Weekly*, 80 (10 September 2016), 34: 1–2

Crichton, Michael, *Travels* (New York & London: Vintage Books, 2014 paperback edition)

Coyle, Bill, *The God of This World to His Prophet* (Chicago: Ivan R. Dee Publishers, 2006)

Cutler, T., 'Dangerous yardstick? early cost estimates and the politics of financial management in the first decade of the National Health Service', *Medical History*, 47 (2003) II: 217–238

Dalrymple, William, *Nine Lives: In Search of the Sacred in Modern India* (London: Bloomsbury, 2009)

Das, Veena, 'The practice of organ transplants: networks, documents, translations', in Margaret Lock, Allan Young and Alberto Cambrosio (eds.), *Living and Working with the New Medical Technologies: Intersections of Inquiry* (Cambridge: Cambridge University Press, 2000), pp. 263–287

Dayell, Tom, 'Westminster scene: to tidy up transplant procedure', *New Scientist* (27 May 1971): 525

Dayell, Tom, *The Importance of Being Awkward: The Autobiography of Tom Dayell with a foreword by Professor Peter Hennessy* (Edinburgh: Birlinn Publishers Ltd, 2012)

Dickenson, Donna, *Body Shopping: The Economy Fuelled by Flesh and Blood* (Oxford: One World Books, 2008)

Dobbels, F., F. Van Gelder, A. Verkinderen, et al., 'Should the law on anonymity of organ donation be changed? The perception of live liver transplants', *Clinical Transplant Journal*, 23 (June–July 2009), 3: 375–381

Dworkin, Gerald, 'The law relating to organ transplantation in England', *Modern Law Review*, 33 (1970), 4: 353–377

Eklund, Anders, Thomas E. Nichols and Hans Knutsson, 'Cluster failure: why fMRI inferences for spatial extent have inflated false-positive rates', *Journal of the Proceedings of the National Academy of Sciences in the United States*, 113 (12 July 2016), 28: 7900–7905

Feenberg, Andrew, Michel Callon, Bryan Wyne, et al., *Between Reason and Experience: Essays in Technology and Modernity* (Cambridge, Mass.: MIT Press, 2010)

Fleischhacker, H. H., 'Hemispherectomy', *The British Journal of Psychiatry*, 418 (January 1954), 100: 66–84

Fischer, Gerhard and Bernhard Greiner (eds.), The *Play-within-the-Play: The Performance of Meta-Theatre and Self-Reflection* (Amsterdam: Rodopi, 2007)

Foucault, Michel, *Discipline and Punish: The Birth of the Prison*, translated by Alan Sheridan (London: Penguin, 1991)

Foucault, Michel, *The Birth of the Clinic* (London: Routledge, 2003)

Foucault, Michel, *Madness and Civilisation* (London: Vintage Books, 2006)

Frank, Arthur W., *The Wounded Storyteller: Body, Illness and Ethics* (Chicago: University of Chicago Press, 1997)

Gangata, Hope, Patheka Ntaba, Princess Akol and Graham Louw, 'The reliance of unclaimed cadavers for anatomical teaching by medical schools in Africa', *American Sciences Education, Journal of the American Association of Anatomists*, 3 (July–August 2010), 4: 174–183

Gattie, W. H., and T. H. Holt-Hughes, 'Note on the Mental Deficiency Act, 1913', *The Law Quarterly Review*, 30 (1914): 202–209

Gawande, Atul, *Being Mortal: Illness, Medicine and What Matters in the End* (London: Wellcome Trust publications, 2015)

Giacomini, Mia, 'A change of heart and a change of mind? Technology and the redefinition of death in 1968', *Social Science of Medicine*, 44 (1997), 10: 1465–1482

Gilbert, Sandra M., *Death's Door: Modern Dying and the Way We Grieve* (London & New York: Norton, 2006)

Gill, P., and L. Lowes, 'Gift exchange and organ donation: donor and recipient of live kidney transplantation', *International Journal of Nursing Studies*, 45 (2008), 11: 1607–1617

Glenday, John, *The Golden Mean* (London & New York: Picador Poetry, 2015)

Goodwin, Michele (ed.), *The Global Body Market: Altruism's Limits* (Cambridge: Cambridge University Press, 2013)

Gorer, Geoffrey, *Exploring English Character* (New York: Criterion Books, 1955)

Gøtzsche, Peter, *Deadly Medicines and Organised Crime: How Big Pharma Has Corrupted Healthcare* (London & New York: Radcliffe Publishing, 2014)

Halewood, Peter, 'On commodification and self-ownership', *Yale Journal of Law & the Humanities*, 20 (2008), 2: 131–162

Hallam, Elizabeth, Jenny Hockey and Glennys Howarth, *Beyond the Body: Death and Social Identity* (London: Routledge, 1999)

Halperin, E., 'The poor, the black, and the marginalized as the source of cadavers in United States anatomical education', *Clinical Anatomy*, 20 (2007): 489–495

Hamilakis, Yannis, Mark Pluciennik and Sarah Tarlow (eds.), *Thinking through the Body: Archaeologies of Corporeality* (New York: Kluwer Academic/Plenum Publishers, 2002)

Hamilton, David, *A History of Organ Transplantation: Ancient Legends to Modern Practice* (Pittsburgh: University of Pittsburgh Press, 2012)

Harding, Mildred Davis, *Air-Bird in the Water: The Life and Works of Pearl Craigie (John Oliver Hobbes)* (Madison, N.J.: Fairleigh Dickinson University Press, 1996)

Harari, Yuval Noah, *Homo Deus: A Brief History of Tomorrow* (London: Harvill Secker Press, 2016)

Hayes, Bill, *The Anatomist: A True Story of Gray's Anatomy* (New York: Bellevue Literary Press, 2009)

Herman, David, Manfred Jahn and Marie-Laure Ryan (eds.), *Encyclopaedia of Narrative Theory* (London: Routledge, 2013)

Higgs, Edward, *The Information State in England: The Central Collection of Information on Citizens since 1500* (Basingstoke: Palgrave Macmillan, 2003)

Hitchens, Christopher, *Hitch-22: A Memoir* (New York and London: Atlantic Books, 2010)

Hitchens, Christopher, *Mortality* (London and New York: Atlantic Books, 2012)

Hobbes, John Oliver and John Morgan Richards, *Life of John Oliver Hobbes Told in her Correspondence with Numerous Friends* (New York: Ulan Press, 1911)

Horden, Peregrine and Richard Smith (eds.), *The Locus of Care: Families, Communities, Institutions and the Provision of Welfare since Antiquity.* Routledge Studies in the Social History of Medicine (New York & London: Routledge, 1988)

Høystad, Ole M., *A History of the Heart* (London: Reaktion Books Ltd, 2007)

Scheper-Hughes, Nancy, 'The ends of the body – commodity fetishism and the global traffic in organs', *SAIS Review*, 22 (2002): 61–80

Hurren, E. T., 'The pauper dead-house: the expansion of Cambridge anatomical teaching school under the late-Victorian Poor Law, 1870–1914', *Medical History*, 48 (2004), 1: 19–30

Hurren, E. T., 'Whose body is it anyway?: trading the dead poor, coroner's disputes, and the business of anatomy at Oxford University, 1885–1929', *Bulletin of the History of Medicine*, 82 (Winter 2008), 4: 775–818

Hurren, E. T., 'Remaking the medico-legal scene: a social history of the late-Victorian coroner in Oxford', *Journal of the History of Medicine and Allied Sciences*, 65 (April 2010): 207–252

Hurren, E. T., '"Abnormalities and deformities": the dissection and interment of the insane poor, 1832–1929', *Journal of the History of Psychiatry*, 23 (2012), 89: 65–77

Hurren, E. T., *Dying for Victorian Medicine: English Anatomy and Its Trade in the Dead Poor, c. 1834–1929* (Basingstoke: Palgrave Macmillan, 2012)

Hurren, E. T., *Protesting about Pauperism: Poverty, Politics and Poor Relief in Late-Victorian England, c. 1870–1900*, Royal Historical Society Series (Woodbridge, Suffolk: Boydell & Brewer, 2015 paperback edition)

Hurren, E. T., *Dissecting the Criminal Corpse: Staging Post-Execution Punishment in Early Modern England* (Basingstoke: Palgrave Macmillan, 2016)

Hurren E. T., and S. A. King, 'Begging for a burial: form, function and meaning of nineteenth century pauper funeral provision', *Social History*, 20 (2005), 3: 1–41

Hurren, E. T. and S. A. King, 'Courtship at the coroner's court', *Social History*, 40 (2015), 2: 185–207

Hurren, E. T. and S. A. King, 'Public and private health care for the poor, 1650s to 1960s', in P. Weindling (ed.), *Healthcare in Private and Public from the Early Modern Period to 2000* (London: Routledge Publishers, 2015), pp. 15–35

Hussain, L. M. and A. D. Redmond, 'Are pre-hospital deaths from an accidental injury preventable', *British Medical Journal*, 308 (23 April 1994): 1077–1080

Innes, J., *Inferior Politics: Social Problems and Social Policies in Eighteenth Century Britain* (Oxford: Oxford University Press, 2009)

Ishiguro, Kazuo, *Never Let Me Go* (New York & London: Vintage Books, 2006)

Jacob, Marie-Andree, *Contemporary Ethnography: Matching Organs to Donors, Legalising and Kinship in Transplants* (Philadelphia: University of Pennsylvania Press, 2012)

Jamie, Kathleen, *Findings* (London: Sort of Books Publisher, 2005)

Jones, Gareth, 'Using unclaimed bodies for dissection draws outcry', *American Medical News* (7 November 2011): 1

Jones, Gareth, 'Unclaimed bodies are anatomy's shameful inheritance', *Scientist*, 2965 (15 April 2014), Comment section, p. 1

Kagarise, Mary Jane and George F. Sheldon, 'Translational ethics: a perspective for the new millennium', *Archives of Surgery, Journal of the American Medical Association* (2000), 135: 39–45

Karpf, Ann, 'The cancer memoir: in search of a writing cure?' in Michael Brennan (ed.), *Theorising the Popular* (Newcastle-up-Tyne: Cambridge Scholars Press, 2017), chapter 4, pp. 61–88

Khan, Peter A., Thomas H. Champney and Sabine Hildebrant, 'The incompatibility of the use of unclaimed bodies with ethical anatomical education in the United States: letters to the editor', *Journal of Anatomical Sciences Education* (December 2016), Letter, p. 1

King, Peter, *Crime and Law in England, 1750–1840: Remaking Justice from the Margins* (Oxford: Oxford University Press, 2010)

Kinkead-Weekes, Mark, *D. H. Lawrence: Triumph to Exile 1912–1922*, volume 2 of *The Cambridge Biography of D. H. Lawrence* (Cambridge: Cambridge University Press, 1996)

Kitamura, Takashi, Sachie K. Ogawa, Dheeraj S. Roy, et al., 'Engrams and circuits crucial for systems consolidation of a memory', *Science*, 356 (7 April 2017), 6333: 73–78

Knights, Sarah, *Bloomsbury's Outsider: A Life of David Garnett* (London: Bloomsbury Reader, 2015)

Kramer, Beverley and Erin F. Hutchinson, 'Transformation of a cadaver population: analysis of a South African cadaver program, 1921–2013', *Anatomical Sciences Education*, 8 (2015), 5: 445

Landecker, Hannah, 'Between beneficence and chattel: the human biological in law and science', *Science in Context*, 12 (1999): 203–225

Langton, Neville, *The Prince of Beggars: Being Some Account of the Beggings of Sydney Holland, 2nd Viscount Knutsford, During his 25 Years as Chairman of the London Hospital* (London: Hutchinson and Co, 1921)

Laqueur, Thomas, *The Work of the Dead: A Cultural History of Mortal Remains* (Princeton: Princeton University Press, 2015)

Latour, Bruno, *Science in Action: How to Follow Scientists and Engineers through Society* (Cambridge, Mass.: Harvard University Press, 1987)

Latour, Bruno, *We Have Never Been Modern* (Cambridge, Mass.: Harvard University Press: English translation, 1993)

Latour, Bruno, *Reassembling the Social: An Introduction to Actor Network Theory* (New York: Oxford University Press, 2005 & 2007 editions)

Latour, Bruno and Michel Callon, 'Don't throw the baby out with the Bath School! A reply to Collins and Yearly', in Andrew Pickering (ed.), *Science as Practice and Culture* (Chicago: Chicago University Press, 1992), pp. 343–368

Latour, Bruno, Steve Woolgar and Jonas Salk, *Laboratory Life: The Construction of Scientific Facts* (Princeton: Princeton University Press, 1986 edition)

Law, John and John Hassard (eds.), *Actor Network Theory and After* (Oxford: Blackwell Books, 1999)

Lederer, Susan, *Flesh and Blood: Organ Transplantation and Blood Transfusion in Twentieth Century America* (Oxford: Oxford University Press, 2008)

Lesaffer, Randall, 'Argument from Roman law in current international law: occupation and acquisitive prescription', *European Journal of International Law*, 16 (2005) 1: 25–58

Lock, Margaret, *Twice Dead: Organ Transplants and the Reinvention of Death* (Los Angeles: University of California Press, 2002)

Longmore, D., *Spare-Part Surgery* (London: Aldus, 1968)

Lopez, Barry, *Crow and Weasel with illustrations* (New York: North Point Press, 1990)

Luckin, B., 'Pollution in the city', in M. Daunton (ed.), *The Cambridge Urban History of Britain*, volume III, *1840–1950* (Cambridge: Cambridge University Press, 2000), pp. 207–228

Luckin, B., 'Demographic, social and cultural parameters of environmental crisis: the great London smoke fogs in the late 19th and early 20th centuries', in C. Bernhardt and G. Massard-Guilbaud (eds.), *The Modern Demon: Pollution in Urban and Industrial European Societies* (Clermont-Ferrand: Blaise-Pascal University Press: 2002), pp. 219–238

MacDonald, Helen, *Human Remains: Dissection and Its Histories* (New Haven: Yale University Press, 2005)

MacDonald, Helen, 'Conscripting organs: "routine salvaging" or bequest? The historical debate in Britain, 1961–75', *Journal of the History of Medicine and Allied Sciences*, 70 (2014), 3: 425–461

MacDonald, Helen, 'Guarding the public interest: England's coroners and organ transplants, 1960–1975', *Journal of British Studies*, 54 (October 2015), 4: 926–946

MacDonald, Helen, 'Crossing the rubicon: death in the "Year of the Transplant"', *Medical History*, 6 (2017) 1: 107–127

Marrus, Michael, *The Nuremberg War Crimes Trial of 1945–6: A Brief History with Documents* (Basingstoke: Palgrave Macmillan, 1997)

Marshall, J. B., 'Tuberculosis of the gastrointestinal tract and peritoneum', *American Journal of Gastroenterol*, 88 (1993) 7: 989

Mason, John N., *Mayday Hospital Croydon, 1885–1985: A History of a Century of Service* (London: Croydon Health Authority, 1986)

Mazyala, Erick J., Makaranga Revocatus, Mange Manyama, et al., 'Human bodies bequest program: a wake-up call to Tanzanian medical schools', *Advances in Anatomy* (2014), 1: 1

McClelland, Shearwood, and Robert R. Maxwell, 'Hemispherectomy for intractable epilepsy in adults: the first reported series', *Annals of Neurology*, 61 (2007), 4: 372–376

McCrae, Niall and Peter Nolan, *The Story of Nursing in British Mental Hospitals: Echoes from the Corridors* (London: Routledge, 2016)

McGauran, Ann, World Report section, 'Regulation of human tissue in the UK', *Lancet*, 388 (17–23 September 2016), 10050: e-4–e-5

Moazam, Farhat, Riffat Moazam Zaman and Aamir M. Jafarey, 'Conversations with kidney vendors in Pakistan: an ethnographic study', *Hastings Center Report*, 39 (May–June 2009), 3: 29–44

Montross, Christine, *Body of Work: Meditations on Mortality from the Human Anatomy Lab* (New York: Penguin Press, 2007)

Moruno, Dolores Martin and Beatriz Pichel, *Emotional Bodies (The History of Emotions): The Historical Performativity of Emotions* (Champaign: University of Illinois Press, 2019)

Munson, Ronald, *Raising the Dead: Organ Transplants, Ethics and Society* (Oxford: Oxford University Press, 2002)

Neville, C., G. Oswald Simon and R. A. Shooter, 'Pneumonia in hospital practice', *British Journal of Diseases of the Chest*, 55 (3 July 1961), 3: 109–118

Noble, Denis, *The Music of Life: Biology beyond the Genome* (Oxford: Oxford University Press, 2006)

Nyhan Julianne and Andrew Flinn, introduction, 'Why oral history?', in *Computation and the Humanities: Towards an Oral History of the Digital Humanities* (Basingstoke: Palgrave, 2016), pp. 21–36

O'Malley, Tom and Olive Soley, *Regulating the Press* (London: Pluto Press, 2000)

Parnia, Sam, *What Happens When We Die?* (Carlsbad, Calif. & London: Hay House, 2005)

Parnia, Sam, *The Lazarus Effect: The Science That Is Rewriting the Boundaries between Life and Death* (London & New York: Rider Books, 2014)

Parnia, Sam with Josh Young, *Erasing Death: The Science That Is Rewriting the Boundaries between Life and Death* (London & New York: HarperOne Books, 2013)

Parnia, Sam et al., 'AWAreness [*sic*] during REsuscitation [*sic*] – a prospective study', *Resuscitation, Official Journal of the European Resuscitation Council*, 85 (December 2014), 12: 1799–1805

Parry, Bronwyn, *Trading the Genome: Investigating the Commodification of Bio-Information* (New York: Columbia University Press, 2004)

Partridge, Burgo, *A History of Orgies* (London: Sevenoaks Publishers, 1958)

Partridge, Francis and Rebecca Wilson (eds.), *Francis Partridge, Diaries, 1939–1972* (London: Phoenix Press, paperback edition, 2001)

Passerini, Luisa, 'Work, ideology and consensus under Italian fascism', *History Workshop Journal*, 8 (1979): 82–108

Perez, Gilberto, *The Material Ghost: Films and their Medium* (Baltimore: John Hopkins Press, 1998)

Pernick, M. S., 'Brain death in a cultural context: the reconstruction of death 1967–1981', in S. J. Youngner, R. M. Arnold and R. Schapiro (eds.), *The Definition of Death: Contemporary Controversies* (Baltimore: Johns Hopkins University Press, 1999), pp. 3–33

Pfeffer, Naomi, *Insider Trading: How Mortuaries, Medicine, and Money Have Built a Global Market in Human Cadaver Parts* (New Haven: Yale University Press, 2017)

Pitman, A., 'Reform of the coroners' service in England and Wales: policy-making and politics', *The Psychiatrist* (2012): 1–5

Plamper, Jan, *The History of Emotions: An Introduction* (Oxford: Oxford University Press, 2017)

Portelli, Alessandro, 'The peculiarities of oral history', *History Workshop Journal*, 12 (1981): 96–107

Prasad, Arathi, *In the Bonesetter's Waiting Room: Travels through Indian Medicine – sponsored by the Wellcome Trust* (London & New Dehli: Profile Books, 2016)

Raleigh, Desmond Mountjoy, 'Character sketches: Part II, in memoriam: Pearl Mary-Teresa Craigie', *The Reviews of Reviews London*, 34 (September 1906): 251–254

Reddy, William, 'Against constructionism: the historical ethnography of Emotions', *Current Anthropology*, 38 (1997): 327–351

Reddy, William, 'Emotional liberty: history and politics in the anthropology of emotions', *Cultural Anthropology*, 14 (1998): 256–288

Reddy, William, 'Sentimentalism and its erasure: the role of emotions in the era of the French Revolution', *Journal of Modern History*, 72 (2000): 109–152

Reddy, William, *The Navigation of Feeling: A Framework for the History of Emotions* (New York: Cambridge University Press, 2001)

Reddy, William, 'Historical research on the self and emotions', *Emotion Review*, 1 (2009): 302–315

Richardson, Ruth, *Death, Dissection and the Destitute* (London: Phoenix Press, 2001)

Riederer, Beat M. and José L. Bueno-López, 'Anatomy, respect for the body and body donation – a good practice guide', *European Journal of Anatomy*, 18 (December 2014), 4: 361–368

Riederer, Beat M., 'Body donations today and tomorrow: what is best practice and why?' *Clinical Anatomy*, 29 (October 2015), 1: 11–18

Roach, Fred, 'A new beginning: memories of a volunteer worker, 1981–1996', *British Cardiac Patients Journal, The Official Magazine of the British Cardiac Patients Association*, 189 (April–May 2013): 13

Roger, Euan C., 'Blakberd's treasure: a study in 15th century administration at St. Bartholomew's Hospital London', in Linda Clark (ed.), *The Fifteen Century XIII: Exploring the Evidence: Commemoration, Administration and Economy* (Woodbridge, Suffolk: Boydell Press), pp. 81–109

Rovelli, Carol, *Seven Brief Lessons on Physics* (New York & London: Penguin Books, 2015)

Rutty, G. N., B. Morgan, C. Robinson, et al., 'Diagnostic accuracy of post-mortem CT with targeted coronary angiography versus autopsy for coroner-requested post-mortem investigations: a prospective, masked, comparison study', *Lancet*, 390 (May 2017), 10090: 145–154

Rycroft, B. W., 'The Corneal Grafting Act', *British Medical Journal*, 37 (1953): 349

Sagan, Carl, *Cosmos: The Story of Cosmic Evolution, Science and Civilisation* (London and New York: Abacas, 1983)

Sakalys, Jurate A., 'The political role of illness narratives', *Journal of Advanced Nursing*, 31 (2000) 6: 1469–1476

Santayana, George, *The Life of Reason and Common Sense; The Phases of Human Progress (1905–6): The Age of Reason*, Volume 1 (New York & London: Scribner's & Constable, 1905)

Santayana, George, *Winds of Doctrine: Studies in Contemporary Opinion* (New York & London: Scribner's & Dent, 1913)

Sappol, Michael, *A Traffic of Dead Bodies: Anatomy and Embodied Social Identity in Nineteenth-Century America* (Princeton: Princeton University Press, 2004)

Scher, Stephen, and Kasia Kozlowska, *Rethinking Health Care Ethics* (Basingstoke: Palgrave Pivot, 2018)

Scholes, Robert, *Textual Power* (New Haven: Yale University Press, 1985)

Schweiger, Elizabeth, 'The risks of remaining silent: international law formation and the EU silence on drone killings', *Global Affairs*, 1 (2015) 3: 269–275

Scott, Michael L., *Programming Language Pragmatics* (New York: Morgan Kaufmann, 2006)

Snell, K. D. M., 'The rise of living alone and loneliness in history', *Social History*, 42 (2017) 1: 2–28

Sohl, P. and H. A. Basford, 'Codes of medical ethics: traditional foundations and contemporary practice', *Journal of Social Science Medicine* 22 (1986), 11: 1175–1179

Sokoll, Thomas, 'The moral foundation of modern capitalism: towards an historical reconsideration of Max Weber's "Protestant Ethic"', in Stefan Berger and Alexandra Przyrembel (eds.), *Moralizing Capitalism, Agents, Discourses and Practices of Capitalism and Anti-Capitalism in the Modern Age* (Basingstoke: Palgrave Macmillan, 2019), pp. 79–108

Stason, E. Blythe, 'The role of law in medical progress', *Law and Contemporary Problems*, 32 (1967), 4: 563–596

Steiner, George, *Grammars of Creation* (New Haven: Yale University Press; London & New York: Faber and Faber, 2001)

Stephens, Trent and Rock Brynner, *Dark Remedy: The Impact of Thalidomide and Its Revival as a Vital Medicine* (New York & London: Perseus Publishing & Basic Books, 2001)

Stone, Richard, 'Counting the cost of London's killer smog', *Science*, 298 (13 December 2002), 5601: 2106–2107

Strange, Julie-Marie, *Death, Grief and Poverty in Britain, 1870–1914* (Cambridge: Cambridge University Press, 2005)

Strange, Julie-Marie, 'Historical approaches to dying', in Allan Kellehear (ed.), *The Study of Dying: From Autonomy to Transformation* (Cambridge: Cambridge University Press, 2009), pp. 123–146

Subaltern Studies Collective work in *Subaltern Studies: Volumes 1–10 as a set: Writings on South Asian History and Society* (Oxford: Oxford University Press, 1999)

Thompson, E. P., *The Making of the English Working Class* (London: Penguin Books, 2002)

Thompson, Paul, *The Voice of the Past, Oral History*, 3rd ed. (Oxford: Oxford University Press, 2000)

Thornicroft, Graham, 'The NHS and the Community Care Act 1990: recent government policy and legislation', *Psychiatric Bulletin*, 18 (1994): 13–17

Titmuss, Richard M., *The Gift Relationship: From Human Blood to Social Policy*, 2nd ed. (London: London School of Economic Books, 1997)

Tomkins, A. and S. A. King, *The Poor in England, 1700–1850: An Economy of Makeshifts* (Manchester: Manchester University Press, 2003)

Tonkin, Richard D., *Lecture Notes on Gastroenterology – Compiled Whilst Consultant Physician at the Mayday Hospital Croydon* (Oxford & Edinburgh: Blackwell Scientific Publications, 1968)

Truong, Robert, 'Is it time to abandon brain death?' *The Hastings Center Report*, 27 (1997), 1: 29–37

Underwood, Emily, 'The polluted brain: evidence builds that dirty air causes Alzheimer's disease', *Science* (26 January 2017), Lead article, p. 2

Underwood, James, 'The future of the autopsy', in Julian L. Burton and Guy N. Rutty (eds.), *The Hospital Autopsy: A Manual of Fundamental Autopsy Practice*, 3rd ed. (London: Hodder Arnold, 2001), chapter 2, pp. 11–18

US State Department, President's Commission for the Study of Ethical Problems in Medicine and Biomedical and Behavioral Research, *Defining Death: A Report on the Medical, Legal and Ethical Issues in the Determination of Death* (Washington, D.C.: US Government Printing Office, 1981)

Vines, Prue, 'The sacred and the profane: the role of property concepts in disputes about post-mortem examination', *Sydney Law Review*, 29 (2007): 235–261

Waddington, K., *Medical Education at St. Bartholomew's Hospital 1123–1995* (Woodbridge, Suffolk: Boydell Press, 2003)

Waldby, Catherine and Robert Mitchell, *Tissue Economies: Blood, Organs, and Cell Lines in Late Capitalism* (Durham, NC: Duke University Press, 2006)

Warraich, Haider, *Modern Death: How Medicine Changed the End of Life* (London: Duckworth Overlook, 2017)

Watson, Katherine, *Poisoned Lives: English Poisoners and Their Victims* (London: Hambledon Continuum Press, 2006)

Weindling, Paul J., *Nazi Medicine and the Nuremburg Trials: From Medical War Crimes to Informed Consent* (Basingstoke: Palgrave Macmillan, 2006)

Weindling, Paul J., *Victims and Survivors of Nazi Human Experiments: Science and Suffering in the Holocaust* (London: Bloomsbury, 2014)

Weindling, Paul J., *From Clinic to Concentration Camp: Reassessing Nazi Medicine and Racial Research, 1933–1945*. The History of Medicine in Context (New York & London: Routledge, 2017)

West, Darrell M., *Biotechnology across National Boundaries: The Science-Industrial Complex* (Basingstoke: Palgrave, 2007)

Whitehead, Anne, 'The medical humanities: a literary perspective – the rise of pathography', in Victoria Bates, Alan Bleakley and Sam Goodman (eds.), *Medicine, Health and the Arts: Approaches to the Medical Humanities* (London & New York: Routledge, 2014), pp. 107–128

Wijdicks, Eelco F. M., 'The neurologist and Harvard criteria for death', *Neurology*, 61 (October 2003): 970–976

Wilson, Duncan, *Tissue Culture in Science and Society: The Public Life of Biological Technique in Twentieth Century Britain* (Basingstoke: Palgrave Macmillan, 2011)

Wilson, Duncan, *The Making of British Bioethics* (Manchester: Manchester University Press, 2014)

Wiltshire, John, 'Biography, pathography, and the recovery of meaning', *The Cambridge Quarterly*, 29 (2000), 4: 409–422

Wise, J., 'Government axes a further 11 health quangos', *British Medical Journal* (2010): 341

Wood, Michael, 'At the movies', *London Review of Books* (16 August 2014): 1
Yovel, Yirmiyahu, *Spinoza and Other Heretics: The Marrano of Reason* (Princeton: Princeton University Press, 1989)

Unpublished Dissertation

Borgstrom, E., 'Planning for death? An ethnographic study of choice and English end-of -life care' (unpublished PhD dissertation, University of Cambridge, 2014), accessed 10/1/2017 at: www.repository.cam.ac.uk/handle/1810/245560

Index

Please note that page numbers in italics direct the reader to images.

.